POISONS
AND
ANTIDOTES

Carol Turkington

Foreword by Shirley K. Osterhout, M.D., Medical
Director, Duke Poison Control Center

POISONS AND ANTIDOTES

Copyright (c) 1994 Carol Turkington

Facts On File, Inc.
460 Park Avenue South
New York NY 10016

Library of Congress Cataloging-in-Publication Data
Turkington, Carol.
Poisons and antidotes / Carol Turkington; foreword by Shirley K. Osterhout.
p. cm.
Includes bibliographical references and index.
ISBN 0-8160-2825-7
1. Toxicological emergencies—Encyclopedias. 2. Poisoning—Encyclopedias. 3. Antidotes—Encyclopedias. I. Title.
[DNLM: 1. Antidotes—handbooks. 2. Poisons—handbooks.
3. Poisoning—handbooks, QV 39 T939p 1994]
RA1224.5.T87 1994
615.9—dc20
DNLM/DLC
for Library of Congress 93-16724

A British CIP catalogue record for this book is available from the British Library.

Facts On File books are available at special discounts when purchased in bulk quantities for businesses, associations, institutions or sales promotions. Please call our Special Sales Department in New York at 212/683-2244 or 800/322-8755.

Jacket design by Catherine Hyman
Composition by Facts On File, Inc.
Manufactured by The Maple-Vail Book Manufacturing Group
Printed in the United States of America

10 9 8 7 6 5 4 3 2 1

This book is printed on acid-free paper.

CONTENTS

Foreword by Shirley K. Osterhout, M.D.   iv

Acknowledgments   v

Introduction   vii

If You Must Call a Poison Control Center   ix

Rescue and Treatment   xi

Entries A to Z   1

Appendix A: Home Testing Kits for Toxic Substances   316

Appendix B: Hotlines   318

Appendix C: Newsletters   319

Appendix D: Organizations   320

Appendix E: Poison Education and Information Materials   324

Appendix F: Poisons by Symptom   328

Appendix G: Regional Poison Control Centers   339

Appendix H: Toxicity Ratings of Poisons   345

References   348

Index   359

FOREWORD

Poisoning can be a problem to everyone, whether by ingestion, inhalation or contact with skin or mucous membranes (including eyes), to adults and children alike, regardless of race or sex. Poisoning can also be a danger to animals at any time.

But what *is* a poison?

A poison is a substance that, on contact with a target, can change basic cellular metabolism in varying degrees of severity.

But what may be a poison resulting in illness under one set of conditions could be healthful under another set of circumstances. Poisoning depends on the form and concentration of a substance, how it makes contact with the body, the length of application, combination with other substances and, of course, the victim.

A substance may be potentially poisonous depending on a person's age, health at the time of contact and other substances to which the victim is exposed.

It is hoped that this book will give readers some insight into the many potentially toxic substances around them—both those found in nature and those made by humans—and will help them learn how to use things appropriately, recognize potential poisons and understand what must be done to prevent illness.

Knowledge, after all, is the major first step in prevention.

—Shirley K. Osterhout, M.D.,
Medical Director, Duke Poison
Control Center

ACKNOWLEDGMENTS

The author would like to thank the librarians at the National Library of Medicine and the medical libraries of Hershey Medical Center, the University of Pennsylvania Medical Center and Reading Medical Center, the staffers at the National Institutes of Health and the countless people from national organizations, services and government agencies around the country concerned with toxicology and poisons.

INTRODUCTION

Since prehistoric times, humans have sought to learn more about the deadly toxins that often look so beautiful and kill so quickly. Ever since the first cave man nibbled on the first poisonous plant or tasted the first tainted meat, people have tried to identify and understand poisons in the natural environment.

The first documented mention of the existence of poison in 1600 B.C. mentions the "use of charms against snake poison." By the time of Christ, the Sumerians, the Indians, the Chinese, the Greeks and the Egyptians all had mastered at least a basic knowledge of natural poisons—especially as instruments of murder.

Unfortunately, poisons today have become part of our everyday life. Deadly toxins are found not only in the plants and animals around us but in the food we eat, the air we breathe, the products we use and the soil on which we stand.

However, most accidental poisonings can be prevented simply by keeping harmful substances out of the reach of children. Other cases of poisoning just take a little knowledge and common sense—don't mix certain common household chemicals, always wear protective clothing when using pesticides or certain paint materials, don't leave antifreeze out where pets can drink it. Still other potentially harmful substances have effects that are not well known to the general public (for example, some brands of artificially sweetened food contain an amino acid—phenylalanine—that can harm the fetus and may cause brain damage in young children).

This book is designed as a guide and reference to a wide range of poisons and antidotes, and to additional information and addresses of consumer products and toxicological groups. *It is not a substitute for prompt medical attention from a poison control center or an experienced physician trained in toxicology.* All cases of suspected poisoning should be immediately reported to a physician or poison control center.

Information for this book comes from the most up-to-date sources available and includes some of the most recent research in the field of toxicology, but readers should keep in mind that changes can occur very rapidly in this field. By its very nature, toxicology is an extremely complex science; because of format and space limitations, it was impossible to include all of the available information. Thus, an extensive bibliography has been provided for readers who seek additional sources of information.

Specific entries include poisonous and toxic substances and their antidotes. All commonly encountered poisonous and toxic substances, plants and creatures have been included, together with a fair representation of more unusual varieties found throughout the world.

To make information more accessible, entries relating to poisonous and toxic substances have been subdivided into "poisonous part" (where applicable), "symptoms" and "treatment." Entries are listed by common names, with Latin names in parentheses; additional common names or nicknames are also provided for all poisonous and toxic entries. All entries are extensively cross-referenced, and several comprehensive appendixes— on home testing kits, hotlines, newsletters, organizations, poisons by symptom, poison control centers, etc.—provide a detailed range of information on safety issues and consumer products.

—Carol Turkington
Morgantown, Pennsylvania

IF YOU MUST CALL A POISON CONTROL CENTER

A poison control center is not a hospital or treatment center; it's basically a library staffed by experts familiar with poisonings. The information it can offer may be crucial to delivering prompt and proper treatment in a poisoning emergency.

If you suspect poisoning, call the nearest poison control center (regional centers are listed in Appendix G). The telephone number is usually listed inside the front cover of the white pages of the telephone directory. If you don't have the number of a poison control center, dial 911 or operator. The best idea is to post the number on your phone *before* you need it. If there is no poison control center in your area, call the nearest hospital emergency room or your doctor. Poison control centers operate 24 hours a day. If you have a poisoning emergency, tell them:

- Your name
- Victim's name
- Victim's age
- Victim's weight
- Kind of poison involved; its name and its ingredient or kind of plant
- How much was swallowed
- When it was swallowed
- Symptoms
- Other medical problems victim may have (diabetes, epilepsy, high blood pressure)
- What medicines are taken regularly.
- Whether victim has vomited
- What you have given to drink
- How long it will take you to reach an emergency room

The poison control center will tell you whether or not to induce vomiting. (Certain poisons should never be vomited up, such as acids and alkalies.) If you do NOT know the identity of the substance swallowed, DO NOT induce vomiting. Poison control may recommend using activated charcoal, Epsom salts or specific neutralizing products in certain circumstances. Always follow the instructions given by a poison control center. Do not trust antidote information on product labels, and do not use mustard or salt to induce vomiting.

Whether vomiting is induced or occurs naturally, make sure that the person does not inhale the vomitus into the lungs. A small child can be held over your knees, face down. A larger person should bend way over, or lie down with head hanging off the side of a bed. The chin should be held lower than the level of the hips. Monitor vital signs. Be alert for changes in the person who has been poisoned. If breathing stops, CPR must be performed. Treat for shock. If the poison has spilled on the person's clothing, skin or eyes, remove the clothing and flush the skin or eyes with water.

IF YOU ARE TOLD TO TAKE THE VICTIM TO THE HOSPI-TAL, TAKE THE FOLLOWING ITEMS WITH YOU:

1. Poison container and any of its remaining contents, or parts of the plant if a plant was involved. Such materials will help doctors identify the poison and estimate how much of it the victim swallowed.
2. If the victim vomited, take a container of the vomit. The vomit can be tested to determine the nature of the poison; if undigested pills are vomited, the doctor may be able to determine how many the victim took.
3. If a plant was involved, taken enough of it for it to be identified (an entire mushroom, a branch with leaves, flowers and berries).
4. Have another person drive while you keep the victim comfortable. If the person is vomiting, have him lie on the side to keep airway clear.

IMPORTANT: Follow the instructions given to you by the poison control center, doctor or emergency room. First aid procedures differ according to the kind of poison involved and how it entered the body, the victim's weight, how long the poison has been working and other factors. Only expert medical personnel can determine the correct procedures. If you attempt to treat the victim yourself without expert advice, you may do further harm.

RESCUE AND TREATMENT

INHALATION

SMOKE, GAS OR CHEMICAL FUMES *Important: Do not light a match, turn on a light switch or produce a flame or spark in any way in the presence of gas or fumes.*

If you're alone, call for help before attempting a rescue. Before entering the area, take several breaths of fresh air, then inhale deeply as you go in. If smoke and fumes are visible in the upper part of the room, stay below them. If auto exhaust or other heavy fumes are visible near the floor, keep your head above them. Remove the person immediately. Don't attempt other first aid until you are in the fresh air.

FIRST AID FOR INHALED POISONS
- Check for breathing; if you're trained in CPR, you can try to resuscitate the person.
- Check eyes and skin for chemical burns. If present, flush thoroughly with water. Seek medical attention immediately, even if the person seems to have recovered.

ABSORPTION

SYMPTOMS Toxic chemicals can burn the skin; plants can cause rash and blisters.
TREATMENT Get victim away from poison. Remove contaminated clothing. Flood skin with large amounts of soap and water for at least 15 minutes.

INJECTION

TREATMENT Remove stinger by scraping; use cold application, ice in towel. Place wound lower than heart, be prepared to give CPR; place constriction band above wound.

Almost all cases of accidental poisoning in the home occur in children under age five. To prevent accidental poisoning:

- Keep all drugs, poisons, insecticides and chemicals out of the reach of children and away from food. In the presence of young children, do not store these products in accessible places (such as under the sink).
- Be sure all poisons are clearly marked.
- Never store poisonous substances in food or beverage containers.
- Never refer to medicine as candy.
- Don't take the medicine in the dark.
- Read all labels and follow "caution" information.

A

AAPCC National Data Collection System   A method of collecting poison data from the American Association of Poison Control Centers, the system has demonstrated steady growth since its inception in 1983. The latest report (issued September 1992) includes 1,837,939 human exposure cases reported by 73 participating poison centers in 40 states during 1991, an increase of 7.3 percent over 1990 poisoning reports. The data represent an estimated 80.4 percent of the human poison exposures. The cumulative AAPCC data base now contains 10.6 million human poison exposure cases. It is estimated that there were 2.3 million human poison exposures reported to all U.S. poison centers in 1991.

acetaminophen   This widely used painkiller is found in many over-the-counter and prescription analgesics and cold remedies. Sold under the trade name Tylenol, Tempra or Panadol, this drug is generally not poisonous unless ingested in large amounts—usually accidentally by children or as a means to commit suicide. While researchers are still unsure as to the key to its painkilling action, it is known that it can damage the kidney and liver in excess amounts. Combined with alcohol, it can cause drowsiness; misuse over a long period of time causes liver toxicity.

Symptoms   If a toxic dose has been taken, symptoms will appear within 24–36 hours and include nausea, vomiting, abdominal pain, lethargy and jaundice at 48 hours or later. The liver may fail if the drug is taken in doses exceeding 140 mg/g in children or 6 g in adults. Chronic toxicity among alcoholics has been reported after daily ingestion of high doses (5–6 g).

Treatment   Empty the stomach as soon as possible. Specific treatment is determined by a blood level of the drug after four hours. The specific antidote is N-acetylcysteine, which must be administered before 12–16 hours have passed, and is given in 17 doses in a hospital. Provide general supportive care for kidney or liver failure; liver transplant may be necessary.

See also ACETYLCYSTEINE.

acetylcysteine   Antidote for acetaminophen overdose and possibly for carbon tetrachloride and chloroform poisoning. Acetylcysteine often causes nausea and vomiting when given by mouth; if the drug is vomited, it should be given again. Rapid intravenous administration can cause a drop in blood pressure, and at least one death has been reported when a child received a rapid intravenous dose.

See also ACETAMINOPHEN.

acids   Acids are chemical substances that have a sour taste, are soluble in water and turn litmus paper red. They produce pain and corrosion to all tissues with which they come in contact. Problems in swallowing, nausea, intense thirst, shock, breathing problems and death can result from ingesting acids.

Acid poisonings should be treated like any other poisoning emergency: Give the person fluids to drink and call the poison control center for specific instructions. DO NOT INDUCE VOMITING.

Acids are identified by their pH value, which ranges from 0 to 14; acidic substances are listed from strongest (0) to weakest (6). Neutral pH is 7; 8 through 14 are alkaline (base).

Many of the foods we eat and drink are slightly acid or base, as are our body's fluids. One of the most common acids is vitamin C (ascorbic acid). Others include:

- sulfuric acid: found in automobile batteries, metal cleaners and polishes
- hydrochloric acid: metal cleaners and polishes
- nitric acid: cleaning solutions
- acetic acid: permanent wave neutralizers, vinegar
- oxalic acid: cleaning solutions, furniture and floor polishes and waxes, bleach
- phosphoric acid: metal cleaners and polishes
- carbolic acid or phenol: antiseptics, disinfectants, preservatives

See also DIMETHYL SULFATE; PHENOL.

aconite   See MONKSHOOD.

aconitine   The chief active ingredient in the dried, powdered root of monkshood (aconite). Aconitine is an unstable alkaloid used in some liniments.

See also MONKSHOOD.

Symptoms   A central nervous system stimulant, aconitine causes a peculiar warm, tingling sensation followed by numbness when absorbed through the mouth. Other symptoms include nausea, vomiting, diarrhea, restlessness, vertigo, slow breathing, low body temperature and convulsions. Heart problems similar to digitalis overdose have also been reported.

Treatment   Symptomatic.

acrylamide   [Other names: acrylamide monomer, acrylic amide, propenamide.] This flaky crystal is a rather strong toxin used to make polyacrylamide, a nontoxic substance used to clear and treat drinking water, to strengthen paper and for other industrial uses. It melts at fairly low heat and dissolves easily in water; it can be swallowed, inhaled or absorbed through the skin.

Symptoms This neurotoxin affects the skin, eyes and nervous system and can cause severe (sometimes permanent) brain damage. Symptoms, which may not appear immediately, include peeling, reddened skin on the hands and feet, a numbness in the feet and legs and sweaty palms and feet. When poisoned with acrylamide, the patient may appear to be drunk, with an awkward, stumbling gait and muted reflexes.

Treatment If there is no vomiting, administer a slurry of activated charcoal followed by gastric lavage with saline cathartics. Daily doses of vitamin B_1 and B_{12} over 45 days may protect the central nervous system. Pilocarpine may cause a temporary improvement in motor activity in some patients, and aspirin or phenylbutazone may be given to ease muscle pain.

Actifed See DECONGESTANTS.

adder Any of several poisonous snakes of the viper family (Viperidae), plus the death adder, a viperlike member of the cobra family. (The name may also be used for the harmless hognose snake.) Adders in the viper family include the common adder, the puff adder and the night adder. No adders are found in the United States.

Although they are related to cobras, adders look more like vipers—thick bodies, short tails and broad heads. They range from 18 to 35 inches long, with gray or brown skins and dark crosswise bands.

Symptoms Within a very short time, victims begin bleeding from the gums, nose and eyes and experience chills, fever, sweating, falling blood pressure, convulsions and death. In cases of a severe bite, the victim will also experience swelling above the elbows or knees within two hours.

Treatment Death from cardiorespiratory failure is unavoidable unless antivenin is given quickly.

See also ADDER, COMMON; ADDER, PUFF; ADDER, NIGHT.

adder, common *(Vipera berus)* This adder is a member of the viper family (also called the European viper) and is the snake that has most commonly made its way into literature. It is found throughout Europe and Asia, ranging north of the Arctic Circle in Norway, where it survives by hibernating through a very long winter. As is typical of the more northerly adders, the common adder is darker than some of its southern cousins; it is usually gray with a black zigzag band on the back, with black spots on the side, and its maximum length is about 30 inches. Its bite is rarely fatal.

This snake is the only venomous snake in the British Isles, where it is regarded with loathing and fear, although responsible for very few fatalities.

Each spring, mating takes place, and ritual fights occur between two males, who twist the front part of their bodies in a vertical column, each trying to push the other over. It is this typical mating behavior that inspired the two entwined snakes on the staff of Hermes the Messenger. This symbol is often confused with the staff of Aesculapius, the Roman god of medicine, which also features a serpent (the Aesculapian snake, a nonpoisonous variety).

Symptoms Within a very short time, victims begin bleeding from the gums, nose and eyes and experience chills, fever, sweating, falling blood pressure and, occasionally, convulsions and death. In cases of a severe bite, the victim will also experience swelling above the elbows or knees within two hours.

Treatment Antivenin is available.

adder, death *(Acanthophis antarcticus)* This highly poisonous snake resembles and behaves like a viper, although it belongs to the cobra family and lives in an area where no vipers are found. It can be found in Australia and New Guinea, has a thick body and a broad, flat, triangular head and is colored gray or brown with dark crossbands. A bite from the death adder is fatal about half of the time without treatment. Its close relative is the desert death adder *(Acanthophis pyrrhus)*, which also has a 50 percent mortality rate.

Symptoms Symptoms appear within 15 minutes to an hour and include nausea, vomiting, faintness, drowsiness, staggering, slurred speech, respiratory distress, hemorrhage and death in about half of untreated cases.

Treatment Antivenin is available, but the specific antiserum must be used. Before it is administered, the victim should be tested for sensitivity.

See also ANTIVENIN; COBRA; SNAKES, POISONOUS.

adder, European See ADDER, COMMON.

adder, night *(Causus)* A member of the viper family and native to Africa, the night adder is a small, thin snake found south of the Sahara. Gray with dark blotches, these snakes grow up to a meter long with small fangs and weak venom that causes pain and swelling. There are no recorded human fatalities.

Nocturnally active, this snake spends the day in its termite mound or hiding under rocks; it is generally slow moving but becomes alert and aggressive when attacked, inflating its body, flattening its neck and huffing and hissing.

Symptoms Within a very short time, victims begin bleeding from the gums, nose and eyes and experience chills, fever, sweating and falling blood pressure. In cases of a severe bite, the victim will also experience swelling above the elbows or knees within two hours.

Treatment Antivenin is available.

See also ANTIVENIN; SNAKES, POISONOUS.

adder, puff *(Bitis)*   There are several poisonous species of puff adder. All members of the viper family, they are found in semiarid savanna and areas of rural human habitation in Africa and Arabia. This is a sluggish snake that tends to lie still rather than flee when approached, but it can strike with amazing speed when aroused and is responsible for numerous snakebites every year. It gets its name from the warning it gives by inflating its body and hissing loudly before striking. This extremely poisonous snake grows from three to five feet long and is gray to brown with thin yellow chevrons on its back.

Symptoms   Within a very short time, victims begin bleeding from the gums, nose and eyes and experience chills, fever, sweating, falling blood pressure, convulsions and death. In cases of a severe bite, the victim will also experience swelling above the elbows or knees within two hours.

Treatment   Death from cardiorespiratory failure is unavoidable unless antivenin is given quickly.

See also ADDER; ADDER, COMMON; ANTIVENIN; SNAKES, POISONOUS.

Advil (ibuprofen) See ANTI-INFLAMMATORY DRUGS.

aflatoxins   A cancer-causing by-product of the *Aspergillus flavus* mold found in peanuts, corn, wheat, rice, cottonseeds, barley, soybeans, Brazil nuts and pistachios. The molds that produce aflatoxin grow in warm, humid climates in the southeastern United States; the mold can also be produced in the field when rain falls on crops, such as corn and wheat, that are left in the field to dry. Aflatoxin-producing mold can even grow on plants damaged by insects, drought, poor nutrition or unseasonable temperatures.

Aflatoxin has been called the most potent natural carcinogen known to humans; rat studies suggest males are more susceptible to cancer following aflatoxin exposure. Poor diet also seems to predispose animals to cancer in the wake of aflatoxin ingestion.

Still, scientists know very little about why or how the aflatoxins are produced by the mold, and because it is sometimes difficult to see, all susceptible crops are subject to routine testing in the United States. Unfortunately, it is not possible to detect the mold with 100 percent accuracy.

While the way agricultural products are stored can affect the mold's growth, the length of time of such storage is also important; the longer agricultural products are stored in bins, the greater the chance that environmental conditions favorable to aflatoxin production will be created. Stored nuts or seeds might accidentally get wet, or the storage bin might not facilitate drying quickly enough to stop the mold from growing.

Aflatoxins are more common in poor-quality cereals and nuts; while most of these low-grade products do not enter the human food market, they are sold as animal feed, which can go on to contaminate animal products (such as meat and milk). For this reason, cottonseed meal (a product often contaminated with high levels of aflatoxin) is banned for use as an animal feed. Cottonseed oil, however, rarely contains aflatoxin, since the toxin sticks to the hulls of the seed.

Milk is commonly contaminated with aflatoxin, and powdered nonfat milk can contain eight times more than the original liquid product, since the aflatoxin adheres to the milk's proteins. In addition, measurable levels of aflatoxin can be found in some baby foods that use dry milk to boost the protein content of the product.

Pasteurization, sterilization and spray-dry processing techniques can substantially reduce aflatoxin contamination of dried milk. Meat products are less often contaminated because little aflatoxin is carried over into the meat, except for pig liver and kidneys. Chicken can also become contaminated with aflatoxin when the bird appears to be only mildly sick.

In humans, aflatoxin is believed to cause liver cancer, according to some east African studies that seem to show a correlation between the two. Epidemiological evidence also suggests men are more susceptible than women, and many scientists believe a poor diet and liver disease also increase susceptibility to liver cancer as a result of aflatoxin exposure. Data from the African studies were strong enough to prompt the Food and Drug Administration and the Environmental Protection Agency to develop strict regulations to control levels in food and animal food sold in the United States.

Aflatoxin can also cause acute poisoning; severe liver disease has been detected in those who ingest highly contaminated food, and children around the world exhibit symptoms similar to Reyes syndrome (fever, vomiting, coma and convulsions) after exposure.

Consumers are urged not to eat moldy food, especially grains or peanuts, and are urged to be cautious about eating unroasted peanuts sold in bulk.

African milk plant *(Euphorbia)*   There are several species of this poisonous African plant family that includes the poinsettia, including *E. candelabrum, E. grantii, E. neglecta, E. giomgiecpstata, E. systyloides* and *E. tirucalli.* The plants, which are reportedly used by African women to eliminate troublesome husbands, are found throughout the continent. While some of the plants are used for medicinal purposes, they are also used as arrow poisons (especially the varieties *E. candelabrum* and *E. neglecta).* While others (notably *E. systyloides)* are used to treat hookworms, too much of the plant can cause delirium, convulsions and death within six hours.

Poisonous part: The latex of some species is poisonous, with the toxic part being complex terpenes.

Symptoms: Irritation of the skin on contact, which may be quite corrosive depending on the species. Ingestion may cause gastritis.

Treatment: For patients experiencing vomiting and stomach upset, provide fluids to offset dehydration.

See also POINSETTIA.

Afrin   Brand name for the nonprescription drug oxymetazoline.
See also DECONGESTANTS.

akee *(Blighia sapida)*   [Other names: ackee, aki, arbre, fricasse, vegetal]
Named for Captain Bligh, captain of the *Bounty*, this tree produces a fruit
that, if eaten unripe and unopened, can cause serious intoxication and death.
The tree grows to 30 or 40 feet tall with long pairs of leaflets and small,
greenish white flowers. A conspicuous red fruit pod splits at maturity, with
shiny black seeds inside. Native to western Africa, akee can be found in the
West Indies, Florida and Hawaii.

Poisonous part   Although the fruit is perfectly edible when eaten ripe
and fully opened, the unripe and the rancid, spoiled fruit are equally
poisonous. Both the fruit capsule and its seeds are poisonous, as is the water
in which the fruit is cooked.

Symptoms   Poisoning reaches epic proportions during the winter
months on the island of Jamaica, where it is called "vomiting sickness," and
it is often fatal. Victims typically experience one of two forms of symptoms:
vomiting with a remission of eight or 10 hours followed by more vomiting,
convulsions and coma—or convulsion and coma present immediately. It
may take from six hours to a day after ingestion for symptoms to appear,
although death can occur within 24 hours after eating. About 85 percent of
victims experience convulsions. In cases of fatal ingestion, hemorrhages can
often be found in the brain.

Treatment   Gastric lavage, fluids, treatment of symptoms and
intravenous glucose to offset severe hypoglycemia (low blood sugar).

Alar (daminozide)   This pesticide has been the focus of massive public
attention since the 1980s in the wake of data suggesting it causes cancer and
tumors and that it commonly remains as a residue on fruits (particularly
apples). Assurances by growers and the Food and Drug Administration that
residue levels are very low were suspect, since the toxic substance cannot be
detected by the FDA's routine testing procedures for pesticide residues,
although specific Alar detection methods are available.

Acceding to public pressure, the manufacturer voluntarily withdrew Alar
from the market in 1990. Although Alar is no longer being sold in the United
States, there are no restrictions on the sale and use of remaining stocks.

A 1987 study by the Natural Resources Defense Council claimed that 38
percent of the U.S. apple crop was treated with Alar (especially varieties
such as Red and Golden Delicious, McIntosh, Jonathan and Stayman).
Residues have not only been detected on fresh produce; the residue also
appears to concentrate in various processed foods, including apple juice,
peanut butter, cherry pie filling and Concord grape juice. In 1989, the
release of a new report by the NRDC pointed out that young children are

at greater risk from residue than adults because they metabolize food differently.

Although often considered a pesticide, Alar is actually a plant growth regulator. It was introduced in 1967 for use on apples, peaches, pears, prunes, cherries, nectarines and peanuts. It has also been used on cantaloupes, brussels sprouts, tomatoes and grapes. The chemical stops fruit ripening, prevents fruit from dropping prematurely and allows the fruit to develop a deeper, more uniform color.

Several studies show that Alar causes cancer, although the data are not complete; a 1987 study by the National Academy of Sciences estimates the risk of benign or malignant tumor formation associated with exposure to Alar to be greater than the one in 1 million risk considered acceptable by the Environmental Protection Agency. There is not enough information to determine whether it causes mutations, birth defects or other problems, although evidence suggests it is not a mutagen or a teratogen. It is of low toxicity when ingested or applied to the skin.

aldicarb   One of the most toxic pesticides in use today, aldicarb has been registered for use since 1970. A carbamate insecticide, it is effective against a variety of insects, mites and roundworms. Because it is an acutely poisonous pesticide, it is not registered for home or garden use, although it is registered for use by certified applicators for a variety of crops (such as sweet potatoes, peanuts, potatoes, oranges, sugar beets, pecans, some seed crops, soybeans and sugarcane).

Several mass poisoning incidents have been reported involving the illegal use of aldicarb on unapproved vegetables and fruits; although it is not approved for use on watermelons, for example, several hundred consumers were poisoned in 1985 after eating watermelon tainted with aldicarb residue.

Aldicarb leaches from the soil and has been found in groundwater in New York, Florida, Wisconsin, Connecticut, Maine, Virginia, Maryland and New Jersey. The problem is especially acute in sandy, acidic soils and warm, moist climates, which help move the poison into groundwater.

The manufacturer has specifically prohibited the use of aldicarb in areas where drinking water has been contaminated. Because it is a systemic insecticide, residues of aldicarb probably cannot be eliminated by washing produce, although heat in cooking may reduce the levels. It is also prohibited for use near habitats of endangered bird species, since aldicarb is highly toxic to birds, honeybees, freshwater fish and invertebrates.

Symptoms   It only takes a very small dose for fatal effects in humans. While it is quickly absorbed in the gastrointestinal tract, most is excreted within two days after exposure. Tests with rabbits suggest it is also readily absorbed through the skin. Symptoms include dizziness, muscle weakness, stomach cramping, diarrhea, excessive sweating, nausea, vomiting, blurry vision and convulsions. Although studies on long-term exposure are inconclusive, there are hints that it may affect the immune system. There is also a potential link to reproductive problems.

Treatment   Atropine is an antidote for aldicarb poisoning, as it is in all carbamate toxicities.

See also CARBAMATE.

Aldomet (methyldopa) This is one of a group of antihypertensive drugs used to lower blood pressure. It is available as a white tablet or liquid. Aldomet's effects are strengthened if it is taken with other antihypertensives; if taken with alcohol, the sedation is deepened and blood pressure falls dangerously low. The effects of a range of other drugs are also increased if taken with Aldomet, including anticlotting drugs, lithium or tolbutamide. Behavior problems may appear if combined with Haldol, and blood pressure will soar if combined with monoamine oxidase (MAO) inhibitors or tricyclic antidepressants.

Symptoms   Within 20 minutes to an hour after ingestion, patients taking an overdose experience drowsiness, headache, dizziness, weakness, tiredness, skin rash, joint/muscle pain, impotence, fever and nightmares.

Treatment   Atropine or caffeine are used to counteract the effects of excessive Aldomet.

aldrin   [Other names: Aldrine, compound 118, octalene] A component of chlorinated hydrocarbon, aldrin is the most toxic substance used as an insecticide dust to control grubs and wireworms and as a spray against caterpillars. Used since the late 1940s, aldrin is a white, odorless crystalline solid that is most poisonous when eaten or inhaled, although chronic skin contact can be fatal. A relative of DDT, it stimulates the central nervous system and is toxic to warm-blooded animals. Along with other chlorinated hydrocarbons, aldrin has been banned by the Environmental Protection Agency since 1974 because of the injurious effects on those exposed to it, but European brands are still used for termite control. Experimental evidence suggests a potential carcinogenic effect.

Symptoms   Symptoms begin within one to four hours and include headaches, dizziness, nausea, vomiting, malaise, convulsions, coma, respiratory failure and death about six hours later. If convulsions begin more than an hour after ingestion, recovery is likely.

Antidote   The body must be decontaminated, and in cases of severe poisoning, an amyl nitrate capsule is given under the nose for 15 seconds of every minute until sodium nitrite and oxygen treatments are started.

See also CHLORINATED HYDROCARBON PESTICIDES; DDT; INSECTICIDES.

alkaline corrosives   The chemical opposites of acids, alkalies can be extremely corrosive. The most dangerous poisons include sodium hydroxide, or lye (found in aquarium products, drain cleaners and small batteries); potassium hydroxide (some small batteries and cuticle remover); sodium phosphate (abrasive cleaners); and sodium carbonate (dye removers and dishwasher soap). Milder alkalies (ammonia or bleaches) generally do not irreparably burn the esophagus, and the burns usually heal without scarring. Mixing alkaline corrosives with ammonia, toilet bowl cleaners or household cleaners can release hazardous gases and is extremely dangerous.

Inquisitive toddlers in particular are vulnerable to injury from alkaline corrosives, which are often kept under the sink or in old soda bottles in many households. Each year, more than 26,000 American children under age six ingest such corrosive chemicals—mostly household products such as detergents and drain openers.

These extremely corrosive substances can eat right through skin. When ingested, they quickly burn through internal tissues, injuring the esophagus; damage can be irreparable for those who survive.

Because of the dangers of ingestion of lye in particular, federal legislation has required safety caps on containers of more than 2 percent concentrations of lye. Since then, there has been a decrease in the occurrence of these types of poisoning.

Symptoms Alkalies cause an immediate reaction upon contact, burning whatever tissues they touch and turning the tissue to a fatty liquid. Upon ingestion, there is severe pain followed by the inability to handle secretions, respiratory problems, collapse and sometimes death.

Treatment *Vomiting is never induced in cases of alkali ingestion, because it brings up the poison and causes more injury.* Administration of an antidote in the case of alkaline corrosive poisoning is controversial, since by the time the person reaches the emergency room, it is too late for an antidote. Instead, immediate treatment at home should only be at the direction of a medical professional or poison control center. Once the alkali enters the stomach, it will usually be neutralized by gastric acids. All persons who ingest alkalies need to be seen as soon as possible in a medical facility. The major problem is constricted esophagus.

While the corticosteroid prednisone has remained the treatment of choice for the past 20 years, several studies have questioned its use. Recent studies at the Children's National Medical Center in Washington, D.C. revealed that those treated with prednisone healed as well as those who were not.

In an editorial published in the *New England Journal of Medicine* (Sept. 6, 1991), Frederick H. Lovejoy of Children's Hospital in Boston writes: "Corrosive injury to the esophagus in children is a completely preventable disease." New studies questioning the role of prednisone have "removed any false security derived from believing that an effective medical treatment exists."

If contamination is on the skin or in the eyes, wash the area with lukewarm water for 30 minutes.

In the ingestion of alkaline disk batteries, there have been reports of gastrointestinal bleeding and perforation of the esophagus; X rays are important in these cases. If the battery gets as far as the stomach and the person reports no symptoms, no further action is required.

See also LYE.

alkaloids   A class of bitter, unpleasant-tasting nitrogen-containing compounds including more than 5,000 types, ranging from very simple to extremely complex. They are found in as many as 10 percent of plant species and in a variety of animals; the compounds can be isolated for use as a drug or poison. Chemically similar to alkalies (bases), alkaloids can have strong effects—both positive and negative—on the human nervous system, and some affect internal organs as well.

Some of the most deadly alkaloids include nicotine, taxine, gelsemine and atropine. While most alkaloids do occur in closely related plants, a few alkaloids are also produced by ladybugs, millipedes, ants, toads and some types of poisonous frogs. Researchers at the University of Chicago have recently uncovered evidence that suggests that at least one variety of bird may also produce alkaloids; a yellow and black bird in New Guinea contains the chemical batrachotoxin, the same chemical found in some types of poisonous frogs. The fingers of anyone who handled the bird immediately became numb as a result of contact with the alkaloid. While there had been no previous evidence of birds containing a chemical defense system, no one had ever looked for such evidence, scientists report.

Symptoms   When ingested, most alkaloids produce a very strong physiological reaction, usually acting on the nervous system in ways that are still little understood.

Treatment   Potassium permanganate.

See also ATROPINE; GELSEMINE; NICOTINE; TAXINE.

Amanita **mushrooms**   A genus of about 100 mushrooms of the family Amanitaceae, between 25 and 35 of which are found in the United States. Some of the *Amanita* mushrooms are extremely poisonous and include the false morel, fly agaric, panther mushroom and—most deadly of all—the destroying angel or death cap *(Amanita phalloides)*. Mycologists disagree about the classification of many of the closely related *Amanita* mushrooms, however, and other sources may differ in these classifications.

Most of the cases of mushroom poisoning in the United States can be traced to the amanitas, particularly *A. muscaria* and *A. phalloides*, which are also sometimes referred to as toadstools (from the German word for "death"). They have been known to be poisonous since ancient times.

Particularly dangerous are the snow-white to pale green or tan amanitas. The amanitas typically have white spores, a ring on the stem slightly below the cap, a veil that is torn as the cap expands and a cup from which the stalk arises.

Poisonous part There are two types of toxic compounds in the amanitas, which cause two separate syndromes in those who consume them. In *A. phalloides*, the substance amanitine is responsible for the major symptoms; phalloidine produces the degenerative changes in the kidney, liver and heart muscles. Cooking the deadly *Amanita* mushrooms does not destroy their toxicity, and it is estimated that just one *A. phalloides* cap can kill an adult. Amanitas that feature amatoxins and phallotoxins include *A. phalloides, A. verna, A. virosa, A. bisporigera, A. ocreata, A. suballiacae and A. tenuifolia.* Amanitas that contain the toxins muscimol and ibotenic acid include *A. muscaria, A. pantherina, A. gemmata, A. cokeri and A. cothurnata.*

Symptoms In *A. muscaria*, rapid poisoning occurs from a few minutes to two hours after ingestion, depending on the amount of toxin present; symptoms include salivation, sweating, cramps, diarrhea, vomiting, circulatory failure, mental disturbances, coma and convulsions. Death is rare from *A. muscaria* poisoning. A more deadly poisoning occurs from *A. phalloides*, whose symptoms never appear before six hours after ingestion. When they do appear, they include the sudden onset of colicky abdominal pain, vomiting and severe diarrhea that may contain blood and mucus. This type of diarrhea is so severe that it is very similar to the symptoms of cholera. Even without treatment, the victim may appear to begin recovering but two to four days after ingestion will experience liver, heart and kidney damage, circulatory failure, convulsions, coma and death.

Treatment Many antidotes to *Amanita* poisoning have been reported, but most of this information has been anecdotal. Some victims of severe *Amanita* poisoning have been treated successfully with a combination of thioctic acid, glucose and penicillin or by filtering the blood through charcoal. Gastric lavage is indicated, if the patient has not vomited already, followed by activated charcoal and saline cathartics.

See also AMATOXINS; DESTROYING ANGEL; FLY AGARIC; MUSHROOM POISONING; MUSHROOM TOXINS; PANTHER MUSHROOM.

amatoxins A group of very toxic peptides found in a few species of poisonous mushrooms, including *Amanita phalloides, A. virosa, A. ocreata, A. verna, Galerina autumnalis, G. marginata* and a few types of *Lepiota.* Amatoxins are among the strongest toxins in the world; the lethal dose is just 0.1 mg/kg, but one *Amanita* mushroom cap may contain between 10 and 15 mg of toxin.

The Meixner test may detect the presence of amatoxins in mushrooms; their presence is indicated by a blue color that appears after one drop of concentrated hydrochloric acid is added to dried juice from the mushroom cap dripped onto unrefined paper. However, this test should not be used to determine whether it is safe to eat a mushroom.

See also AMANITA MUSHROOMS; MUSHROOM POISONING; MUSHROOM TOXINS.

ammonia   This colorless, strong-smelling poison gas is formed by blowing steam through incandescent coke. Extremely toxic when inhaled in concentrated vapors, ammonia is irritating to both eyes and mucous membranes. It is one of the top five most common inorganic chemicals produced in the United States, where it is used in refrigerants, and to manufacture detergents, permanent wave lotions and hair bleaches, and cleaning agents. It is also used in the manufacture of explosives and synthetic fabrics, herbicides, fertilizers and pesticides.

Ammonia has been shown to produce skin cancer in humans in doses of 1,000 mg/kg of body weight. It also irritates the lungs and can cause swelling of lung tissue. It may even cause explosions if mixed with silver or mercury.

Ammonium hydroxide (ammonia water) is a weak alkali formed when ammonia dissolves in water. This clear, colorless liquid contains between 10 and 35 percent ammonia and is used as an alkali in metallic hair dyes, hair straighteners and protective skin creams; it is also used in detergents, stain removers and ceramics.

Symptoms   Ammonia fumes can irritate the eyes and upper respiratory tract, causing vomiting, conjunctivitis and inflammation of the lips, mouth and throat. Toxic cases of inhalations cause airway obstruction, pulmonary irritation with swelling, cyanosis, bronchitis and pneumonia. Ammonia can damage cells directly, and skin contact can lead to dermatitis; ingestion can burn the esophagus.

Treatment   The ammonia is diluted or neutralized with water or milk, but the victim should not vomit, as the substance could burn the mouth or throat—especially in concentrations greater than 5 percent. For eye contamination, wash the eyes with running water for 15 to 20 minutes. If ammonia is inhaled, move the victim to fresh air and give artificial respiration.

amphetamines   [Other names: beans, bennies, black beauties, black mollies, copilots, crank, crossroads, crystal, dexies, doublecross, hearts, meth, minibennies, pep pills, roses, speed, thrusters, truck drivers, uppers, wake-ups, whites. Trade names: Aktedron, Benzedrine, Elastonon, Orthedrine, Phenamine, Phenedrine.] This white powder (or colorless liquid) is a highly addictive stimulant, once widely prescribed as a diet pill—but this use has now been banned by the Food and Drug Administration.

Amphetamines were also used to treat Parkinson's disease and similar symptoms, depression, alcohol withdrawal, premenstrual tension and hyperactivity. Today, they are strictly controlled and seldom administered because of serious withdrawal problems and dangerous side effects.

Usually taken in pill form, amphetamine can also be injected when in solution.

(A form of amphetamine commonly known as "speed" or "meth"—methamphetamine—is usually injected intravenously, although speed also comes in oral doses.)

Symptoms Amphetamines can stimulate both the sympathetic and central nervous systems, and are toxic in levels only slightly above usual doses, although a degree of tolerance can develop over time. Symptoms appear within 30 minutes to an hour, and when these drugs are taken in too large a dose, the symptoms can include sleeplessness, restlessness, tremors, palpitations, nausea, vomiting, diarrhea, anorexia, delirium, hallucinations, euphoria, nervousness, confusion, irritability, short temper, depression, cyanosis, sweating, convulsions, coma and cerebral hemorrhages. Brain damage or death may result from ventricular arrhythmia or stroke. When amphetamines are taken in only a mild overdose, symptoms include fatigue, mental depression and high blood pressure. Those who chronically abuse amphetamines may develop heart problems and behavioral abnormalities (such as picking at the skin) and appear paranoid and anorexic. In fact, appetite suppression in long-term addicts can continue for up to two months after amphetamine use has stopped.

Treatment Isolate the victim in a quiet, darkened room to avoid overstimulation and possible heart failure. Gastric lavage may be helpful if the person is awake, but emesis is not induced because of the risk of abrupt onset of seizures. Administer activated charcoal and a cathartic. Other symptoms are treated, and Valium may be given to slow the heartbeat.

amyl nitrite An antispasmodic, this is an antidote of cyanide and ergot that is also used medically to dilate the coronary vessels and lower blood pressure. It has been used as a vasodilator in angina therapy for a long time and has also been used as an industrial chemical and perfume scent. The increasing abuse of amyl nitrite "poppers" led to their restriction and the increased popularity of butyl and isobutyl nitrites (related volatile compounds sold over the counter as room odorizers under such names as "Locker Room.") These are inhaled to produce highs and intensify sexual orgasms and are sometimes sprayed in discos to stimulate dancing.

Symptoms Inhaling the volatile nitrites dilates blood vessels, causing low blood pressure lasting about 90 seconds. Other symptoms include pulsating headache, rapid flushing of the face, dizziness, confusion, vertigo, restlessness, weakness, blue skin, nausea and vomiting. In addition, butyl nitrite sniffing has caused mild methemoglobinemia in otherwise healthy patients. Chronic abuse of amyl nitrite can cause anemia.

Treatment Administration of methylene blue may be effective in treating methemoglobinemia. Other treatment is symptomatic.

Anaprox See NONSTEROIDAL ANTI-INFLAMMATORY DRUGS.

anectine (succinylcholine) This extremely fast-acting drug is also known as curare and is one of a group of neuromuscular blocking agents that affects skeletal muscles. It is used to promote muscle relaxation during surgical anesthesia and is sometimes given to control convulsions. It is generally used in the operating room during lung procedures, as it stops normal breathing and allows the patient to be placed on a respirator. Many physicians also use it before surgery as a muscle relaxant because it cuts down on the amount of anesthesia needed. It is also an antidote for strychnine poisoning and an anticonvulsant treatment for tetanus (lockjaw). An effective dose can be fatal if breathing is not maintained artificially. This bitter, white powder dissolves easily in water and can be administered either in the muscle or in the veins.

Symptoms Almost immediately upon injection, anectine produces respiratory paralysis by blocking the neuromuscular transmissions. Symptoms will continue for one to 10 minutes after the injection is discontinued. Cardiac arrest has occurred during the administration of anectine after a head injury.

Treatment There is no antidote—it works too quickly.

See also CURARE; NEUROMUSCULAR BLOCKING AGENTS.

anemone, sea One of the most abundant of the coelenterates, these immobile flowerlike creatures range in size from a few millimeters to about one and a half feet with long tentacles. Anemones are tube-shaped animals usually fixed to a firm surface, with a mouth slit on top and a range of tentacles around the mouth.

There are thousands of varieties of anemones, which differ from one another in every way. They do share one trait in common, however: the ability to sting and paralyze a victim with specialized cells lining their tentacles, which—while not usually fatal in itself—can cause drowning. Some varieties are poisonous to eat as well as capable of delivering a venomous sting.

While not all sea anemones are poisonous, the Matamalu samasama from Samoa *(Radianthus paumotensis, Rhodactis howesii)* is poisonous when eaten raw or cooked and causes respiratory failure. The *Actinia equina* floats along the eastern Atlantic, in the Mediterranean Sea, the Black Sea and the Sea of Azov; the hell's fire sea anemone *(Actinodendron plumosum)* is found in tropical waters of the Pacific Ocean and the Great Barrier Reef off Australia; and the rosy anemone *(Sagarita elegans)* inhabits the waters off Iceland to the Mediterranean Sea and the coast of Africa.

Symptoms Effects of the sea anemone sting are usually local, causing itching, burning, swelling and reddening followed by sloughing of the skin. The tissues may then slough off followed by a long period of purulent discharge, and multiple abscesses may occur. More generalized symptoms include fever, chills, abdominal pain, nausea, vomiting, diarrhea, headache, thirst and prostration.

Treatment Soak the stung area in water as hot as possible without scalding the person for up to one hour, using hot soaks while on the way to the doctor. Observe for signs of shock. The ulcers resulting from a sea anemone sting are usually slow to heal and can be resistant to treatment. Baking soda in a paste with water should be applied to the sting to relieve pain. Calamine lotion will also help ease the burning sensation, and painkillers may help with the stinging pain. (Other local remedies for pain used around the world include meat tenderizer, sugar, ammonia and lemon juice.)

anesthetics, gaseous/volatile   These drugs include ether, chloroform, ethylene and cyclopropane. They are also found as gases, including ethylene, cyclopropane and nitrous oxide.

All these anesthetics produce general anesthesia; at cold temperatures, they are volatile liquids before they become gases and can be inhaled or ingested.

Symptoms   Overdose stops respiration and interferes with the action of the autoimmune system, causing unconsciousness, respiratory failure, cyanosis and heart irregularities.

Treatment   Remove gas, maintain respiration and keep warm. In the event of fever, lower temperature with wet towels.

See also CHLOROFORM; CYCLOPROPANE; ETHER.

anesthetics, local   These drugs are used to numb one particular area of the body either by injection or by topical skin application (and include epidural, spinal and regional nerve blocks). No two act the same, and their effect on patients varies from one person to another depending on the person's physical makeup. These drugs are all related to cocaine and are synthetic versions of the coca bush alkaloids. Local anesthetics include procaine, lidocaine, marcaine, monocaine, nesacaine, nupercaine, duranest, xylocaine, carocaine, oracaine, unacaine, citanest and novocaine. Of these, procaine is considered the most dangerous and has caused numerous fatalities; shock can occur with only very small doses, and it enhances the action of muscle relaxants.

All of the local anesthetics are colorless (either liquid or gel) and are injected.

Symptoms   Local anesthetics work by blocking the nerve signals, providing a local loss of sensation. When the drugs are given in overdose, these actions may cause central nervous system and cardiovascular toxicity. Toxic levels can result from a single excessive injection, from a series of smaller injections or by accumulation of drug level by repeated doses. Symptoms of systemic poisoning affect primarily the central nervous system and include giddiness, feelings of oppression, severe collapse, coma, convulsions, dizziness, cyanosis, low blood pressure, tremors, coma, irregular and weak breathing, bronchial spasm and heart failure. Repeated skin applications of local anesthetic can cause hypersensitivity, including itching, redness, swelling and blistering.

Treatment   First, the injected drug must be removed from the body and absorption from the injection site lessened by using a tourniquet or ice pack. Treat symptoms, maintain airway and give artificial respiration with oxygen to control convulsions and central nervous system depression.

See also LIDOCAINE; PROCAINE.

aniline (amino benzol)   A colorless, oily fluid that turns brown when exposed to air, used in inks for stamp pads, printing and cloth marking, in addition to dyes, paint removers and paint. Aniline can be ingested or absorbed as a gas, powder or liquid.

Occasionally, aniline dye poisonings do occur among infants and young children; newborns have been poisoned by touching—and inhaling fumes from—diapers freshly stamped with aniline dye. It is also possible to become poisoned from absorbing shoe polish that contain aniline dyes. Fortunately, there are few poisonings from this substance today.

Symptoms   Aniline interferes with the transportation of oxygen throughout the central nervous system, and within two hours after exposure, moderate exposure may cause cyanosis of the lips, ears and cheeks. In more severe cases, symptoms of cyanosis are much more marked, together with headaches, shallow breathing, vertigo, chills, nausea and vomiting. Infants are apathetic and may exhibit convulsions, coma and death. Direct contact of aniline dye with the skin will cause dermatitis. Chronic poisoning in the wake of inhalation or skin absorption causes mild cyanosis, anorexia, weight loss, weakness, headache, vertigo, irritability and anemia.

Treatment   Remove victim to fresh air. If the skin has been contaminated, wash thoroughly with vinegar followed by soap and water. If aniline has been ingested, administer gastric lavage followed by liquid petrolatum and a saline cathartic. Oxygen, doxapram and blood transfusions may also be necessary. In very severe cases, hemodialysis should be used.

Antabuse   (disulfiram)   This drug is used to treat alcoholics, who experience an extremely unpleasant side effect if they drink alcohol while taking it. Long-term use of Antabuse can damage the peripheral nerves.

Symptoms   An acute overdose may cause vomiting, clumsiness, lethargy, seizures and coma. Several deaths have been reported as a result of liver failure. Ingestion of alcohol (including some types of cough syrup or other alcohol-containing products) while taking Antabuse can cause flushing, throbbing headache, anxiety, vertigo, vomiting and convulsion; the severity of the reaction is tied to the amount of Antabuse and alcohol ingested. It generally takes at least one day on the drug before the interaction will set off this reaction, but the reaction will also occur up to several days after the last dose of Antabuse has been taken.

Treatment There is no specific antidote. For overdose of Antabuse: Induce vomiting or perform gastric lavage; administer activated charcoal and a cathartic. For interaction of Antabuse and alcohol: Once symptoms appear, there is not much that can be done; if the victim drank a large amount of alcohol, gastric lavage and activated charcoal should help.

antianxiety drugs A group of drugs used to relieve symptoms of anxiety; benzodiazepines and beta adrenergic blockers are the two main types. Among them are Xanax (alprazolam), Librium (chlordiazepoxide), Tranxene (chlorazepate), Valium (diazepam), Dalmane (flurazepam), Ativan (lorazepam), Serax (oxazepam), Centrax (prazepam) and Halcion (triazolam). Most are addictive.

Symptoms Overdose can bring on drowsiness, weakness, double vision, clumsiness, lethargy, convulsions, coma, cyanosis and breathing problems. Chronic abuse can cause skin rash, gastric upset, headaches and blurred vision. Most reports of fatalities with antianxiety drugs involve multiple drug ingestions.

Treatment Induce vomiting or perform gastric lavage followed by the administration of activated charcoal and a saline cathartic. Follow with supportive measures, including monitoring of blood pressure and fluid levels.

See also BENZODIAZEPINES; BETA ADRENERGIC BLOCKERS; DALMANE.

antiarrhythmic drugs Prescribed to control unwanted variations in heartbeat, the most famous of these is digitalis. Certain recent varieties are classified as beta adrenergic blockers or calcium channel blocking drugs. Other examples of antiarrhythmic drugs include quinidine, procainamide (Pronestyl) and disopyramide (Norpace). All three may be toxic in doses only slightly above the recommended dose and may prove fatal.

Symptoms Toxicity with antiarrhythmic drugs primarily affects the cardiovascular and central nervous systems. Symptoms include heartbeat irregularities, dry mouth, dilated pupils, delirium, seizures, coma and respiratory arrest. Quinidine often causes nausea, vomiting, diarrhea and, with chronic doses, cinchonism (ringing in the ears, vertigo, deafness and visual disturbances). Procainamide may cause upset stomach and a lupuslike syndrome with chronic use.

Treatment Heart problems are treated with hypertonic sodium bicarbonate and possibly insertion of a pacemaker; treat symptoms and monitor vital signs. Do not induce vomiting because of the risk of rapid onset of seizures; perform gastric lavage followed by activated charcoal and a cathartic.

See also BETA ADRENERGIC BLOCKERS, DIGITALIS, QUINIDINE.

anticoagulants Drugs used to keep the blood from clotting too quickly and reduce mortality asociated with blood clots. They include warfarin, dicumarol, phenprocoumon and phenindione and work by interfering with the production in the liver of a number of clotting factors depending on vitamin K. Warfarin sodium (Coumadin) is the least toxic, and most widely used, anticoagulant. A wide range of factors can influence a person's response to anticoagulants, including changes in diet, environment and medication.

Symptoms   Sudden rush of blood hemorrhaging of the larynx, trachea or lungs, bloody stools, hemorrhages in other organs, bruising and bleeding into joint spaces, skin rash, vomiting, fever and kidney damage. Repeated use leads to acute poisoning. Fatalities from kidney and liver damage have been reported after repeated doses, and death may not occur until several weeks after the drug has been discontinued.

Treatment   Complete bed rest; medication is administered to prevent internal bleeding.

See also WARFARIN.

antidepressants   A class of drugs used to treat depression and anxiety; the two main types of antidepressant drugs are the tricyclic antidepressants (TCAs) and, less popular, monoamine oxidase (MAO) inhibitors. TCAs are widely used to treat depression and are also one of the most common types of drugs involved in intentional overdoses.

Symptoms   A tricyclic antidepressant overdose acts on the central nervous system, causing confusion, hallucinations and lethargy progressing to seizures or coma. Its most serious effect is on cardiac conductivity, resulting in multiple heart arrhythmias, which may result in death. Acute overdose of MAO inhibitors causes slow heartbeat, confusion, hallucinations, agitation and convulsions. High blood pressure may quickly reverse to low blood pressure, which is an indication of a very serious prognosis. Beer, wine and cheese eaten with MAO inhibitors can cause very serious symptoms, including intracranial bleeding, circulatory failure and death.

Treatment   The victim should be under medical supervision, since induced vomiting could cause seizures or arrhythmias. At a hospital, gastric lavage is followed by administration of activated charcoal and a cathartic. For cases of severe overdose of TCA, physostigmine salicylate may be used as an antidote. Hospitalization is strongly recommended. Patients receiving good supportive care will recover within four days.

See also MONOAMINE OXIDASE (MAO) INHIBITORS.

antifreeze   Most types of antifreeze contain ethylene glycol or methanol, both of which are poisonous to drink. About 50 deaths occur each year in the United States from antifreeze poisoning, most of which are among alcoholics who turn to antifreeze as an alternative to alcohol; some people attempt to commit suicide by this method. Antifreeze poisoning is also a problem for household pets, who are attracted by the sweet taste. According to Dr. Steve Hansen of the National Animal Poison Control Center, it only takes one teaspoon of undiluted antifreeze/coolant to kill a seven-pound cat.

Poisonous part Antifreeze containing ethylene glycol is extremely toxic because of its breakdown products and resulting acidosis.

Symptoms In small amounts, antifreeze poisoning resembles intoxication from alcohol; large doses cause vomiting, seizures and coma within a few hours, followed by acute kidney failure within 24 to 36 hours. The lethal dose of ethylene glycol is considered to be 100 ml for an adult, although recovery has been noted after ingestions ranging up to 970 ml. Antifreeze containing methanol can also cause blindness.

Treatment The victim should be taken to a medical care facility immediately. Do not attempt home treatment unless advised by a medical professional. If the eyes are contaminated, immediately rinse with warm running water for 15 to 20 minutes. Hospital treatment may include gastric lavage and the administration of diuretic drugs, in addition to intravenous alcohol and intravenous bicarbonate. Alcohol may be given orally every four hours for one to three days.

For antifreeze poisoning in pets, owners should first feed the pet soft food (milk or canned pet food) and then induce vomiting using syrup of ipecac. *If the pet is found within one hour of poisoning,* alcohol (such as whiskey) may be given as an antidote after vomiting—one or two ounces for smaller dogs and up to three or four ounces for larger breeds. If more than five hours have elapsed since poisoning, emergency home treatment will be fruitless. *Animal ingestion of antifreeze is a serious emergency that requires immediate, intensive veterinary care. Vomiting and alcohol should be administered at home only when veterinary care is not immediately available.* For emergency advice in an animal poisoning emergency, call the National Animal Poison Control Center at (900) 680-0000 ($2.95 per minute) or at (800) 548-2423 ($30 per call). The center's phones are staffed by trained veterinarians 24 hours a day, seven days a week.

See also METHANOL; NATIONAL ANIMAL POISON CONTROL CENTER; PETS AND POISONING.

antihistamines A group of drugs that block the effects of histamine, a chemical released during an allergic reaction. While harmless in normal amounts, they can be fatal when taken in massive overdose (as in a suicide attempt or accidental ingestion by young children). Antihistamines are being used more and more, not only to treat allergies and respiratory infections but also for motion sickness and as sedatives. Many are available over the counter.

Symptoms Antihistamines are a central nervous system depressant, causing drowsiness, dizziness and clumsiness; symptoms also resemble atropine poisoning, including dry mouth, fixed dilated pupils, fever and flushed and reddened face. Children are particularly susceptible to the stimulating effects of antihistamines and can show excitement, hallucinations, toxic psychosis, delirium, tremors and convulsions followed by respiratory or cardiac arrest.

Treatment Supportive. Induce vomiting followed by the administration of cathartics and activated charcoal. Perform gastric lavage for cases in which vomiting is not indicated, such as with poisoning with phenothiazine-type antihistamines, which are less responsive to ipecac-induced vomiting.

antihypertensive drugs Medications prescribed to lower high blood pressure, they are also classified as belonging to one of several drug families according to the way they work. The subdivisions include drugs that increase the rate at which the body eliminates urine and salt (diuretics); beta adrenergic blockers, drugs that block many of the effects of epinephrine (adrenaline) in the body; drugs that block the entry of calcium into the walls of the small arteries (calcium channel blockers); and drugs that block formation of a natural body chemical and dilate small arteries (angiotensin-converting enzyme inhibitors).

Antihypertensives include Aldomet (methyldopa), Catapres (clonidine), Minipress (prazosin hydrochloride), procainamide (procainamide hydrochloride), quinidine (cinchonan-9-ol and others) and sodium thiocyanate.

Symptoms In general, overdose causes a generalized depression of the sympathetic nervous system, including lethargy, pinpoint pupils, slow heartbeat, low blood pressure, low fever, apnea and coma. Onset of symptoms is usually within 30 to 60 minutes; full recovery occurs within 24 hours.

Treatment Treatment for antihypertensive overdose includes induced vomiting or gastric lavage followed by the administration of activated charcoal and a cathartic.

See also ALDOMET; BETA ADRENERGIC BLOCKERS; CATAPRES; DIURETICS; EPINEPHRINE; MINIPRESS; QUINIDINE.

anti-inflammatory drugs These medications are used to reduce inflammation and include a wide variety of corticosteroids and nonsteroidal anti-inflammatory drugs (NSAIDS), such as aspirin and ibuprofen. Inflammation is one of the body's defense mechanisms in response to infection and certain chronic diseases such as rheumatoid arthritis. But as inflammation increases blood flow, it causes swelling, redness, pain and heat. Anti-inflammatory drugs are designed to combat this inflammation.

On their own, anti-inflammatory drugs are not very toxic, but persons with gastrointestinal tract disease, peptic ulcers or poor heart function or those on anticoagulants should avoid them.

Anti-inflammatory drugs include diflunisal (Dolobid), ibuprofen (Motrin, Rufen, Advil, Haltrain, Medipren, Nuprin, Trendar), fenoprofen (Nalfon), meclofenamate (Meclomen) and naproxen (Anaprox, Naprosyn). None of these should be taken with other nonsteroid analgesics, or with warfarin or other oral anticoagulants, because bleeding time may be prolonged while on anti-inflammatory pain relievers. Antacids, however, may sometimes reduce the effects of an anti-inflammatory drug.

Symptoms   If a person is allergic to aspirin or other analgesic drugs, using another anti-inflammatory medicine could be fatal. Anti-inflammatory drugs become toxic when given to those with kidney problems, since the kidneys cannot cleanse the blood. Overdose causes kidney failure and severe liver reactions, including fatal jaundice.

Normally, anti-inflammatory overdose produces mild stomach upset, with nausea and vomiting plus abdominal pain and internal bleeding. Occasionally, other symptoms might include sleepiness, lethargy, nystagmus (involuntary oscillation of the eyeball), tinnitus (ringing in the ears) and disorientation. However, with some of the more toxic drugs and significant overdose of ibuprofen (in excess of 3,200 mg per day), symptoms can include seizures, coma, metabolic acidosis, kidney and liver failure and cardiorespiratory arrest.

Treatment   There is no antidote. Maintain symptomatic treatment together with antacids for mild stomach problems; perform gastric lavage, followed by administration of activated charcoal and a cathartic.

antimony   This silvery white soft metal is a popular hardening agent used in the production of soft metal alloys and rubber, as a coloring agent and in flameproofing compounds. It is also contained in a wide variety of products, including batteries, foil, safety matches, ant paste, ceramics, textiles, glass, enamels, typesetting metals and alloys. It is also used medicinally as an emetic and to combat worms. It is present in the dust and fumes produced during mining and refining, and from the discharge of firearms. Stibine (antimony hydride) is a colorless gas produced as a by-product when ore containing antimony is treated with acid.

A strong tissue irritant, antimony is lethal in doses of between 100 and 200 mg. Fatal poisonings from antimony are usually from drug overdoses, not from industrial exposure to vapors or dust. This is an extremely rare toxin in the 1990s.

Poisonous part   The toxic mechanism of both antimony and stibine is unknown, but its chemical action is similar to that of arsenic and arsine. It is believed that antimony compounds probably inactivate key enzymes in the body; stibine, like arsine gas, may destroy red blood cells.

Symptoms   While death is rare following the ingestion of antimony if the patient survives the initial gastroenteritis, symptoms are unpleasant and include nausea, vomiting and bloody diarrhea, with hepatitis and kidney problems. Chronic antimony poisoning is quite similar to chronic arsenic toxicity, causing itchy skin, conjunctivitis, laryngitis, headache, anorexia, weight loss and anemia. The inhalation of stibine causes headaches, weakness, nausea, vomiting, jaundice, anemia and kidney failure.

Treatment There is no specific antidote. As in arsenic poisoning, treatment for ingestion involves gastric lavage followed by the administration of activated charcoal (although there is no evidence that this is effective). Do not use cathartics. Dimercaprol (to hasten the excretion of metals such as arsenic, gold and mercury as well) may be administered, as well as narcotics for pain. Hospitalization is recommended. In stibine poisoning, a blood transfusion may be necessary after massive destruction of red blood cells.

See also ARSENIC; ARSINE GAS.

antipsychotic/psychometric drugs These drugs are used to treat psychosis and agitated depression and are a common choice for suicide. They include chlorpromazine (Thorazine), ethopropazine, fluphenazine (Permitil), mesoridazine (Serentil), perphenazine (Trilafon), prochlorperazine, promethazine, thioridazine (Mellaril), trifluoperazine (Stelazine), chlorprothixene, thiothixene (Navane), haloperidol (Haldol), loxapine, molindone and trimethobenzamide.

These drugs are mainly found as pills, though a few are injectable. Most of them are used to treat schizophrenia and manic-depression with psychotic manifestations. They may also be used before surgery to ease fears, to treat tetanus and to relieve behavior disorders in children.

Symptoms These drugs seldom cause death because it takes a high dosage to reach toxic levels. There is also tolerance to the sedating effects, and patients on chronic therapy may tolerate much larger doses than normal. Therefore, the toxic dose after acute ingestion is quite variable. Severe intoxication may cause coma, seizures and respiratory arrest. There may also be jaw muscle spasm, rigidity and tremor. Further, patients on long-term antipsychotic medication may develop a neuroleptic malignant syndrome (rigidity, high fever, sweating, lactic acidosis).

Treatment There is no specific antidote. Some experts recommend bromocriptine in the treatment of neuroleptic malignant syndrome, although other treatments for high fever are successful. Induce vomiting or perform gastric lavage if victim is seen within 30 to 60 minutes or if the overdose is substantial (gastric lavage is preferred).

See also THORAZINE.

antiseptics and disinfectants Both products are designed to kill microorganisms; antiseptics are applied to living tissue and disinfectants to inanimate objects. Despite the fact that they have never been proven to kill germs, they are widely used in both home and medical applications. Among the best known are hydrogen peroxide and hexylresorcinol. All of these agents are generally used in diluted solutions and cause very little toxicity. Still, skin contact and vapors can be irritating to skin and the respiratory system. These products are more hazardous when used in aerosol form, since the mist can be inhaled through the nose and mouth.

See also HYDROGEN PEROXIDE; IODINE; ISOPROPYL ALCOHOL.

antivenin   A specific treatment for snake, scorpion, spider or other venomous animal bites. It is produced by inoculating animals (usually horses) with venom from a poisonous animal, which stimulates the production of antibodies in the horse to neutralize the poisons in the venom. A preparation with the antibodies (or antivenins) can then be produced from samples of the horse's blood. When given to a snakebite victim, the antibodies bind to and neutralize circulating venom proteins.

Commercial antivenins are available for bites from all types of pit vipers (rattlesnakes, cottonmouth and copperhead snakes) and the coral snake. Antivenins for treating the bites of scorpions, spiders, fish and jellyfish—or snakes that originate outside the United States—can be obtained at zoos and from veterinarians. However, black widow spider antivenin is available in hospitals within the United States; antivenin for the stings of poisonous fish and jellyfish are generally not available in this country.

Experts do warn that the two commercially marketed antivenins for snakebite available in this country cause painful and sometimes serious reactions in the vast majority of treated snakebite victims. While neither poses a life-threatening risk, both trigger a generalized and sometimes severe immunological reaction called "serum sickness" in about 75 percent of individuals.

The most difficult aspect of producing antivenin lies in the purification—that is, extracting protein from the horse's blood that has the antibodies but not the other, useless proteins. These "useless" proteins from the horse are what trigger the serious reactions when injected into humans, since the human immune system recognizes them as foreign. In response to these foreign substances, a few people go into anaphylactic shock, a life-threatening immune response characterized by flushing and itching, nausea, breathing problems and lowered blood pressure.

It is possible to test a snakebite victim's sensitivity to horse protein, but the skin test itself can trigger anaphylactic shock, and a positive response would then require a physician to choose between a potential severe reaction to antivenin and death or amputation from the snakebite. And in about 3 percent of cases, victims with negative skin tests go on to have severe reactions to the antivenin anyway.

Recent research suggests that high-tech purification techniques using sheep's blood or chicken eggs instead of horse serum may result in a better antivenin. Chicken-based antibodies cannot trigger the highly inflammatory allergic reaction in humans that horse proteins can (unless there is a history of severe egg allergy); sheep antibodies also seem to cause fewer allergic reactions in humans.

See also ANTIVENIN, BLACK WIDOW SPIDER; ANTIVENIN, CORAL SNAKE; ANTIVENIN, RATTLESNAKE; SNAKES, POISONOUS.

antivenin, black widow spider   The antidote for the bite of the black widow spider, this antivenin is produced by injecting horses with venom and collecting some of the blood, which then contains antibodies to the poison. The antivenin should be given to victims of black widow spider bite in the presence of uncontrolled severe high blood pressure or if the victim is pregnant. Black widow spider bites in pregnant women may cause an abdominal spasm so severe that it sets off a miscarriage or early onset of labor.

As with other types of antivenin produced from horse serum, immediate allergic reaction is possible and a skin test for hypersensitivity should be performed.

See also ANTIVENIN; BLACK WIDOW SPIDER.

antivenin, coral snake   The antidote to the bite of the poisonous eastern coral snake (*Micrurus fulvius*) or the Texas coral snake (*M. fulvius tenere*). It is not effective against the bite of the Arizona or Sonora coral snake (*M. euryxanthus*).

The antivenin is produced by injecting horses with venom and then collecting some of the blood, which contains antibodies to the poison. As with other types of antivenin produced from horse serum, immediate allergic reaction is possible, and a skin test for hypersensitivity should be performed.

See also ANTIVENIN; CORAL SNAKE, ARIZONA; CORAL SNAKE, EASTERN.

antivenin, rattlesnake   The antidote for rattlesnake bite is produced by injecting horses with the pooled venoms of the eastern diamondback rattlesnake, the western diamondback, the cascabel, or tropical, rattlesnake and the fer-de-lance. The blood serum from the horse then contains a combination of several antibodies against venom constituents.

When given intravenously to the victim of rattlesnake bite, the antivenin binds to the venom throughout the body. However, it is possible to have an allergic reaction to the antivenin, causing anaphylactic shock even in those who tested negative for horse serum allergy.

See also ANTIVENIN; RATTLESNAKES.

apomorphine   This powerful emetic is an alkaloid salt derived from morphine. It has been used to induce vomiting in cases of oral poisoning, but at the moment, it is rarely used in either adult or childhood poisoning cases because it also strongly depresses breathing. Naloxone is used to treat the respiratory depression that occurs following apomorphine use. Apomorphine is popular, however, in veterinary medicine.

See also NALOXONE.

apple of Sodom *(Solanum sodomeum)* This common Hawaiian weed is also known as Dead Sea apple. It is a member of a very large genus of 1,700 species, most of which have not been evaluated toxicologically.

Poisonous part Human poisoning is usually attributed to immature fruit, which contains the toxin solanine glycoalkaloid.

Symptoms While there is little danger of fatal poisoning in adults, children may ingest a fatal amount of this plant. Symptoms appear several hours after ingestion and include gastric irritation, scratchy throat, fever and diarrhea. (Solanine poisoning is often confused with bacterial gastroenteritis.)

Treatment The same general supportive care that would be given in gastroenteritis cases; fluid replacement may be required.

apricot pit See PRUNUS.

aquarium products According to numerous reports at poison control centers around the country, a wide range of fairly nontoxic products sold for the upkeep of home aquariums may end up in the hands of young children, who may inadvertently ingest them. In addition, adults may find them in medicine cabinets and use them mistakenly for eye, ear or nose drops.

These products include antichlorine compounds (sodium thiosulfate), pH indicators, vitamins, copper sulfate, aquarium salts and a range of antimicrobials used to combat algae and fungi. Most are not very toxic, with the exception of some pH kits that contain sodium hydroxide (lye).

See also ALKALINE CORROSIVES.

arrow poison frogs (Dendrobatidae and *Phyllobates*) This tree frog (also called "dart poison frogs") of the Colombian rain forest is one of a group of brightly colored amphibians of South and Central America.

Once captured by the native people, it is carried back to camp, impaled on a sharpened stick and slowly roasted over an open fire; as it dies, the frog secretes a highly toxic mucus from the pores of its skin. This poison will later be applied to the tips of the Indians' blowgun darts and arrows. One specimen in this group is so toxic that one frog contains enough poison to kill about 100 people; handling this frog with bare hands could be fatal.

A supposed source of hunting magic in the rain forest, another type of this frog provides ointment used in prehunt ceremonies in which hunters burn themselves and then rub a stick coated with this frog's chemical on their wounds. According to legend, they awake with much keener senses the next morning. South American natives also rub frogs on wounds and cuts because the frog's skin contains potent antibiotic peptides.

Secretions from still another type of toxic frog will change the color of parrots; rubbing a bit of frog secretion over the spot of a plucked feather will cause a new feather to grow back in a different color.

Some poison frogs grow no bigger than a fingernail, whereas others vary so much in color that even frog experts mistake cousins as separate species. They all are rain forest inhabitants and live on land away from water, as long as there is enough water to lay their eggs. Most of these frogs have only slight water requirements, and some can be found living in the tiny water sac of bromeliad plants high above the forest floor. Most, however, prefer to live among the leaves that litter the rain forest floor, not in trees.

All the arrow poison frogs are very small and beautifully colored and can be handled carefully without danger—as long as they don't get excited. While there are many hundreds of different species, only a few are actually used to treat arrows; it takes up to 50 of them to coat the tips of a quiver. The most common of the poisonous arrow-tippers are:

Flat-spined Atelopus (Atelopus planispina), a gold and green Ecuadoran mountain frog with white spots and black markings.

Zetek's frog (Atelopus zeteki), a Panamanian golden frog; males have black blotches.

Yellow-spotted arrow poison frog (Dendrobates flavopictus), a black central Brazilian frog from the uplands, with bright yellow spots and lines.

Boulenger's arrow poison frog (Atelopus boulengeri), a black mountain frog from Peru and Ecuador with creamy spots.

Three-striped arrow poison frog (Dendrobates trivittatus), a South American black and yellow striped frog.

Two-toned arrow poison frog (Phyllobates bicolor), a vivid red frog with black markings from northern South America.

Gold arrow poison frog (Dendrobates auratus), a small gold and green frog from Nicaragua through Panama to Columbia.

Poisonous part   Of the family Dendrobatidae, four genera have skins with alkaloid compounds capable of killing a human if the toxin enters the blood (as from an arrow wound), and more than 50 poisonous species have been documented so far. Herpetologists suspect that the frog alkaloids are a by-product of metabolism.

Symptoms   While the toxin of the arrow poison frogs can be deadly if it enters the bloodstream (and one species, *Phyllobates horribilus*, can be fatal if chewed), skin contact with the frogs causes an irritating skin reaction, with swelling, reddening and blistering.

Treatment In cases of skin contact, wash secretions immediately with soap and water. If a person touches the skin and rubs an eye, the eye should be immediately rinsed with water or a saline solution. Significant skin reactions may require a doctor's care and treatment of dermatitis-type reaction; steroids may be helpful.

arsenic [Other names: arsenic trihydride, arsenic trioxide, arsenous oxide, metallic arsenic, white or gray arsenic] The 20th most common element that occurs naturally in pure form, arsenic is present in all human tissue and is a fairly accessible poison. It is used in the manufacture of ceramics, enamels, paint, wallpaper, weed killer, insecticide, rat poisons and pesticides. In its natural state, arsenic is a gray metal. While arsenic has been used intentionally to murder, poisoning also occurs as a result of industrial accidents or accidental ingestion.

In addition, arsenic (present throughout the earth's crust) contaminates the groundwater around the world. According to California's Environmental Protection Agency in Berkeley, drinking this arsenic-contaminated water has recently been found to pose a far more serious toxic threat than had been previously believed. In fact, new tests suggest that lifetime consumption of water with levels at the current federal limit (50 parts per billion) presents a one-in-100 cancer risk. Toxicologists have recommended that California lower its 50-ppb drinking water standard to just two parts per trillion, which corresponds to an overall cancer risk of roughly one in one million.

Symptoms Most toxicologists believe arsenic combines with enzymes to interfere with cellular function, causing severe gastric distress, esophageal pain, vomiting and diarrhea with blood. The skin is cold and clammy, and blood pressure plummets followed by convulsions and coma.

Arsenic poisoning can be chronic, occurring over a long period of time, and in such cases causes weakness, tiredness, scaly skin and changes in skin pigmentation, followed by swelling of the lining of the mouth and finally a degeneration of nerves, causing tingling and numbness and moments of paralysis; death comes eventually from heart failure, bone marrow failure or infection.

Poisoning may also result from a single large dose (acute poisoning), in which case death can come within a day, and sometimes after only a few hours. In acute cases, the arsenic affects the intestinal lining, quickly producing painful symptoms—nausea, vomiting, diarrhea, sweating and burning of the throat, followed by collapse and death. Individual susceptibility to arsenic poisoning varies, and some individuals can develop a tolerance to doses of arsenic that would kill others.

Because arsenic is an element and cannot be broken down any further, traces remaining in a person's hair, fingernails and urine can be identified upon urinalysis or autopsy.

Treatment In acute arsenic poisoning, the patient should be transported to a medical facility. Gastric lavage and fluid replacement are vital, together with the administration of dimercaprol for two or three days followed by penicillamine until the arsenic level in the urine drops. The victim should also be treated for dehydration, shock, pulmonary edema and liver damage and may be put on a kidney dialysis machine after the dimercaprol. Chronic poisoning is also treated with dimercaprol.

arsine gas This arsenic compound is an extremely poisonous, colorless inflammable gas (AsH_3) composed of arsenic and hydrogen, which occurs when metals containing arsenic are exposed to acids. The gas, also called arsenic hydride, is used as a military poison gas, but most cases of arsine poisoning occur in the metallurgic industries during the refining process and during galvanizing, soldering and lead plating.

According to the American Conference of Environmental Industrial Hygienists, 0.05 part per million is the maximum safe concentration for prolonged arsine exposure.

Arsine gas has a disagreeable odor, similar to that of onions or carbide.

Symptoms Inhalation causes vomiting, cramps and nausea; decreased or cessation of urine output, which is often stained red four to six hours after exposure, followed by the appearance of jaundice. Effects of exposure to arsine gas include damaged kidneys and destruction of red blood cells; chronic exposure leads to gradual loss of strength, diarrhea or constipation, scaling of the skin that can become malignant, paralysis, confusion and anemia.

Treatment Physicians advocate early exchange transfusions and the administration of dimercaprol, which is usually not effective. Those with less than fatal doses of gas will recover; those who receive a fatal dose cannot be saved despite treatment. The only true solution to arsine gas poisoning is prevention.

See also ARSENIC.

artane See TRIHEXYPHENIDYL.

asbestos A mineral fiber found in rocks and manufactured into heat- and friction-resistant materials. Asbestos is one of the most widely recognized sources of environmentally produced disease. It was used in a wide variety of ceiling materials, insulation, roofing, shingles and siding, hair blowers, some vinyl floor tiles and vinyl sheet flooring, stoves and furnaces, appliance insulation, walls and pipes.

Unfortunately, the toxic nature of asbestos (it causes lung and stomach cancer) was not realized until the demand for its use resulted in its incorporation in most buildings and vessels constructed for an entire generation. And even though it has been accepted that asbestos can cause disease in those exposed to it, there is considerable controversy about the dose required to produce disease.

Occupations most at risk for asbestos exposure include insulators, shipyard workers, construction workers and pipe fitters.

Exposure to asbestos leads to an accumulation of the mineral in the lung, which then migrates to other regions in the body. It can cause asbestosis, a disease characterized by a pulmonary fibrous reaction to the inhalation of asbestos fibers with progressive restriction of lung capacity. Other diseases associated with asbestos exposure include lung cancer and mesothelioma (a rare tumor originating in the cells lining the chest and abdominal cavity).

Asbestos-like fibers are commonly found in drinking water sources throughout the United States originating from rock areas in watersheds, from refuse dumps and in asbestos-containing water pipes. There is no evidence, however, that ingesting these fibers causes disease in humans.

If asbestos is found and must be disturbed, handle it carefully wearing a filtered mask. If at all possible, experts recommend that a trained contractor remove it.

ascorbic acid   *(vitamin C)* This is a powerful reducing agent used in treating methemoglobinemia in conjunction with methylene blue following poisoning with benzene, lead or arsenic poisoning, nicotine intoxication, bacterial toxins and anaphylaxis.

See also BENZENE; LEAD POISONING; ARSENIC; NICOTINE.

asp See COBRA, EGYPTIAN.

aspartame   Sold under the trade names NutraSweet and Equal, aspartame is an artificial sweetener discovered by accident in 1965. It is a synthetic combination of two amino acids (phenylalanine and aspartic acid).

Although it was kept off the market for many years because one animal study suggested a high incidence of brain tumors, other studies failed to duplicate these results. Eventually it proved to taste better than many alternatives on the market, and it was subsequently approved for use as a food additive after being subjected to one of the most rigorous scientific safety testings.

After more than 100 studies, however, there is still controversy over its safety. Critics say that many of the studies used by the Food and Drug Administration (FDA) to approve the use of aspartame are tainted by excessive food industry support. But FDA reviews show no adverse health effects among laboratory animals tested.

Yet complaints about aspartame account for 80 percent of the telephone calls received on the FDA food additives hotline, second only to sulfites.

The most common complaint is that it causes severe headaches among sensitive users, but the FDA cannot prove this is the case, although it did find some consumers who break out in hives after ingesting aspartame. In addition, aspartame can cause severe problems for people with phenylketonuria (PKU) disease.

Critics are most concerned about aspartame because it contains phenylalanine and aspartic acid, which in large doses excessively stimulate the brain, similar to the effect of monosodium glutamate (MSG). This overstimulation can damage the brain, perhaps leading to neurological diseases. Studies done on animals also suggest that children, especially infants, could be particularly vulnerable to brain damage caused by aspartate-induced overstimulation of brain cells. For this reason, some scientists recommend that pregnant women avoid using aspartame since studies suggest that—at least in animals—infants are particularly vulnerable to brain damage caused by aspartate's excess stimulation to the brain.

Because of a child's small body weight, aspartame doses per pound of body weight can easily be two to three times higher than that of an adult drinking, for example, the same amount of artificially sweetened soft drink.

As a condition of FDA approval, aspartame manufacturers are required to monitor the consumption of aspartame in food products. Products using aspartame must carry a label to warn people with PKU disease that the product contains phenylalanine.

While the long-term safety of aspartame has yet to be determined, large acute ingestions require only supportive therapy, if any.

Aspergillus flavus   A species of mold that produces the very toxic substance aflatoxin.

See also AFLATOXINS.

aspirin (acetylsalicylic acid)   This common painkiller and antipyretic (fever reducer) is a slightly bitter white powder usually sold in tablet form and, in correct dosages, is not poisonous. However, in large doses (such as a child would take in swallowing a bottle of pills) it can cause acid-base imbalance, convulsions, coma and, occasionally, respiratory failure.

Salicylic acid was first isolated from willow bark in 1838, but it was another 60 years before aspirin found its way into clinical practice. Since then, aspirin and other salicylates have been the most widely used medicines in the country. Because of this extensive use, it is not surprising that a large number of overdoses—both acute and chronic—have been recorded.

In the United States, more than 200 different products contain acetylsalicylic acid (aspirin), sodium salicylate and salicylate acid itself. Salicylates are also found in a number of products designed for topical application, where they can lead to poisoning through absorption through the skin.

There are a number of ways in which salicylate poisoning can occur.

Because the metabolic pathways in young children are soon saturated by repeated excessive doses of salicylates during illnesses accompanied by fever, it is fairly easy to give too much aspirin to young children. For this reason and because of the association between aspirin given during certain illness and Reye's syndrome, pediatricians usually prefer the use of acetaminophen with young children. Frequent application of teething gels containing salicylates an also cause toxicity. In addition, deliberate suicide attempts by overdosing on aspirin are common in persons between ages 15 and 35 and sometimes occur in those as young as 8 or 10.

However, according to the poison experts, the incidence of salicylate poisoning is decreasing; the proportion of salicylate poisoning to others below age five fell from 21.7 to 3.4 percent between 1967 and 1977. Toxicity is decreasing, experts believe, primarily because less aspirin is being used by children and adults and because of child-resistant containers. Unfortunately, there has been a parallel trend of an increase in poisoning with acetaminophen, probably because of increased use of this medicine.

Symptoms A central nervous system stimulant, aspirin in large doses can cause pain in the abdomen, lethargy, tinnitus (ringing in the ears), acid-base imbalance, fever, dehydration, restlessness, convulsions, coma and respiratory failure. Chronic poisoning may cause bleeding.

Treatment Unless breathing is slow, give a glass of water and induce vomiting with syrup of ipecac if within two hours of ingestion. Then administer activated charcoal to diminish the absorption of salicylate. This is most effective if given immediately, as it will only work within two hours after ingestion. Diuresis (increasing production of urine) may be induced; in those who have ingested a large amount, hemodialysis may be a very efficient method of eliminating the salicylate from circulation. Management is usually determined by a salicylate level at six hours.

See also SALICYLATES.

atropine An alkaloid frequently found in different species of nightshade that can cause problems in swallowing or speaking, rapid heartbeat, dilation of pupils and very high fever and delirium. Atropine is extracted from deadly nightshade (belladonna) for medicinal purposes—as a premedication before general anesthesia to lessen lung secretions, or as an emergency treatment for an abnormally slow heartbeat. Most homes, in fact, have medications containing atropine, since they are widely used for eye, skin, rectal and gastrointestinal problems.

The fatal dose of atropine is unknown; while there is wide variance in tolerance from one person to another, estimates suggest that more than 20 mg is fatal to children and more than 100 mg fatal to adults. Jimsonweed—especially the seeds—is the plant most commonly ingested, usually to obtain a "high."

Symptoms Symptoms of atropine poisoning include dry, burning mouth; difficulty swallowing; thirst; blurred vision; hot, dry skin; fever; and tachycardia. Fever can spike to 109°F in infants. Urinary problems, confusion, mania, delirium and psychotic behavior may continue for hours or days. With severe overdose, death can occur following circulatory and respiratory collapse.

Treatment The treatment for atropine poisoning involves the administration of physostigmine.

See also ALDICARB; ALDOMET; ALKALOIDS; ANTIHISTAMINES; BENZTROPINE; BETEL NUT SEED; CATAPRES; CHRISTMAS ROSE; CLIMBING LILY; COLOCYNTH; DEATH CAMAS; DIGITOXIN; FLY AGARIC; HENBANE; INDIAN TOBACCO; JIMSONWEED; MANDRAKE, AMERICAN; MUSCARINE; NIGHTSHADE, BITTERSWEET; NIGHTSHADE, DEADLY.

azalea See RHODODENDRON.

B

Bacillus thuringiensis (Bt)   A popular botanic insecticide, Bt is a species of bacterium sold in a variety of strains and kills soft-bodied insects or those in their larval form. The most widely used strain kills larval caterpillars of many moths, including the gypsy moth, the cabbage moth and the berry moth. Newly developed strains are aimed at beetle larvae (such as bean beetles and potato beetles), while others are aimed at borers. Some Bts from specialty stores combine the different strains into one superpesticide.

Bt will also kill some beneficial insects, but only in the soft-bodied larval stage. It is considered safe for humans, other mammals and birds.

See also BOTANIC INSECTICIDES; PESTICIDES.

BAL   (2,3-dimercaptopropanol, dimercaprol, British anti-lewisite) An antidote for mercury, copper, arsenic, gold, nickel, lead and antimony poisoning, but less effective for silver poisoning. It may make iron, selenium or cadmium poisoning worse, since BAL complexes act on the liver. It is best given as soon as possible following ingestion of the toxic substance.

baneberry *(Actaea)*   [Other names: black baneberry, cohosh, doll's eyes, European baneberry, herb-Christopher, necklaceweed, snakeberry, western baneberry] This plant of the buttercup family includes eight species of perennial herbs that grow less than two feet tall in richly wooded areas, boasting oversize leaves each with two or more leaflets. In warm weather (usually spring) this herb is adorned with distinct bunches of pearly white flowers at the tips of the stems. The fruit matures in late summer or early fall.

The white baneberry *(A. pachypoda* or *A. alba)* has snow-white fruit and is native to North America. The red baneberry or red cohosh *(A. rubra)* is another North American native and bears a red or ivory fruit. Cohosh or herb-Christopher *(A. spicata)* resembles *A. rubra* and has dark purple fruit sometimes used to make dye.

A. pachypoda thrives from Nova Scotia, Canada south along the east coast of the United States as far as Georgia, west to Missouri and north to Minnesota. *A. rubra* grows throughout Canada and the United States. *A. spicata* is cultivated in Canada and the United States.

Poisonous part   Only the red or white berries, foliage and roots contain the unknown toxin, which is a fast-acting and deadly poison acting on the heart. The root is a violent purgative, irritant and emetic. In mountain forests, the black berries are often confused with blueberries. While no loss

34

of life has been reported in the United States, European children have died after eating baneberry fruit.

Symptoms   Prolonged contact with the skin causes skin rash. If the plant is eaten, symptoms begin within several hours to a few days, with excruciating pain and inflammation followed by blisters or open sores of the lips, tongue, mouth and throat. Larger amounts of the plant cause vomiting streaked with bright-red blood; severe diarrhea and relentless abdominal cramps; excessive, blood-tinged urine; dizziness; fainting; and mental confusion or hallucinations. In critical cases, there are grand mal seizures.

Prognosis is guarded; often, the electrolytes and fluids of the body are depleted, and the kidneys and nervous system can sustain permanent damage if the symptoms are severe or prolonged. Death may follow if the poison is not cared for immediately.

Treatment   The irritating effects of this plant usually limit the amount ingested. Gastric lavage should be performed followed by the administration of milk or egg white as a demulcent. Renal function and fluid and electrolyte levels should be monitored.

Barbados nut   *(Jatropha curcas)*   [Other names: curcus bean, kukui haole, physic nut, purge nut] This small, spreading shade tree grows to about 15 feet and is found in southern Florida and Hawaii, Africa, Mexico, Asia, and Central and South America. Its flowers are small and green-yellow, with three to five lobed leaves; it also produces a sticky sap. A resinous substance produced by insects feeding on the leaves is used to make a varnish for guitars. *Jatropha* is a genus of the spurge family found in both the Old World and New World, containing about 125 species of herbs, shrubs and trees.

Unfortunately, while the seeds contained in the nut of this tree are extremely tasty, they contain more than 55 percent of an oil more potent than castor oil. In tropical areas the seeds are still used by folk healers, although they are quite dangerous.

Poisonous part   All parts of the Barbados nut contain the poison jatrophin, which is a harsh purgative. The poison kills by interfering with the synthesis of protein in intestinal wall cells. The seeds can be eaten if thoroughly roasted to remove the poison.

Symptoms   This plant is quickly fatal; within 15 to 20 minutes, symptoms appear: burning throat, bloating, dizziness, vomiting, diarrhea, drowsiness, leg cramps, difficulty breathing. May be fatal to children.

Treatment   Gastric lavage (unless there has been a great deal of vomiting already). Rehydration.

See also CORAL PLANT.

barbiturates   A group of sedative drugs including pentobarbital (Nembutal), phenobarbital (Luminal or "downers"), secobarbital (Seconal or "reds"), thiopental (Pentothol) and amobarbital (Amytal), that work by depressing brain activity. Overdosing on barbiturates is a common cause of death from suicide. Because these drugs are highly addictive and often abused, their use today is strictly controlled. Overdose—particularly when used with alcohol—is common. The toxicity of a particular type of barbiturate depends on how quickly it is designed to act. All cause unconsciousness, and their effects depend in part on how well the liver metabolizes them.

Symptoms Within 30 minutes (usually much sooner) sedation begins, followed by dizziness, headache, confusion, heart irregularities, low blood pressure and then coma, which may last up to several days. While the toxicity level for barbiturates is high, they can be fatal in combination with alcohol.

Treatment Barbiturates are quickly absorbed in the system, so gastric lavage needs to be performed no later than the first few hours after ingestion if treatment is to be effective. Even when it is performed quickly, however, often little of the drug is retrieved this way. This may be followed by repeated doses of activated charcoal. Fatality from barbiturate overdose ranges between 5 and 7 percent, but many people attempt suicide again using barbiturates. For this reason, follow-up mental health care is strongly recommended.

barium While barium poisonings are not common, they are usually due to accidental contamination of food or a result of suicide. Water-soluble barium salts (barium acetate, carbonate, chloride, hydroxide, nitrate, sulfide) are extremely toxic, but the insoluble salt barium sulfate is not because it cannot be absorbed. The soluble barium salts are used in fireworks, depilatories and rat poisons and are used to manufacture glass and to dye textiles.

Symptoms Within minutes to a few hours after ingestion, victims experience muscle weakness, followed by paralysis of the limbs and lungs, with additional heart problems. There may also be gastroenteritis with watery diarrhea, impaired vision and central nervous system depression. However, victims usually remain conscious.

Treatment Symptomatic treatment, with the administration of potassium chloride. Induce vomiting or perform gastric lavage; administer activated charcoal and a cathartic.

bee stings For most Americans, a bee sting is a minor annoyance and can be fatal only if occurring in large numbers (hundreds in an adult). But between one million and two million Americans are severely allergic to the inflammatory substances in the venom of bees, wasps, hornets and yellow jackets—which means they have been sensitized by the venom from a sting in the past, so that a single subsequent sting could provoke a severe allergic reaction.

Bee stings cause three to four times more deaths in the United States compared with snake bites, but the deaths are related to an individual's sensitivity, not the relative toxicity of any one insect poison. About 50 to 100

Americans die each year from bee stings. Since the bee venom toxicity is related to an individual's sensitivity and not to the venom itself, there is no bee antivenin available.

While hornets and wasps usually do not attack unless their nest is threatened, yellow jackets are very aggressive and quick-tempered. Of all the stinging insects, the most lethal is the wasp. The vicious hornet or yellow jacket (striped yellow and black) is so aggressive that it both stings and bites. Honeybees have round, smooth abdomens; bumblebees are two to three times larger than honeybees and have round, furry abdomens. Hornets, yellow jackets and wasps have long, slender abdomens and are all usually striped yellow and black.

A bee sting activates the body's immune system, which releases antibodies that counteract the harmful effects of germs and toxins. However, some individuals release too much of this antibody, which can become life threatening.

Allergic reactions to bee stings, therefore, are more common in adults than in children because adults have had more of a chance to develop a serious allergy to the stings. Each subsequent sting usually results in a more serious allergic reaction in those already sensitized.

The severity of a sting also depends on where it is located on the body: A sting to the neck can affect breathing, and swallowing a bee can cause strangulation if the bee stings the inside of the throat.

Certain types of clothing can be good protection against a bee sting; white or light-colored clothing with a smooth finish is less likely to excite bees to attack. Leather is particularly irritating to bees, but they will also become disturbed with brightly colored, dark, rough or wooly material. Bees also seem to become irritated over perspiration odors, perfumes, suntan lotions and hair sprays.

It is always better to remain motionless than to run in order to avoid being stung (unless being pursued by a colony of bees). Do not swing at a bee but slowly retreat, with your face protected with your hands and fingers outstretched. Or, if possible, lie face down on the ground.

Symptoms   When stung, allergic individuals experience soreness and swelling not only at the site of the sting but on other parts of the body as well. Symptoms in those allergic to bee stings include fever, chills, light-headedness, hives, joint and muscle pain, swelling of the lymph glands and bronchial constriction. Other severe reactions include a sudden drop in blood pressure with loss of consciousness, difficulty breathing, shock and, occasionally, death within one hour. Multiple stings—30 or 40 insects—will cause a reaction even in an unsensitized individual, including chills, fever, vomiting, pulmonary edema, difficulty breathing, drop in blood pressure, and collapse.

Treatment   A bee will often leave its sting sac in the wound; thus to treat a sting, remove the stinger by scraping it away with a fingernail or the edge of a knife blade. Grasping it with tweezers will simply squeeze more venom into the wound. Wash the wound with soap and water and apply antiseptic and a cold compress; ice will help reduce swelling.

Pain and irritation can be relieved by applying a paste made from either baking soda and water, or meat tenderizer and water. The meat tenderizer, developed to break down meat protein, also neutralizes bee venom. For stings in the mouth or throat, give victim ice cubes to suck while seeking medical attention.

Those who have had a severe reaction should carry an emergency self-treatment kit, available only with a doctor's prescription, containing anti-histamine tablets, alcohol swabs and a preloaded syringe with epinephrine, which counteracts the allergic response of the sting. Diphenhydramine (Benadryl) can stop or slow symptoms, but it must be given immediately.

In addition, highly sensitized individuals may consider taking immuno-therapy, but since this procedure carries a risk of anaphylactic shock, it should only be administered by a physician with access to epinephrine.

bellyache bush *(Jatropha gossypiifolia)*   This annual found throughout the New World is a member of a large genus of shrubs or small trees with a three-sided seed capsule.

Poisonous part   The seeds are poisonous and contain a variety of toxins and cathartic oils. Ingestion of just one seed can be serious. The toxins inhibit protein synthesis in cells of the intestinal wall and may cause serious or fatal poisoning.

Symptoms   The onset of symptoms (nausea, vomiting and diarrhea) occurs rapidly, unlike poisoning with other plants with toxic lectins.

Treatment   Treat symptoms; give fluids.

benzene   This simple aromatic hydrocarbon is a common household solvent used as a cleaning agent for rubber, fats, grease paints and lacquers and is a known carcinogen. Because of this, it has widely been replaced by toluene in many industrial products. It is no longer available for home or private use. Benzene is obtained from coke-oven gas or from petroleum, and it is highly toxic. Long-term exposure may lead to acute leukemia and aplastic anemia. Most cases of benzene poisoning are caused by skin contact or breathing fumes in poorly ventilated rooms; recent cases have been reported of fatalities following cleaning of tank cars. It may even occur after sniffing gasoline with a high benzene content.

Symptoms   Symptoms are caused by stomach irritation and benzene's depressive action on the body's central nervous system and bone marrow. Breathing these solvent fumes can cause headache, eye irritation, dizziness, visual disturbances, nausea and euphoria; more toxic cases include tremors, delirium, unconsciousness, coma and convulsions. In extreme cases, inhaling these fumes can be fatal.

Chronic cases of breathing benzene fumes cause a diminished production of all blood components and can lead to weakness, anorexia and anemia, with abnormal bleeding. In cases of chronic poisoning, symptoms may not appear until months or years after contact—even after exposure to benzene has ceased.

Treatment Call the poison control center before attempting any treatment. If fumes have been inhaled, get the victim into fresh air and give artificial respiration if needed. For skin contamination, rinse in running water for at least 15 minutes.

benzene hexachloride [Other names: gammahexane; 1,2,3,4,5,6-hexachlorocyclohexane; BHC; DBH; HCCH; HCH; trade name Streunex] This synthetic pesticide is found in a white crystalline, wettable powder, emulsion, dust and solution in organic solvents. Both benzene hexachloride and lindane are moderately toxic when inhaled or absorbed and extremely poisonous if ingested. Disagreeable in odor, benzene hexachloride does not dissolve in water but is readily soluble in fats or oils and is therefore particularly dangerous if ingested after a fatty meal. Benzene hexachloride is widely used by veterinarians to combat fleas and ticks.

Symptoms Benzene hexachloride affects the central nervous system and may cause liver and kidney damage. Symptoms appear within 30 minutes to three hours, although it may take as long as six hours before reactions appear. When benzene hexachloride is ingested, mucous membranes that touched the poison become irritated, followed by vomiting, diarrhea and convulsions. Poisoning may be fatal, usually as a result of pulmonary edema. Bread tainted with HCH has sickened some people, including infants breastfed by women who have eaten the bread. Because benzene hexachloride is rapidly excreted by the body, chronic poisoning is unlikely.

Treatment Symptomatic treatment.

benzodiazepines A class of drugs containing compounds that vary widely in their strength, duration and clinical use. In general, they are given as muscle relaxants, to relieve short-term anxiety due to stress or trauma, to relieve the unpleasant delirium of alcohol withdrawal and to help induce sleep. Fatalities from overdose of a benzodiazepine is rare, unless the drug is used with other central nervous system depressants (such as alcohol or barbiturates).

Benzodiazepines include Ativan (lorazepam), Centrax (prazepam), Dalmane (flurazepam), Librium (chlordiazepoxide), Serax (oxazepam), Tranxene (chlorazepate) and Valium (diazepam). Newer potent short-acting agents include Halcion (triazolam), Xanax (alprazolam) and Versed (midazolam).

Symptoms Most benzodiazepines are addictive, and all can be either taken by mouth or injected; a few are available as suppositories. In general, overdose symptoms include drowsiness, weakness, crossed eyes, double vision, uncoordination and lassitude, followed by convulsions, coma, cyanosis and breathing problems. Chronic abuse can produce a skin rash, stomach problems, headaches and blurred vision. In all of these drugs, symptoms can appear within a few minutes to several hours. Respiratory arrest is more common with the shorter-acting drugs (Xanax, Versed and Halcion).

Treatment Symptomatic treatment. It has been reported that the benzodiazepine antagonist flumazenil can quickly reverse a coma caused by benzodiazepine overdose, although it is not yet commercially available in the United States. Perform gastric lavage; induce vomiting except in those patients who have ingested one of the short-acting drugs. Follow this with the administration of activated charcoal and a cathartic.

See also DALMANE; DIAZEPAM; MIDAZOLAM.

benztropine (Cogentin) This is an antidote to many of the extrapyramidal side effects (wobbly gait, slurred speech, foaming at the mouth, forgetfulness, drooling, stiffness) sometimes seen with large doses of psychiatric drugs. It is pharmacologically similar to atropine.

See also ATROPINE.

beta adrenergic blockers These "beta blockers" slow the heart rate and reduce the force of the heart muscle's contraction and are used to treat high blood pressure, arrhythmias, angina, migraine headaches and glaucoma. There are a wide variety of beta blockers, including Tenormin, Lopressor, Visken and Inderal.

Symptoms Unfortunately, the response to beta blockers varies from patient to patient, depending on overall health and other medications; it is possible to have a fatal reaction to even a normal dose. Ingestion of only two or three times the therapeutic dose should be considered to be potentially fatal for any patient. In addition, the sudden withdrawal of beta blockers can cause heart failure, especially in patients who have problems with the aorta. Many patients who overdose on beta blockers may also be taking other cardioactive drugs or have an underlying heart problem, both of which may worsen the effects of the overdose. Overdoses with beta blockers all have similar symptoms and toxicity ratings.

Treatment Symptomatic treatment; perform gastric lavage (vomiting is not recommended because of the danger of seizures and coma). Administer activated charcoal and a cathartic.

betel nut seed *(Areca catechu)* This poisonous seed is chewed for its narcotic effects by native peoples in central and southwest Asia and South America, but too large an amount can be toxic.

Poisonous part   The seeds are considered extremely poisonous and contain the toxic alkaloid arecain and other poisons.

Symptoms   Within 20 minutes of ingestion, patients experience vomiting, diarrhea, difficulty breathing, impaired vision, convulsions and death.

Treatment   Antidote is atropine.

birth control, botanical   From earliest times, people have searched for an herbal remedy for unwanted pregnancy; unfortunately, most plants capable of killing a fetus are also capable of killing the mother. The Amazon Indians chew the leaves of several jungle plants for contraceptive purposes, and the Chinese have used abortifacients since the ninth century.

According to Aristotle, oil from the cedar and olive prevent conception; in medieval times, onion juice smeared on the penis was supposed to work. Abortifacients over the centuries include thyme, rue, mugwort, ergot, iris and pennyroyal; a chemical from the English yew was so widely used for abortion that the plant was known as the "bastard killer."

See also ERGOT; PENNYROYAL OIL; YEW.

birth control pills   Medication containing progesterone or estrogen (or derivatives) used for the prevention of pregnancy. At present, they are not considered toxic when ingested accidentally by children.

black locust *(Robinia pseudoacacia)* [Other names: bastard acacia, black acacia, false acacia, green locust, pea flower locust, post locust, silver chain, treesail, white honey flower, white locust, yellow locust.] The towering locust tree can grow to be 80 feet tall and is found particularly in the eastern United States from Pennsylvania through Georgia, in the Smoky Mountains and the Ozarks.

Its compound leaves have a series of leaflets one inch long and a pair of woody thorns where the leaf stem emerges from the branch. The fragrant white flower clusters produce a flat, reddish brown fruit pod that remains over the winter months.

Poisonous part   The poison is a phytotoxin called "robin," a plant lectin (toxalbumin) that interferes with the synthesis of protein in the small intestine. It is particularly prevalent in the inner bark, seeds and leaves.

Symptoms   Appearing within one or more hours, symptoms include nausea, vomiting, diarrhea, stupor, weak pulse and gastroenteritis. Poisoning may be followed by shock, convulsions and death, although these are uncommon.

Treatment   Gastric lavage; fluid and electrolyte level correction; oral administration of magnesium sulfate.

See also PHYTOTOXINS.

black snake, Australian *(Pseudeschis porphyriacus)*   The most common of the poisonous Australian snakes, the black snake has a blue-black body with a small head and a red belly and is found in marshy areas of Australia. Others in the same group include the spotted black snake (*P. guttatus*) and the mulga (*P. australis*). Note: The Australian black snake should not be confused with the American black snake, a common—and nonpoisonous—snake.

Poisonous part   Its venom is a powerful anticoagulant.

Symptoms   Within 15 to 30 minutes symptoms appear: pain, swelling, a drop in blood pressure, confusion, slurring of speech, dilation of the pupils, strabismus (abnormal deviation of one eye in relation to the other), drooping of the upper eyelid and muscle weakness. The respiratory muscles are affected last, and respiratory muscle paralysis is the most common cause of death.

Treatment   Australian black snake antiserum should be used.

See also ANTIVENIN; SNAKES, POISONOUS.

black widow spider   [Other names: button spider (South Africa), karakurt (Russia), katipo (New Zealand), malmignatte (Mediterranean).] One of two species of poisonous spiders found in the United States, the black widow has a globe-shaped, shiny black body with a red or orange hourglass-shaped mark on its belly. On some spiders, there are several triangles or spots instead of the well-known hourglass shape. Male spiders, much smaller than the female, may have only a small, reddish dot on their belly and are not considered dangerous. Reluctant to bite humans, black widows are responsible for about three deaths in the United States each year. All six species of black widow are venomous, but none are usually fatal.

In the past, however, they were responsible for a number of deaths—particularly during swarms, recorded in Spain in 1833 and 1841 and in Sardinia in 1833 and 1839, when many people were bitten and some died. In addition, the Gosiute Indians of Utah mixed the venom of the black widow and the rattlesnake to coat their arrowheads.

Black widow spiders build their messy, tangled webs under or between rocks, under loose bark, around outdoor water faucets, and in woodpiles, garages, basements, garbage cans and sheds. They also hide in cushions and under toilet lids, so that the most common and deadly bites are on the genitals. Although they are found throughout the United States and Canada, most inhabit warmer regions of the United States. They are also found in Mexico, Central America and the Antilles, and the western part of South America.

The brown widow (*L. geometrieus*) lives in the tropics and bears the same markings as the black widow, but it rarely bites humans.

Poisonous part   The venom of the black widow spider is a neurotoxin that acts on the nerve endings, destroying peripheral nerve endings and causing an ascending paralysis, usually affecting muscles in the thigh, shoulder and back first.

Symptoms   The bite of a black widow is not extremely painful and may not be felt at all. There may be slight swelling and two tiny puncture marks at the wound site, and following the bite there is a dull, numbing pain increasing in intensity, peaking in one to three hours and continuing up to 48 hours. Within 10 to 40 minutes after the bite, the venom attacks the nerves, causing abdominal or chest muscles to become rigid and flulike symptoms to appear. At the same time, there is stomach pain and muscle spasms in the extremities, along with difficulty in breathing and swallowing, chills, urinary retention, sweating, convulsions, paralysis, delirium, nausea, vomiting, drooping eyelids, headache and fever. When death occurs, it is due to cardiac failure. Most victims recover without serious complications.

Treatment   Antivenin is available, but most people can be managed without using the equine-derived antivenin. However, it may be needed for elderly patients and children, who do not respond to more conventional therapy for high blood pressure, muscle cramps or respiratory distress, or for pregnant women threatening premature labor. Cleanse the wound and treat infection, give a tetanus shot if needed and monitor for at least six to eight hours. Muscle cramping may be treated with intravenous calcium or muscle relaxants; pain may be treated with morphine. Keep the victim warm and quiet and call a physician immediately.

bleach   See ALKALINE CORROSIVES.

blister beetle   Any of the more than 2,000 species of the insect family Meloidae, found throughout the Midwest and the eastern United States. These beetles secrete an irritating substance called cantharidin, collected from the European species *Lytta vesicatoria* (or Spanish fly). Powdered cantharidin is used as a topical skin irritant to remove warts and is also intensely irritating to the mucous membranes. Although Spanish fly has a reputation as an aphrodisiac, it is in fact deadly poisonous and often fatal.

Poisonous part   Blister beetle venom contains large amounts of cantharidin, which produces painful blisters and reddening when it comes in contact with the skin.

Symptoms   A large, painful blister with erythema following contact with the toxic substance secreted by the blister beetle.

Treatment   Ice packs to relieve pain; corticosteroid cream is helpful. See also CANTHARIDIN.

bloodroot *(Sanguinaria canadensis)*   This bitter-tasting perennial herb is considered to be very toxic and is found from southern Canada to Florida and as far west as Texas. It has shiny white poppylike flowers that appear in early spring and when squeezed can produce a red juice. Bloodroot is usually found in woodlands and along fence rows.

Poisonous part   All parts of the plant contain the poison sanguinarine, which reduces the heart's action and muscle strength and is a nerve depressant. All parts are toxic when eaten; the red sap can cause a painful skin rash upon contact.

Symptoms Appearing within one to two hours after ingestion, symptoms include violent vomiting, thirst, burning and soreness in the throat, heaviness of the chest, breathing problems, dilated pupils, faintness and cardiac paralysis resulting in death.

Treatment Gastric lavage and symptomatic treatment.

blowfish See PUFFERFISH.

boomslang *(Dispholidus typus)* Found in Africa, this is a dangerously venomous snake of the family Colubridae, the only rear-fanged colubrid that is dangerous to humans. Its venom is lethal in even the smallest quantities.

The boomslang lives in savannas throughout sub-Saharan Africa and easily blends into its surroundings, changing its skin and eye color, which makes it difficult to spot. When looking for prey, it can lie in a bush or tree, partly extended into the air for long periods of time. When provoked, the boomslang hisses and inflates its neck, showing the dark skin between the scales, and then strikes. However, it is normally a mild-mannered and placid snake that spends all its time in trees. It comes in two colors: a brownish gray and a vivid green.

Symptoms Pain, swelling, hemorrhage, bleeding from nose and mouth, headache, vomiting, collapse and death. The venom of the boomslang is fatal in tiny amounts.

Treatment Antivenin is available.

See also ANTIVENIN; SNAKES, POISONOUS.

boric acid This white, crystalline powder is used as an antiseptic and, in diluted amounts, to treat eye irritations. It is also used as a roach poison, food preservative and a buffer in talcum powder. The use of boric acid in large amounts on broken skin or mucous membranes is toxic. It is no longer added to baby powders, and the use of boric acid should be strongly discouraged in any products for infants.

While boric acid is fairly safe when used appropriately, it can be extremely dangerous and is toxic to all cells—especially those in the kidneys.

Symptoms Primary symptoms are reddened, flaking skin, weight loss and hair loss, together with symptoms similar to those of toxic shock: fever, vomiting, dehydration, anuria and convulsions.

Treatment For ingestion, immediately perform gastric lavage followed by the administration of cathartics. For skin contamination, thoroughly wash the skin. Symptomatic treatment, including phenobarbital or diazepam to control convulsions.

botanic insecticides   Insecticides prepared from plant sources. Although many people choose "organic" botanic insect controls because they somehow seem safer than inorganic chemicals, they can still be poisonous. Because they have natural sources, botanic insecticides break down quickly in the environment and are consumed by soil microbes or—in the case of insect diseases—dissipate when there is no longer anything to infect. But they are still poisons; in fact, many of these compounds are extremely toxic—some more so than their manufactured "chemical" cousins. Most are deadly to a wide range of insects (both the "good" and "bad" insects); and some are toxic to birds, other animals and humans. Botanic insecticides include nicotine, pyrethrin/pyrethrum, rotenone, Bacillus thuringiensis (BT) and sabadilla. Because they are derived from plants, contact with some of these (such as pyrethrins) can result in an allergic reaction.

See also BACILLUS THURINGIENSIS; NICOTINE; PYRETHRIN; PYRETHRUM; ROTENONE.

botulin   The toxin produced by the single-celled botulinum bacterium; it is the most poisonous substance in the world—six million times more toxic than rattlesnake venom. When ingested, it causes botulism, a form of food poisoning that can cause muscle paralysis and death.

Despite its deadly reputation, however, botulin is also used in small doses to treat a whole area of human illness called dystonias (uncontrollable muscle spasms that may be caused by involuntary electrical brain impulses). Every dose of botulin ever administered was created by 84-year-old professor and biochemist Ed Schantz, professor emeritus at the Food Research Institute of the University of Wisconsin at Madison. Because the dystonias are rare, and because of the extreme toxicity of botulin, drug companies are not particularly interested in manufacturing the toxin.

See also BOTULIN ANTITOXIN; BOTULISM; BOTULISM, INFANT; FOOD POISONING.

botulin antitoxin   The antidote to poisoning by the various strains of *Clostridium botulinum* (A, B and E) that cause botulism. The antibodies bind and inactivate freely circulating botulin toxins, but they do not remove toxin that has already bound to nerve terminals and will not reverse paralysis that has already begun. Therefore, treatment within 24 hours of the onset of symptoms may shorten the course of the poisoning and may prevent total paralysis. Botulin antitoxin is not recommended in the treatment of infant botulism.

See also BOTULIN; BOTULISM; BOTULISM, INFANT; FOOD POISONING.

botulism   The most serious type of food poisoning, poisoning by the *Clostridium botulinum* toxin is rare and very deadly—two-thirds of those afflicted die, and the rest face a long recovery period. Botulism is more common in the United States than anywhere else in the world owing to the popularity here of home canning; there are about 20 cases of food-borne botulism poisoning each year. Botulism got its name during the 1800s from *botulus,* the Latin word for sausage, in the wake of poisoning from contaminated sausages.

The *C. botulinum* toxin is found in air, water and food as inactive spores that are harmless—until the spores are deprived of oxygen, such as inside a sealed can or jar. If conditions are favorable, the spores will begin to grow, producing one of the most deadly toxins known to humans—seven million times more deadly than cobra venom.

Cases of botulism from commercially canned food are rare because of strict health standards enforced by the Food and Drug Administration, and most incidences of botulism occur during errors in home canning. Still, it is easy to prevent, since botulism is killed when canned food is boiled at 100°C for one minute or if the food is first sterilized by pressure cooking at 250°F for 30 minutes.

While the tightly fitted lids of home-canned food will provide the anaerobic environment necessary for the growth of botulism toxins, the spores will not grow if the food is very acidic, sweet or salty, such as canned fruit juice, jams and jellies, sauerkraut, tomatoes and heavily salted hams. Canned foods that are highly susceptible to contamination include green beans, beets, peppers, corn and meat. Although the spores can survive boiling, the ideal temperature for their growth is between 78°F and 96°F. They can also survive freezing.

Even though botulism spores are invisible, it's possible to tell if food is spoiled by noticing if jars have lost their vacuum seal; when the spores grow, they give off gas that makes cans and jars lose the seal. Jars will burst or cans will swell. Any food that is spoiled or whose color or odor doesn't seem right inside a home-canned jar or can should be thrown away without tasting or evening sniffing, since botulism can be fatal in extremely small amounts. Botulism can also occur if the *C. botulinum* bacteria in the soil enters the body through an open wound.

Symptoms   Onset of symptoms may be as soon as three hours or as late as 14 days after ingestion, they include nausea, vomiting, diarrhea, stomach cramps, weakness, blurred vision, headache, difficulty in swallowing, slurred speech, drooping eyelids, dilated pupils and paralysis progressing to the respiratory muscles. The earlier the onset of symptoms, the more severe the reaction. Symptoms generally last between three and six days; death occurs in about 70 percent of untreated cases, usually from suffocation as a result of respiratory muscle paralysis. In infants, symptoms may go unrecognized by parents for some time until the poisoning has reached a critical stage. Infant botulism symptoms include constipation, facial muscle flaccidity, sucking problems, irritability, lethargy and floppy baby syndrome.

Treatment   Prompt administration of the antitoxin (type ABE botulinus) lowers the risk of death to 25 percent. The Centers for Disease Control in Atlanta, Georgia is the only agency with the antitoxin, and it makes the decision to treat. Local health departments should be called first for this information. Emesis is indicated immediately following ingestion of food known to contain botulism toxin. But since emesis may not be complete and the disease can occur with a small amount of toxin, botulism may still develop. Patients with symptoms should not have lavage or an emetic. Enemas may be necessary. Patients are usually put on a respirator to ease breathing difficulties. In infant botulism, if symptoms are present, it is often too late to administer antitoxin, since the damage probably has already been done by the toxin. However, it is still possible to try.

See also BOTULIN; BOTULIN ANTITOXIN; BOTULISM, INFANT; FOOD POISONING.

botulism, infant   Unlike botulism in adults, which occurs after eating contaminated food, infant botulism is caused by the production of toxin produced by *C. botulinum* in the infant's intestinal tract. While it is believed that adults, children and infants consume *C. botulinum* spores on a regular basis—since they are present in a wide variety of foods, house dust, etc.—for some reason the intestinal tracts of some infants under age one are susceptible to the spores. In particular, there appears to be a link between spores and honey; infants have died from eating honey contaminated with the spores, and for this reason, children under age one should never be fed honey.

Since researchers have not yet discovered why some infants appear to be susceptible to the botulism spores, parents are advised to keep rooms dust free and not to feed honey or corn syrups. Commercially prepared foods that are sterilized and contain low acid are botulism free. Research also suggests that mother's milk may also provide some immunological protection against infant botulism, although this has not yet been proven.

See also BOTULIN; BOTULIN ANTITOXIN; BOTULISM; FOOD POISONING.

brewer's yeast   Once an antidote for thallium ingestion (found in depilatories and rat poison); it is no longer routinely used.

See also THALLIUM.

bromates (potassium bromate) A corrosive poison once widely used (between the 1940s and the 1970s) in the neutralizer solutions of home permanent kits. While less toxic substances have now been substituted for products offered to consumers in the home, poisonings do still occur from products used by professionals. Bromates may still be found in commercial bakeries (bromate salts improve bread texture) and in the production of some types of explosives.

Poisonous part   Bromate is usually found as a 3 percent solution with water and must be taken orally to be toxic. It becomes poisonous when the hydrochloric acid in the stomach turns the potassium bromate into hydrogen bromate, an irritating acid.

Symptoms   Within five to 20 minutes after ingestion, bromates can cause vomiting, collapse, diarrhea, abdominal pain, lethargy, deafness, coma, convulsions, low blood pressure, kidney damage and a skin rash.

Treatment   Gastric lavage or an enema, with solutions containing sodium bicarbonate; sodium thiosulfate is given intravenously as an antidote.

bromide   This former sedative was once found in over-the-counter products ranging from Bromo-Seltzer and Dr. Miles' Nervine, but today it is rarely used because of its potential toxicity. It can be found occasionally in well water and in some bromide-containing hydrocarbons. Because bromide affects not just the skin and stomach but the brain, and thus can cause a variety of aberrant behaviors, bromide exposure in the past was responsible for a number of admissions to psychiatric hospitals.

Symptoms   Nausea, vomiting, gastric irritation, lethargy, confusion, hallucinations, psychosis, weakness, stupor, coma, anorexia, constipation and rashes.

Treatment   There is no specific antidote, but because bromide is excreted entirely by the kidneys, intravenous administration of sodium chloride will enhance elimination. Induce vomiting or perform gastric lavage if ingestion has been recent.

bronchial tube relaxers   Also called bronchial tube dilators, these drugs are used to alleviate asthma, bronchitis and emphysema and to relieve spasms and tightness in the chest. They can be fatal if used in excessive amounts. Bronchial tube dilators also cause serious side effects if taken with or soon after another bronchial tube relaxer or decongestant pills or liquid. These drugs are dangerous when taken with antihypertensives, epinephrine and lithium. If taken with beta blockers, the effect of both drugs is diminished.

Symptoms   In large doses, bronchial fluid builds up and causes inflammation, pounding heartbeat, dizziness, nervousness, bad taste in the mouth, dry mouth, headache, insomnia, anxiety, tension, blood pressure changes, flushing, sweating, angina and arm pain. Overdoses can cause convulsions, low potassium levels, hallucinations, serious breathing problems, fever, chills, vomiting, clammy skin, spike in blood pressure and stroke.

Treatment   Administer oxygen and treat symptoms as needed.

brown recluse spider   *(Loxosceles reclusa)*   [Other names: fiddleback or violin spider.] The brown recluse is one of two species of poisonous spiders found in the United States and is by far the most dangerous of the spider family—ounce for ounce, its venom is more deadly than that of many poisonous snakes.

Native to Central and South America, the brown recluse is thought to have been inadvertently imported to the United States in crates of fruit and vegetables within the last 50 years. Since then, it has been making its way steadily north and westward and is now found ranging to Texas and Arkansas and as far north as Massachusetts.

Its brown or fawn-colored body is about 1/2 inch long and has a dark, violin-shaped mark on its back. Although brown recluse spiders are some-times found outdoors, most live in houses, spinning their webs in dark areas inside homes or outbuildings. They get their name from their habit of hiding in closets, dresser drawers, the folds of clothing, garages, attics and sheds. Brown recluse spiders are not aggressive and will try to escape, not attack; but if trapped, they will bite. The venom of females is more deadly than that of males.

Symptoms   The bite of a brown recluse causes little pain, but within two to eight hours the pain will be severe and the area of the bite will become red. Any place on the skin the spider has bitten will necrose and die. Brown recluse venom contains a substance that is very destructive to tissue and causes a large, spreading sore that eventually turns into a blister, becoming dark and hard within four days. In some cases, this sore becomes star-shaped and deep purple and within two weeks forms an open ulcer, although the venom does not necessarily kill. As this ulcer heals, it often becomes infected; in a very small percentage of victims the ulcer does not heal for an extremely long time.

The bite can also cause a range of systemic reactions, including fever, chills, weakness, nausea, vomiting, joint pain and sometimes a generalized rash or reddish spots. Death, when it does come, is caused usually within the first 48 hours as a result of renal failure because of blood coagulation.

Treatment   There is no specific antivenin, although antivenin for other species of brown spiders of South America should give protection. Since this antivenin contains norepinephrine, administration of phentolamine may help head off swelling and necrosis. Antihistamines, muscle relaxants and adrenocortical steroids may provide some relief. Exchange transfusion may be attempted. Immediate excision of the bite area may be the only way to prevent the massive necrosis caused by the brown recluse venom, although not all experts agree on this treatment. Most physicians will not touch the lesion until all destruction has been done, sometimes as long as 40 weeks after the bite. Skin grafts may be necessary to heal the ulcer. If the bite of a brown recluse is suspected, a physician should be called at once.

See also ANTIVENIN; SPIDER, POISONOUS.

brown snake *(Demansia textilis)*   Found in Australia, the brown snake includes any of several species named for their primary color, ranging from light brown to dark green. This slender member of the cobra family can be about 7 feet long and is extremely bad tempered and poisonous. When threatened, it will rear and strike repeatedly. It is responsible for more deaths in Australia than any other snake. Brown snakes found in the New World are sometimes also called grass snakes, ranging from Canada to Honduras, and are harmless.

Symptoms Symptoms can take up to 12 hours to appear and include abdominal pain, staggering gait, problems in swallowing, stiff jaws, respiratory distress, coma, cardiac failure and death.

Treatment Copperhead antivenin is used for this snakebite.

See also ANTIVENIN; COBRA; SNAKES, POISONOUS.

brown spider   See BROWN RECLUSE SPIDER.

bryony *(Bryonia dioica, B. alba* or *B. cretica)* Also called the devil's turnip or British mandrake, bryony is considered to be very toxic (fewer than 40 berries will kill an adult). A common climbing plant in public gardens with pretty red berries and black and yellow seeds, bryony blooms in the summer and is found in England, Wales and other northern countries. The entire plant has a foul-smelling milky juice, and its fleshy white roots can be mistaken for turnips or parsnips. When the berries are distilled, the resulting beverage can cause abortions. Medically, it can be used as a diuretic.

Poisonous part Roots and berries contain the poisons glycoside, bryonin and bryonidin.

Symptoms Within several hours after ingestion, victims experience burning mouth, nausea, vomiting, diarrhea, convulsions, paralysis and coma; death follows because of respiratory arrest. The juice can also irritate the skin and cause a rash.

Treatment Perform gastric lavage, while keeping the victim warm and quiet. Replace fluids and monitor electrolyte levels, and provide pain medication as needed.

See also GLYCOSIDE.

buckeye *(Aesculus)* [Other names: conquerors, horse chestnut, fish poison.] These trees—consisting of about 13 species—have white, pink, yellow and red clusters of flowers and compound leaves. The seed pod is leathery, with glossy brown seeds bearing a brown scar. The trees are found in the central and eastern temperate zones to the Gulf Coast and California and in parts of Canada.

Poisonous part Flowers, nuts, sprouts and twigs are toxic and contain a mixture of cytotoxic saponins known as aescin.

Symptoms Because the saponins are not well absorbed, poisoning is generally not fatal unless as a result of frequent exposure. In addition, the unpleasant taste usually prohibits ingestion in large enough quantities to kill. Generally, symptoms are limited to severe gastroenteritis, inflammation of mucous membranes, depression, weakness and paralysis. However, there have been reports of fatalities among children.

Treatment   Gastric lavage, general treatment for gastroenteritis, with fluid and electrolyte replacement and administration of oral magnesium sulfate.

See also SAPONIN.

buckthorn   *(Karwinskia humboldtiana)*   A shrubby tree that grows up to 6 feet tall; its berries turn black when mature. It is found in western Texas and New Mexico.

Poisonous part   The fruit is poisonous and contains anthracenones.

Symptoms   Chronic ingestion may cause ascending paralysis; weakness occurs after a latent period of several weeks; paralysis may progress for a month or more.

Treatment   Supportive. If victims survive respiratory paralysis, they will completely recover.

bushmaster   *(Lachesis muta)*   One of the larger and most dangerous South American pit vipers is the bushmaster, which is found in tropical forests from Costa Rica to the Amazon Basin. The longest venomous snake in the New World (it can grow up to 12 feet long), the bushmaster can be either tan or pink with dark diamond markings, and while this snake is rarely seen, its bite is potentially lethal.

The bushmaster is the only American pit viper that lays eggs.

Symptoms   Within a very short time, victims begin bleeding from the gums, nose and eyes and experience chills, fever, sweating, falling blood pressure, convulsions and death. In cases of a severe bite, the victim will also experience swelling above the elbows or knees within two hours.

Treatment   Death from cardiorespiratory failure is unavoidable unless antivenin is given quickly.

See also ANTIVENIN; PIT VIPERS; SNAKES, POISONOUS.

buttercup *(Ranunculus)*   [Other names: bassinet, blister flower, buttercress, butter daisy, butterflower, crowfoot, devil's claws, figwort, gold-balls, goldweed, horse gold, hunger weed, lesser celandine, pilewort, ram's claws, St. Anthony's turnip, sitfast, spearwort, starve-acre, water crowfoot.] Annual or perennial herbs that grow in wet, moist or swamp places throughout the United States and Canada. They range in height from a few inches to three feet tall, with yellow, red or white flowers.

Poisonous part   The sap and roots are toxic and contain protoanemonin, a direct irritant and vesicant of the skin and mucous membranes.

Symptoms After ingestion, symptoms include severe pain, swelling and blisters in the mouth, followed by bloody diarrhea and painful abdominal cramps. The toxin, which affects the central nervous system, also causes systemic symptoms including dizziness and sometimes convulsions.

Treatment Because of the intense pain following ingestion, large amounts of this plant are generally not eaten. If this is the case, gastric lavage is recommended followed by the administration of demulcents (such as milk); give plenty of fluids and monitor kidney function.

C

cadmium   Found in sulfide ores (together with zinc and lead), cadmium is used in electroplating, as a pigment and stabilizer in plastics, in soldering and welding and in nickel-cadmium batteries. Solder made of cadmium used for water pipes, and cadmium pigments in pottery, can contaminate water and acidic food.

Symptoms   Cadmium fumes and dust are at least 60 times more toxic than other forms, causing chemical pneumonitis and pulmonary edema and hemorrhage, in addition to coughs, wheezing, headache and fever. Symptoms appear within 12 to 24 hours after inhalation. Ingested cadmium, on the other hand, affects the gastrointestinal tract and the kidneys, causing nausea, vomiting, cramps, diarrhea and death as a result of shock or acute kidney failure.

Treatment   There is no evidence that chelation therapy is effective. In cases of inhalation poisoning: Monitor blood and general condition; remove the victim from exposure and give supplemental oxygen if necessary. For ingestion: Treat fluid loss; perform gastric lavage but do not induce vomiting because cadmium salts are an irritant; and administer activated charcoal (but do not give cathartics in the presence of diarrhea).

caffeine   This alkaloid is one of the most widely consumed drugs in the United States and is contained in a wide variety of products, including coffee, chocolate, medications and over-the-counter stimulants.

In one recent study, about 30 percent of Americans said they drank between five and 10 cups of coffee a day, resulting in a daily dose of 500 to 600 mg of caffeine daily. It is also becoming a popular "street drug" in some areas; for example, the Duke University Poison Control Center in Durham, North Carolina reports deaths from accidental overdose.

Caffeine can be found naturally in kola nuts, cocoa beans, tea leaves and coffee beans. This white, odorless, crystalline powder was first extracted from plants in 1820. Caffeine is quickly absorbed orally, rectally and through the skin and is rapidly metabolized and excreted. At one time, it was often combined with aspirin and phenacetin in a wide range of prescription and over-the-counter medications, and it is still included today in many analgesics, stimulants and cold preparations available without a prescription.

It is believed that caffeine affects the synthesis and release of catecholamines (especially the stress hormone norepinephrine), and after ingestion, it quickly disperses throughout all organ systems, crossing both the blood-

AMOUNTS OF CAFFEINE IN COMMON PRODUCTS

Source	Amount[*]	Dose
Beverages		
Brewed coffee	85–120 mg	cup
Instant coffee	60–100 mg	cup
Cola[**]	25–60 mg	glass
Tea	30–75 mg	cup
Cocoa	6–42 mg	cup
Decaffeinated coffee	2–6 mg	cup
Medications		
migraine drugs	50–100 mg/dose	
analgesics	15–40 mg/dose	
cough/cold	15–125 mg/dose	
over-the-counter stimulants	65–250 mg/dose	

* Approximation based on range gathered from several sources
** Caffeine-containing colas only

brain barrier and the placenta. At high doses, it affects blood vessels, breathing, the brain and the spinal cord.

In newborns, however, the metabolism of caffeine is markedly delayed, which contributes to caffeine toxicity in infants exposed to the substance.

Symptoms   Caffeine toxicity can be chronic or acute, but despite its extreme popularity, few deaths have been recorded. The acute lethal dose of caffeine in adults may be as low as 6 g, although the dose is much lower for children. One gram can cause symptoms of toxicity.

Chronic "caffeinism" is caused by constantly consuming products containing caffeine, such as colas and chocolates. The effects might include headache, indigestion, insomnia, restlessness, nervousness, confusion, tremors, constipation, fever and sensory disturbances.

Toxic symptoms can appear in adults after one gram of oral caffeine. Victims of caffeine toxicity often complain of irregular heartbeat and nervousness, together with sleeplessness, excitement and mild delirium. In severe cases of overdose, symptoms include loss of consciousness, rapid heartbeat, irregular heart rhythms, seizures and caffeine-induced psychosis. A number of deaths have reportedly occurred following caffeine-induced seizures. There have also been cases in which caffeine has worsened the symptoms of persons already suffering from schizophrenia or manic-depression. The most widespread and chronic symptom of caffeine is a severe headache upon withdrawal, although the reason behind this is not known.

Treatment   Gastric lavage, with supportive and symptomatic treatment including withholding further caffeine. To control seizures, diazepam and phenobarbital can be administered. Cardiac evaluation is essential, as death is most commonly due to arrythmia. Specific treatment may be necessary.

calcium   Necessary for the normal function of a wide variety of enzymes and organ systems in the body, calcium is used in the treatment of poisoning by fluoride, oxalate, phosphate or the intravenous anticoagulant citrate. It is also helpful in the treatment of muscle cramping or rigidity following black widow spider bites.

See also BLACK WIDOW SPIDER; FLUORIDE; OXALATES; PHOSPHATE ESTERS.

calcium EDTA   This chelating agent is used in the treatment of acute and chronic lead poisoning and may also be helpful to treat poisoning with manganese, zinc, chromium, nickel or heavy radioisotopes. It is not effective in the treatment of mercury, gold or arsenic poisoning.

See also ARSENIC; LEAD POISONING; MERCURY.

California mussel *(Mytilus californianus)*   These mollusks become poisonous to eat because of feeding on toxic one-celled animals called dinoflagellates.

See also DINOFLAGELLATES; PARALYTIC SHELLFISH POISONING; SHELLFISH POISONING.

camphor   This respiratory aid and mild local anesthetic is found in mothballs and liniments; the related compound camphorated oil (a 20 percent solution of camphor in oil) is highly toxic but was banned by the Food and Drug Administration in 1982. Both the ingestion of camphor and the prolonged inhalation of camphor vapors can be toxic. Because of its strong medicinal odor, camphor is included in a large number of over-the-counter products. Camphor is rated as very toxic, with a lethal dose of 50 to 500 mg/kg. According to the Food and Drug Administration, in 1979 alone there were 768 cases of camphor poisoning and more than 20 fatalities. All of these fatalities were the result of either a child accidentally ingesting a product not labeled as toxic that was intended for topical use, or the accidental substitution of a camphor-containing medicine instead of the proper drug (most commonly, camphor for castor oil or cod liver oil).

Symptoms   Appearing within 15 to 60 minutes after ingestion or prolonged vapor inhalation, symptoms include headache, excitement, a feeling of warmth, clammy skin, weak pulse, nausea, vomiting, burning in the mouth and throat and delirium. Camphor can also be smelled on the breath. Twitching and muscle spasms may be followed by convulsions and circulatory failure.

Treatment   Gastric lavage followed by administration of activated charcoal via tube. Vomiting is not induced because of the danger of seizures. Valium may be used to control convulsions; hemodialysis may help eliminate the drug from the body.

cantharidin   A powder obtained from the blister beetle, cantharidin is used to remove warts and is extremely irritating to the mucous membranes. Nicknamed "Spanish fly," it is popularly believed to be an aphrodisiac; it is in fact a deadly poison that is responsible for many fatalities. When ingested, Spanish fly is highly toxic.

Symptoms   Ingestion of Spanish fly causes burning in the throat and sloughing of the upper gastrointestinal tract. Kidney failure can occur, and death often follows.

Treatment   Dilute with 4 to 8 ounces of water. Do not induce emesis. Treatment is also supportive; hemodialysis may be necessary if the kidneys fail, and treatment of the throat injury is similar to that for lye ingestion. Also, treat gastrointestinal bleeding.

See also BLISTER BEETLE.

cantil snake   *(Agkistrodon bilineatus)* Also called a Mexican moccasin, this pit viper is a brightly colored but extremely dangerous snake found in the low regions of the Rio Grande all the way to Nicaragua. Related to the cottonmouth (or water moccasin), this snake has a yellow or red tail that contrasts with the dull appearance of the rest of the body.

Pit vipers seem to be extremely highly evolved snakes very well designed for capturing, killing and eating fairly large, warm-blooded prey, with retractable hollow fangs in the front of the upper jaw. The fangs can be folded back and then positioned forward as the mouth opens to strike. The pit viper's name comes from the heat-sensitive pits located on each side of the head between the nostril and the eye, which are used to locate its prey.

Seriousness of the bite depends on a wide variety of variables, including the snake's size (usually the larger, the more venomous) and whether the snake is hungry or alert. The angle of the bite and its depth and length also affect the seriousness of the bite. In addition, the size of the victim can be important (children and infants are at greater risk), and the health of the victim at the time of the bite will also affect the outcome. Persons with diabetes, hypertension or blood coagulation problems and the elderly are particularly sensitive to snake venom, and menstruating women may bleed excessively following the bite of a pit viper. Several cases of miscarriage have been reported when pregnant women have been bitten.

Finally, the location of the bite itself is crucial to its seriousness; venomous snake bites on the head and trunk are twice as serious as those on the extremities, and bites on the arms are more serious than those on the legs.

Poisonous part   The venom of the pit vipers is a mixture of proteins that acts on a victim's blood. Even snakes that appear to be dead by the side of the road have been reported to bite. The size of the snake can give an idea of its potential dangerousness and can be judged by the distance between the fang marks. Fang marks less than 8 mm would be a small snake; between 8 to 12 indicates a medium-size snake, and more than 12 mm suggests a large venomous snake. Even snakes that have been "de-fanged" can be dangerous, since all snakes grow new fangs from time to time.

Symptoms Swelling, internal bleeding, changes in red blood cells; central nervous system symptoms sometimes include convulsions, psychotic behavior, muscle weakness and paralysis. In addition, there are general systemic symptoms of fever, nausea, vomiting, diarrhea, pain and restlessness. Tachycardia and bradycardia can develop, and kidney failure has been reported.

Treatment Within the first 30 to 45 minutes after the bite of a pit viper, apply a venous tourniquet a few inches above the bite, loosening it every 15 to 30 minutes and reapplying it above the level of progressive swelling. Keep the victim quiet, lying down to decrease metabolic activity (which affects the spread of the venom). The wound area (especially if it is an arm or leg) should be kept lower than the heart. Within 30 minutes, trained individuals can incise the wound area and apply suction. Antivenin is available but should be administered within four hours; antivenin is rarely helpful if given more than 12 hours after the bite. Tetanus prophylaxis is advisable; other treatment might include blood transfusions, intravenous fluids, treatment for convulsions and antihistamines to control itching. In addition, broad-spectrum antibiotics may be administered, since snakebites are notorious for becoming infected. If antivenin has not been administered (or was given hours after the bite), sloughing of the skin around the bite is common. Some individuals may be sensitive to the antivenin, so skin testing is advised.

While certain anecdotal reports in the popular press have reported that some individuals become immunized after many bites of the pit viper, scientifically controlled attempts to develop immunity in human beings have failed.

See also, ANTIVENIN; PIT VIPER; SNAKES, POISONOUS.

carbamate A group of synthetic pesticides made up of carbon, hydrogen, oxygen and nitrogen. They include carbaryl, chlorpropham, carbofuran, aldicarb, pirimicarb, bufencarb, isolan, maneb, propoxur, thiram, Zectran, zineb and ziram. Atropine is the antidote for most carbamate poisonings.

See also CARBARYL; ORGANOPHOSPHATE INSECTICIDES.

carbaryl (Sevin) This derivative of carbamic acid (H_2N-COOH) is used as an herbicide, insecticide and medicinal agent and is one of the carbamates, a relatively new class of contact insecticides that supplement the organophosphates.

Symptoms Carbaryl poisoning resembles parathion intoxication, although it is much less toxic. Symptoms include nausea, vomiting, abdominal cramps, diarrhea, excess salivation, sweating, lassitude, weakness, tightness in the chest, blurring of vision, eye pain, loss of muscle coordination, slurred speech, muscle twitches, breathing problems, blue skin, incontinence, convulsions and coma. Death occurs from respiratory arrest and paralysis of the respiratory muscles. It is an eye and skin irritant and does not accumulate in the tissues. It is poisonous through ingestion or skin absorption.

Treatment Give atropine immediately; some reports suggest atropine is dangerous in the presence of anoxia (loss of oxygen); correct cyanosis (blueness of skin) before giving atropine. Give oxygen, artificial respiration as needed. Perform gastric lavage or administer syrup of ipecac if vomiting is not prompt. Wash contaminated skin with soap and water (or 95 percent ethyl alcohol). Irrigate affected eyes with water or saline. Administer isotonic saline to counteract dehydration and electrolyte imbalance.

See also CARBAMATE; ORGANOPHOSPHATE INSECTICIDES.

carbolic acid   See PHENOL.

carbon monoxide   A colorless, odorless poisonous gas that occurs during the incomplete burning of organic substances (local, wood, kerosene, paper, oil, cooking gas or gasoline). Carbon monoxide is also found in the exhaust of internal-combustion engines, including car engines.

Carbon monoxide gas is extremely poisonous, and recent research has shown that there are many mechanisms of toxicity. It doesn't irritate or damage the skin but kills by binding with hemoglobin (the oxygen-carrying molecule in red blood cells) and preventing it from carrying oxygen. When this happens, the tissues cannot get oxygen and asphyxiation occurs. Continuing inhalation of the gas can lead to permanent brain damage and death. Breathing air that contains as little as 0.1 percent carbon monoxide by volume can be fatal; a concentration of about 1 percent can cause death within a few minutes. Car exhaust contains 1 to 7 percent carbon monoxide and is a common method of attempted suicide.

Common sources include gas cooking ranges, hot water heaters and dryers, wood- or coal-burning stoves and fireplaces, oil burners and kerosene heaters. Gas water heaters and dryers and oil burners must have stacks that move the carbon monoxide outside. Wood-burning stoves and fireplaces must have chimneys that vent the gas outside. Unvented kerosene heaters spread carbon monoxide gas indoors; therefore a window must always be open slightly when you use a kerosene heater. Cooking with a charcoal grill in an enclosed area can also release carbon monoxide; for this reason, such grills should never be used indoors.

Symptoms Initial symptoms (which can be confused with food poisoning) include headache, dizziness, drowsiness, weakness, nausea with possible vomiting, rapid breathing and flushed skin. In chronic cases, carbon monoxide poisoning may interfere with the development of the fetus. As the level of gas in the blood rises, the individual may become confused and have impaired judgment, dulled sensation, clumsiness and dim vision. Loss of consciousness and death quickly follow. Carbon monoxide poisoning has the same effect on a heart patient as strenuous exercise and has caused fatal heart attacks. The toxicity is caused by interfering with the ability of red blood cells to carry oxygen, prohibiting the transportation of oxygen from the lungs to the tissues.

Treatment   It is essential to get the victim into fresh air immediately; then call for help. If the victim isn't breathing or is breathing irregularly, artificial respiration should be given, and the victim should be kept warm and quiet to prevent shock. Administration of oxygen, often with 5 percent carbon dioxide and sometimes under high pressure, is often given. A physician should be consulted to check for long-term effects, even if the victim seems to have recovered.

carbon tetrachloride   A colorless, volatile liquid with a characteristic odor, this once-common household solvent is used to clean metals, in dry cleaning and to remove oil, grease, wax and paint. An ingredient in fire extinguishers and insecticide sprays, it is also used in the manufacture of Freon propellants and refrigerants. Consumers can no longer buy carbon tetrachloride; it is available only for industrial or commercial use. This dangerous chemical can cause liver and kidney damage if inhaled or drunk.

Symptoms   Breathing these solvent fumes can cause headache, eye irritation, dizziness, visual disturbances and nausea. In extreme cases, inhaling these fumes can be fatal. If this chemical is drunk, symptoms include headache, nausea, pain in the abdomen and convulsions.

Treatment   Victim should vomit unless unconscious or having convulsions. If fumes were inhaled, the victim should be taken into fresh air and given artificial respiration if necessary. Skin contamination should be treated with running water for at least 15 minutes. Drinking large amounts of this substance has been reported to be fatal in 90 percent of cases, but with early intervention prognosis is good.

carbutol   See BARBITURATES.

cardiac glycosides   One of the toxic glycosides in the plant kingdom that affect the heart, cardiac glycosides remain one of the major therapies for congestive heart failure. There are more than 400 different types, but the most common is digitalis, which is found in the foxglove *(Digitalis purpurea)* and other "digitoxins" (similar to digitalis) found in *Nerium oleander* and the lily family.

Most cardiac glycosides come from the figwort, lily and dogbane families. In therapeutic amounts, they will act directly on the heart to increase the force of contractions and decrease the heartbeat—but no one knows how. Overdoses produce nausea, dizziness, blurred vision and diarrhea. It is suspected that there is a relationship between the cardiac glycosides and plant toxicity. Poisonous plants containing cardiac glycosides include pheasant's-eye, dogbane, lily of the valley, foxglove and oleander.

See also FOXGLOVE; GLYCOSIDE; LILY OF THE VALLEY; OLEANDER.

carneum   A variety of chrysanthemum used in the production of the botanic insecticide pyrethrum.

See also BOTANIC INSECTICIDES; PYRETHRUM.

Carolina horse nettle *(Solanum carolinense)* [Other names: ball or bull nettle, ball nightshade, sandbriar, tread softly.] This member of the Solanum family grows from Nebraska to Texas, east to the Atlantic and in extreme northern Ohio, southern Ontario and southern California. It is a member of a very large genus with 1,700 species, most of which have not been evaluated toxicologically.

Poisonous part   Human poisoning is usually attributed to immature fruit, which contains the toxin solanine glycoalkaloid.

Symptoms   While there is little danger of fatal poisoning in adults, children may ingest a fatal amount of this plant. Symptoms appear several hours after ingestion and include gastric irritation, scratchy throat, fever and diarrhea (solanine poisoning is often confused with bacterial gastroenteritis).

Treatment   The same general supportive care that would be given in gastroenteritis cases; fluid replacement may be required.

cascabel   See RATTLESNAKE, CASCABEL.

cassava *(Manihot esculenta)* [Other names: bitter cassava, juca, manioc, manioc tapioca, sweet potato plant, yuca.] Found in the tropics, this is a tuberous edible plant of the spurge family and is cultivated for its roots, from which cassava flour, breads, tapioca, laundry starch and alcoholic beverages are made. It is believed that cassava was once cultivated by the Maya in Yucatan. Tapioca is the only cassava product on sale in northern markets.

If improperly prepared and cooked, cassava can cause poisoning to those who eat it, although there is no danger if it is prepared properly. Cassava meal and tapioca are made from the tuberous plant, but the plant must be heated and the poison dissolved out before the plant is edible. The two kinds of cassava (bitter and sweet) are often confused, but the bitter variety is more poisonous. Both require careful preparation.

Cassava appears in many varieties, with usually large fan-shaped leaves very much like the castor bean. The varieties range from low herbs to tall, slender trees and are found in dry areas as well as along riverbanks in Guam, Hawaii, the West Indies, Florida and the Gulf Coast states.

Poisonous part   Cyanogenetic glycosides (linamarin and lotaustralin) are broken down in the body to produce hydrocyanic acid; they occur in different amounts in most varieties. The roots are the most poisonous, although the leaves also contain variable amounts. Primitive people were able to remove the poison by grating, pressing and heating the tubers. The poison amygdalin in the juice breaks down into hydrocyanic acid, which can cause cyanide poisoning and has been used for darts and arrows.

Symptoms   Experts differ as to how rapidly death can occur, with times ranging from within minutes to hours. Symptoms can include nausea, respiratory problems, twitching, staggering, convulsions, coma and death.

Treatment   Gastric lavage followed by a 25 percent solution of sodium thiosulfate.

castor bean   *(Ricinus communis)*   [Other names: African coffee tree, castor oil plant, gourd, koli, man's motherwort, Mexico weed, palma Christi (from the shape of its leaves, resembling Christ's hand), steadfast, wonder tree.] This is considered by some sources to be the most dangerous plant in the United States. It is the source of castor oil and is also used as a mosquito repellent and a cathartic. Castor bean is grown for commercial and ornamental use in the United States and the tropics and has become naturalized in Florida, along the Gulf and Atlantic coasts, in southern California and in Hawaii.

A member of the spurge family, castor bean is a large annual that grows up to 15 feet high and has hollow stems that bear blue-green leaves up to three feet across. It produces bronze-red clusters of flowers in June followed by spiny seed pods containing plump seeds; the pods are often removed because of the highly toxic content concentrated in their seeds.

Early Americans made a laxative from the beans. Native to Africa, the plant is now naturalized throughout the tropics. *R. communis* is the only species in its genus, but there are hundreds of varieties.

Poisonous part   All parts of the plant (especially the seeds) contain the poison ricin, a plant lectin (toxalbumin) that is one of the world's most toxic substances. While the toxic mechanism of ricin is not well understood, it is thought that it inhibits the synthesis of protein in the intestinal wall. Small amounts of castor oil are also present in the seeds. If the beans are swallowed whole, the hard seed coat prevents absorption and therefore inhibits poisoning, but two to six beans can be fatal if well chewed. In a child, one or two seeds can be fatal.

Symptoms   Usually developing after several hours, symptoms include a burning sensation in the mouth, throat and stomach, nausea, vomiting, severe bloody diarrhea, abdominal cramps, dulled vision, convulsions, trouble in breathing, paralysis and death from within hours up to 12 days. One to six well-chewed seeds may be fatal to a child. Castor beans can also induce labor.

Treatment   There is no known antidote for ricin poisoning, so treatment is primarily supportive and symptomatic. Perform gastric lavage immediately, with bismuth subcarbonate or magnesium trisilicate to line the stomach. Fluids and electrolytes must be monitored. Administration of activated charcoal can be successful, since charcoal binds ricin well.

Catapres (clonidine)   One of a group of antihypertensive drugs designed to lower blood pressure, Catapres is considered to be supertoxic in either its tablet or injectable form. Once it is administered to control blood pressure, an abrupt withdrawal of the drug can precipitate a dangerous spike in blood pressure, psychosis, hyperexcitability, irregular heartbeats and death.

Symptoms   Wtihin 30 minutes after ingestion, an overdose causes slow heartbeat, drowsiness, stomach upset, rash, low blood pressure, depressed breathing, coma and heart failure.

Treatment   Atropine is administered, while monitoring the cardiorespiratory system and kidney function.

See also ANTIHYPERTENSIVE DRUGS.

catfish (*Siluriformes*)   Related to carp and minnows, the catfish gets its name from the four to five long whiskers on the upper jaw; many also have spines in front of the dorsal and pectoral fins that may cause painful stings, especially by young catfish. There are about 2,500 species of catfish in about 30 families mostly living in fresh water, although a few live in the sea. Those who make their homes in fresh water are found throughout the world and are generally bottom swimmers, scavenging on animal or vegetable matter during the night. Catfish stings are common and can be very painful; they are usually the result of handling the fish while removing it from hook or net. While most varieties cause only a painful sting, the venom of one species, *Plotosus lineatus* (found in the Indo-Pacific), can be lethal.

Symptoms   While death is rare, the sting of the catfish causes an immediate severe stinging or throbbing pain, which may stay at the site of the wound or spread throughout the body and last for several hours or days. There may be redness and swelling at the site of the sting, and the area may become numb.

Treatment   Flush the wound with fresh or salt water, and then soak the affected area in hot water or put hot compresses on it. The water should be very hot (122°F), so that the heat will deactivate the poison. Continue applying hot water for 30 minutes to an hour. These common stings often become infected, and removal of the barb is essential. X rays can determine whether the barb has actually been removed; if not, the wound should be opened and the spine taken out. Both antibiotics and tetanus prophylaxis are indicated.

centipedes   While small centipedes from temperate zones are harmless, the larger varieties found in the tropics can cause pain by injecting venom through their claws. The biggest is the giant centipede *(Scolopendra gigas)*, which ranges from the Southern United States to the West Indies. Centipedes are found in loose soil and leaf litter and under stones and may not have 100 feet—despite their name.

Poisonous part   These insects inject toxic substances into the skin from a pair of hollow jaws that act like fangs. The venom is relatively weak. The giant centipede is the only one in the United States dangerous to humans.

Symptoms   Generally a mild inflammation at the wound site with mild swelling of the lymph nodes. The bite of the giant centipede causes inflammation, swelling and redness and systemic symptoms that fade within five hours.

Treatment   Apply cool compresses at wound site; for the bite of the giant centipede, use cool saline compresses with painkillers or sedatives as required.

charcoal, activated   This substance, which absorbs a wide variety of toxins and renders them ineffective, is an indispensable part of any first aid kit. Activated charcoal is made from coal, lignite or waste from paper manufacturers, and soft organic material like vegetables. It is used to prevent the absorption of toxins in the gastrointestinal tract within a few minutes of administration.

Activated charcoal can be effective with most chemicals and is considered one of the best, cheapest and most practical emergency antidotes. For maximum effectiveness, activated charcoal should be administered within the first hour of poison ingestion. The sooner it is given, the more poison it is capable of absorbing.

According to some reports, the recommended dosage of activated charcoal is 30–50 grams in 4 ounces of water for children and 50–100 grams in 8 ounces of water for adults—a dose far larger than those included in most home poison kits.

Activated charcoal will inactivate syrup of ipecac and should not be given at the same time.   It should be administered only after vomiting has been successfully induced. It is nontoxic and is inert if aspirated, and there are contraindications to its use. It is not used when a neutralizing agent is administered by mouth (such as to treat iodine ingestion or mercury, iron, strychnine, nicotine or quinine poisoning).

In addition, it is not used when a patient is vomiting blood, nor is it effective with certain heavy metals such as iron salts or lithium. Activated charcoal is also poorly effective with products involving alcohol and petroleum distillates and is contraindicated after ingestion of strong acids or strong alkalies. It should not be given if analysis of gastric contents is necessary, or if the contents need to be viewed (to tell the color or number of pills, etc.).

Caution: Giving artificial charcoal too fast usually causes vomiting.

See also IPECAC SYRUP.

charcoal briquettes   A type of compressed fuel intended for outdoor use in charcoal grills and hibachis. However, in enclosed areas with little ventilation, the burning charcoal releases fatal amounts of carbon monoxide gas. At least 40 fatalities have been reported in recent years because of the indoor use of such charcoal in campers, trailers, tents, boats, apartments, and other enclosed areas.

See also CARBON MONOXIDE.

chelating agent   Chemicals used to treat poisoning by metals such as arsenic, mercury, lead or iron, these agents combine with the metal to form a less poisonous substance, which is then more quickly excreted in the urine. Penicillamine is a common chelating agent.

The word *chelate* is derived from the Greek *chele*, which refers to the claw of a lobster; this describes the pincerlike binding ability of metal ions.

See also ARSENIC; LEAD POISONING; MERCURY.

cherries, wild and cultivated *(Prunus)*   Although the cherry tree is widely cultivated for its fruit, the pits and leaves of the tree are poisonous.

Poisonous part   The pits contain cyanogenic glycosides (amygdalin), a substance that, when eaten, releases hydrocyanic acid.

Symptoms   Some hours may pass before symptoms appear, since the glycosides are not released until they are hydrolyzed in the gastrointestinal tract. When they do appear, symptoms include shortness of breath, vocal cord paralysis, abdominal pain, muscle twitches, vomiting, lethargy, sweating and weakness. In severe poisoning, symptoms progress to seizures, unconsciousness, stupor and coma.

Treatment   Gastric lavage (if conscious) followed by a 25 percent solution of thiosulfate. If the victim unconscious, acidosis is corrected and shock treated, together with the administration of oxygen and a cyanide antidote.

See also CYANOGENIC GLYCOSIDES.

cherry pit   See PRUNUS.

chinaberry *(Melia azedarach)*   [Other names: African lilac tree, bead tree, China tree, false sycamore, hog bush, Indian lilac, Japanese bead tree, paradise tree, Persian lilac, pride of China, pride of India, Texas umbrella tree, West Indian lilac, white cedar.] Found in the southern United States from Virginia to Florida west to Texas, in Hawaii, the West Indies and Guam, the chinaberry tree grows as high as 50 feet, with two-inch-long serrated leaves and fragrant purple flower clusters. The yellow fruit contains up to five smooth black seeds.

Poisonous part   Fruit and bark contain tetranortriterpene neurotoxins and unidentified gastroenteric toxins; toxicity varies considerably depending on the concentration of toxin in the plant.

Symptoms   Following a fairly long latency period, symptoms include faintness, confusion, stupor, vomiting, and diarrhea, which can lead to shock. Breathing problems may be followed by convulsions, paralysis and, very rarely, death. While six to eight fruits can be lethal to a child, human exposures in the United States are generally limited to severe gastroenteritis.

Treatment   Replace fluids and electrolytes and treat symptoms. Kidney and liver function should be monitored.

chinchonism   A syndrome produced by overdose of quinine, salicylates and cinchophen, consisting of ringing in the ears, hearing and balance problems, blurred vision, photophobia, headache, nausea, vomiting, diarrhea, flushed skin, sweating, fever and skin rash.

See also CINCHOPHEN; QUININE; SALICYLATES.

chloral hydrate   The well-known "Mickey Finn" or "knockout drops" popularized in the detective fiction of the 1930s, chloral hydrate is the oldest prescription sleeping pill available today. It was introduced in 1862 as a derivative of chloroform and quickly became a popular drug of abuse during those years; it is one of five sedative-hypnotic drugs introduced before 1900.

Symptoms   A central nervous system depressant, chloral hydrate in therapeutic doses produces drowsiness within 30 minutes after ingestion, followed by a sound sleep within an hour. Unlike with other sedatives, under normal conditions there is rarely a hangover afterward. However, doses larger than 2 g can cause poisoning, and the reported fatal dose is between 5 and 10 g. The toxicity of chloral hydrate does vary considerably but in general acts in three ways: depressing the central nervous system, corroding the skin and mucous membranes and affecting some major organs. Ingested in large amounts, chloral hydrate causes sleepiness, confusion, clumsiness, slow and shallow breathing, weakness, low blood pressure, cyanosis and a deep coma within 30 minutes of ingestion. It may be fatal in a few hours—or even sooner, as a result of respiratory collapse. In addition, there may be kidney and liver damage.

Chloral hydrate can also cause chronic poisoning, resulting in a skin rash, confusion, dizziness, drowsiness, depression and a wide range of behavioral abnormalities, including irritability, poor judgment and a general lack of interest in personal appearance.

Chloral hydrate is radiopaque, and diagnosis of overdose can be confirmed with an abdominal X ray.

Treatment There is no known antidote to chloral hydrate poisoning. Treatment is similar to poisoning with other narcotics: gastric lavage (only if begun soon after ingestion, because of this drug's rapid absorption in the gastrointestinal tract). Since onset of action is so rapid, induced vomiting could be dangerous. Afterward, administer activated charcoal and provide demulcents (such as milk). Provide supportive treatment (including oxygen). Hemodialysis may also be effective.

chloramine gas   A deadly gas that results from the combination of ammonia and cleaners containing hypochlorite salts. For this reason, two different types of household cleansers should never be mixed.

Symptoms Breathing these fumes can cause headache, eye irritation, dizziness, visual disturbances and nausea.

Treatment Remove victim from contaminated air; observe for breathing problems.

Chloramine-T (sodium *p*-toluenesulfochloramine) This drinking water disinfectant and deodorant contains 12 percent chlorine, which is slowly released on contact with water; as a solution, it is used as a mouthwash. It is also used to remove odor from cheese.

Symptoms It is believed that this compound works by transforming chloramine-T into a derivative of cyanide, resulting in cyanosis, respiratory failure, collapse and frothing at the mouth. Death follows within a few minutes. It is suspected of causing rapid allergic reactions in hypersensitive victims.

Treatment Gastric lavage, followed by the administration of sodium nitrate and sodium thiosulfate. Patients who survive 24 hours are expected to recover.

chlorate poisoning   Chemicals used in some defoliant weed killers and in industries to make dyes, explosives or matches can cause kidney, liver and intestinal damage and can be fatal in small doses, especially in children.

Symptoms Ulcers in the mouth, abdominal pain and diarrhea.

Treatment If spilled onto skin or eyes, wash off immediately with water. If ingested, seek medical help immediately.

chlordane (1,2,4,5,6,7,8,8   octachloro-4,7-methano-3a,4,7,7a-tetrahydroindane; chlordan octachlorotetrahydro methano indane) [Trade names: CD-68, Dowklor, Octa-Klor, Ortho-Klor, 1068, Toxichlor, Velsicol 1068.] One of a group of synthetic organochlorine pesticides, chlordane is a viscous liquid with a chlorine odor ranging from colorless to amber. Introduced in 1945, it has been banned from most commercial use in 1975 because it does not disperse in the environment but instead accumulates in biological systems. Some uses are still permitted, including pest control in some fruit and to remedy some pest control problems in some parts of the country.

It dissolves in both water and fat and is available as a powder, dust, emulsion concentrate and a concentrated solution in oil. Skin absorption is rapid, but reports of human poisonings are limited.

Symptoms Chlordane is a fairly quick acting chemical and less toxic than similar pesticides, but still toxic; violent convulsions appear suddenly within 30 minutes to three hours after ingestion. The first 12 hours are the most dangerous, and death—if it is likely to occur—will usually take place within this time frame. It is possible, however, that a person will live up to 20 days after ingestion before finally succumbing. Other symptoms include liver damage and congestion in the brain, lung, heart and spinal cord. The estimated lethal oral dose of chlordane in an adult is 3–7 g. It has been implicated in acute blood abnormalities.

Treatment There is no specific antidote. Perform gastric lavage, but do not induce vomiting because of the risk of sudden onset of seizures; administer activated charcoal and a cathartic. Irregular heartbeat may respond to propranolol. If convulsions last for some time, recovery is unlikely.

See also CHLORINATED HYDROCARBON PESTICIDES.

chlorinated hydrocarbon pesticides This group of insect-fighting chemicals was once widely used in agriculture and malarial control programs around the world from the 1940s through the 1960s. However, environmental contamination has led to their disfavor; DDT and chlordane, for example, are banned from commercial use because they do not disperse in the environment and because they accumulate in biological systems. Some have been shown to cause cancer in humans, including chloroform, vinyl chloride, aldrin, chlordane, dieldrin, heptachlor, lindane, toxaphene and carbon tetrachloride. Instead, organophosphates (such as malathion and diazinon) have more or less replaced the chlorinated hydrocarbons, since they control insects, are biodegradable and (according to their manufacturers) do not contaminate the environment.

The most highly toxic of the group are aldrin, dieldrin, endrin and endosulfan; moderately toxic are chlordane, DDT, heptachlor, kepone, lindane, mirex and toxaphene; slightly toxic are ethylan (perthane), hexachlorobenzene and methoxychlor.

As a group, these insecticides interfere with the transmission of nerve impulses throughout the body (especially the brain), causing behavior changes, involuntary movements and depressed respiratory system. They may also cause liver or kidney damage and may also be carcinogenic. In general, the route of poisoning is through the skin (especially with aldrin, dieldrin and endrin).

Symptoms Soon after these chemicals are ingested, symptoms of nausea and vomiting appear followed by confusion, tremor, coma, seizures and respiratory depression. There have been reports of delayed and recurrent seizures and irregular heartbeat.

Treatment There is no specific antidote for chlorinated hydrocarbon poisoning. Treat symptoms and perform gastric lavage, but do not induce vomiting. Then administer activated charcoal and a cathartic.

See also CHLORDANE; DDT; DIELDRIN; ENDRIN; LINDANE; MIREX.

chlorine This yellow-green gas with an irritating odor is widely used to manufacture chemicals, as a swimming pool disinfectant and cleaner and as a bleach. Chlorine and chlorine-containing compounds are also found in table salt (sodium chloride), plastics (polyvinyl chloride), aerosol propellants (chlorofluorocarbons) and pesticides, as well as throughout the body in all nerve and muscle tissues.

Chlorine was also used briefly as a chemical weapon during World War I, but it was subsequently replaced by other chemicals. Current toxic exposures come from accidental spills and the improper use of household products. A derivative of chlorine's derivative, hypochlorite, is found in most household bleaches in solutions of 3 to 5 percent; adding ammonia to this hypochlorite solution may release chloramine, which can cause unconsciousness, especially if the area is small and unventilated. However, a person would need to be in the fumes for more than an hour for serious problems to develop. Adding an acid to hypochlorite solution releases chlorine gas.

A natural chemical element and a gas at room temperature, chlorine is easily liquefied under pressure. Pure chlorine rarely occurs in nature, except in volcanic eruptions—and even then, the quantities released are small.

Accidental spills or leaks of chlorine gas during transport or storage are the greatest exposure hazard today; in the event of such a spill, whole neighborhoods or towns may be evacuated. Chlorine and hydrochloric acid rank first and third respectively in causing injuries and deaths from large accidents involving industrial chemicals, although the actual number of incidences is small.

Symptoms When in contact with moist tissue (such as the eyes and upper respiratory tract), chlorine gas is a strong irritant and causes corrosive injury; aqueous solutions of chlorine also cause corrosive injury to eyes, skin and gastrointestinal tract. Inhaling chlorine gas causes immediate burning of eyes, nose and throat, with coughing and wheezing. More serious poisoning results in croupy cough, hoarseness and upper airway swelling to the point of obstruction. In quite severe cases of poisoning, pulmonary edema may result. Skin or eye contact with either the gas or the concentrated solution causes corrosive burns. Ingestion of 3–5 percent hyperchlorite solution is not particularly serious, causing an immediate burning in the mouth and throat but no further injury. More concentrated solutions may result in serious esophageal and gastric burns, together with drooling and severe throat, chest and abdominal pain and with perforation of the esophagus or stomach.

There is a slight increase in the risk of bladder cancer and possibly colon and rectal cancers in longtime users of chlorinated water supplies.

Hypochlorite in bleach is a corrosive substance that can damage skin, eyes and other membranes. According to poison control centers, a high number of children each year accidentally swallow laundry bleach, although relatively few fatalities are reported (probably because of the vomiting that bleach causes). However, damage to the esophagus and stomach can occur.

Treatment While many experts recommend administration of corticosteroids in an attempt to limit esophageal scarring, this treatment is unproven and may be harmful in those with perforations or serious infection. For the inhalation of chlorine gas, give humidified supplemental oxygen, and observe for signs of upper airway obstruction. Treat symptoms. For ingestion of hyperchlorite solution greater than 10 percent (or with symptoms of corrosive injury), check for serious esophageal or gastric injury with a flexible endoscope. A chest X ray will also reveal a perforated esophagus.

For contaminated skin and eyes, flush exposed skin with water; irrigate eyes with water or saline. For ingestion of hypochlorite solution, immediately give water or milk by mouth. Do not induce vomiting; perform gastric lavage after concentrated liquid ingestion. Do not use activated charcoal, since it may interfere with the endoscopist's view.

See also CHLORINE GAS.

chlorine gas   This yellow-green gas is used in the manufacture of plastics, purified water, cloth and paper and usually causes poisoning after a leak in a storage tank. The damage following exposure to chlorine gas depends on its concentration, duration of exposure and the water content of the exposed tissue, but it is capable of causing rapid and extensive tissue destruction. Chlorine gas is 30 times more toxic to cells than hydrochloric acid.

Symptoms Skin contact causes severe burns; inhalation of gas at greater than 3 to 6 parts per million causes conjunctivitis, keratitis, sore throat, burning chest pain and coughing. A moderate exposure causes immediate, severe irritation of the mucous membranes of the nose, throat and eyes, with a distressing cough. Excessive exposure results in a severe, productive cough, difficulty in breathing and cyanosis. There may be prolonged vomiting, restlessness and anxiety, followed by lack of oxygen and heart attack.

Treatment Remove the victim from the environment. Wash eyes with saline after the application of topical anesthesia. Burns should be washed with saline; hospitalization may be necessary. Bronchodilators and humidified oxygen will alleviate breathing problems, together with the administration of steroids.

See also CHLORINE.

chlorobenzene derivatives   These chemicals are a type of synthetic organic insecticide and include DDT, TDE, DFDT, DMC, neotrane, ovotran, and dilan. They are soluble in fat (not water), and according to reports, the amount of these chemicals present in the body fat of individuals in the United States is higher than in Canada, England, France and the former West Germany. In those preparations that are still legally available, the commercial solutions are sold in dry mixtures or in solutions of one or more inorganic solvents (kerosene, benzene, etc.), which are also toxic in themselves.

Symptoms   These compounds affect the central nervous system and result in restlessness, irritability, muscle spasm, tremor and convulsions followed by depression, collapse and breathing problems due to respiratory failure. Absorption through the skin or by inhalation causes eye, nose and throat irritation, blurred vision, pulmonary edema and skin problems. Chronic poisoning symptoms include loss of weight, liver and kidney damage and disturbances of the central nervous system.

Treatment   Gastric lavage followed by saline cathartics. Avoid all fats and oils (including milk), since they increase the rate of absorption of chlorinated hydrocarbons. Administer phenobarbital sodium for tremors, and barbiturates for convulsions, and provide oxygen if necessary. If the skin has come in contact with these insecticides, wash with soap and water immediately to head off skin problems and systemic absorption. Remove contaminated clothing.

See also DDT; INSECTICIDES.

chloroform   (trichloromethane) This chlorinated hydrocarbon solvent is used in the production of Freon and as a solvent in the chemical and pharmaceutical industries; it is a direct central nervous system depressant.

It was discovered independently and simultaneously in 1831 in Germany, France and the United States, and accounts of its abuse were reported in the United States in that same year. Dentist Horace Wills, the first person in the United States to use nitrous oxide in surgery, died from complications resulting from his own chronic chloroform abuse. Chloroform was introduced as an anesthetic during surgery in 1847; it became so popular that Queen Victoria knighted its discoverer, Dr. James Simpson, after he delivered her eighth child.

However, as other anesthetics were discovered and the number of overdoses of chloroform rose, its medical use lost favor. It has since been abandoned because of the toxic effects on the liver, which can progress to fatal cirrhosis. In addition, about 10 percent of the population have a genetic response to chloroform that results in an uncontrolled high fever (over 110°F) during or after anesthesia.

Chronic low levels of the chemical may still be found in some municipal water supplies.

Symptoms In addition to its effects on the central nervous system, chloroform may also cause heartbeat irregularities and damage the liver and kidneys. Chloroform is also toxic to the fetus and is a suspected carcinogen. Ingestion or inhalation causes a mild to moderate systemic toxicity, including headache, nausea, vomiting, confusion and drunkenness followed by coma, respiratory arrest and heartbeat irregularities. Kidney and liver failure may be discovered up to three days after exposure.

Treatment If skin or eyes have come in contact with chloroform, remove affected clothing and wash with soap and water; irrigate eyes with tepid water or saline. If inhaled, remove the victim from the area and give oxygen. If ingested, perform gastric lavage, but do not induce vomiting (chloroform is rapidly absorbed and may depress the central nervous system). Administer activated charcoal and a cathartic; provide supportive treatment. Acetylcysteine may help prevent kidney and liver damage.

See also ANESTHETICS, GASEOUS/VOLATILE.

chlorthion See ORGANOPHOSPHATE INSECTICIDES.

choke cherry pit See PRUNUS.

Christmas rose *(Helleborus niger)* Also called black hellebore or winter rose, this very poisonous plant of the buttercup family is found in the northern United States and Canada and blooms from late fall through early spring—often in the snow. Its groups of evergreen leaflets resemble fingers on a hand; its flowers are white to pinky green and appear during Christmas in milder climates. The Christmas rose is found in damp, shady places and is closely related to the later-blooming Lenten rose *(H. orientalis)*.

Poisonous part All parts of the plant contain the digitalis-like glycosides helleborin, hellebrin; and the direct irritants saponins and protoanemonin.

Symptoms Within 30 minutes after ingestion, the poison will blister the mucous membranes in the mouth, with abdominal pain, severe diarrhea, vomiting and death from cardiac arrest. The amount ingested will determine the length of time between ingestion and the appearance of symptoms; generally, poisoning symptoms include conduction defects and sinus bradycardia.

Treatment Amyl nitrate, strychnine and atropine are often used as cardiac and respiratory stimulants. Perform gastric lavage or induce emesis, and activated charcoal may be given repeatedly.

See also BUTTERCUP; GLYCOSIDE; SAPONIN.

chromium   This silver metal is used by electroplaters, welders, lithographers and metal or textile workers and can be toxic by skin contact, inhalation or ingestion.

Poisonous part   Trivalent chromium compounds (chromic oxide, chromic sulfate) and chromate salts of lead, zinc, barium, bismuth and silver do not readily dissolve in water and, because they are poorly absorbed, are not very toxic. Hexavalent compounds (chromium trioxide, chromic anhydride, chromic acid and dichromate salts) do dissolve in water and are more easily absorbed by the lungs, gastrointestinal tract and skin. Some of the hexavalent compounds are also carcinogenic.

Symptoms   Skin/eyes: Contact with the skin may cause severe burns; contact with the eyes can cause serious corneal injury. There have been reports of fatalities after skin contact causing only 10 percent burned surface area, because the skin burns enhance absorption. Inhalation: Symptoms (which may appear several hours after exposure) include upper respiratory tract irritation, wheezing and pulmonary edema. Ingestion: There may be immediate gastroenteritis, with massive fluid and blood loss leading to shock and kidney failure. Other symptoms include hepatitis and cerebral edema. Serious poisoning has occurred from ingesting as little as 500 mg of hexavalent chromium.

Treatment   Treat symptoms; chelation therapy is not effective. Skin/eyes: Wash exposed area with soap and water (for eyes, flush with tepid water or saline). Inhalation: Give supplemental oxygen if necessary. Ingestion: (of hexavalent compounds) Ascorbic acid may be administered; give milk or water to dilute corrosive effects, and perform gastric lavage, but do not induce vomiting because of the potential for corrosive injury. Administer activated charcoal.

ciguatera   The most common clinical syndrome caused by certain tropical marine reef fish that become toxic at certain times of the year. It is believed to be caused by a type of dinoflagellate *(Gambierdiscus toxicus)* that is eaten by reef herbivores, which in turn are eaten by larger fish. Ciguatera occurs most often in the Caribbean Islands, Florida, Hawaii and the Pacific Islands. Recent reports cited 129 cases over a two-year period in Dade County (Florida) alone. It appears to be occurring more often, probably because of the increased demand for seafood around the world and its recurrence in edible fish.

Ciguatera occurs in about 300 species of fish, including barracuda, kingfish, dolphinfish, wrasses, triggerfish, moray eels, surgeon fish, filefish, grouper, red snapper, herring and pompano.

Poisonous part   The toxin believed to be involved in ciguatera is ciguatoxin, a fat-soluble, odorless, tasteless poison that cannot be destroyed by heat or freezing.

Symptoms   Ingestion of ciguatoxin causes both gastrointestinal and neurological symptoms, which may develop quickly or slowly. Victims often report a type of sensory reversal—for example, they would report a burning-hot sensation when picking up a cold glass. Other symptoms include a tingling sensation in the lips and mouth followed by numbness, nausea, vomiting, abdominal cramps, weakness, headache, vertigo, paralysis, convulsions, skin rash, coma and death in about 12 percent of cases. After the acute phase of poisoning, patients may complain of weakness for several weeks. Researchers note that subsequent episodes of ciguatera may be more severe.

Treatment   Recent research suggests that pralidoxime chloride (a cholinesterase reactivator) is an effective antidote. Other treatment is symptomatic and supportive.

See also DINOFLAGELLATE; SHELLFISH POISONING.

cimetidine   (Tagamet) An ulcer-healing drug related to the antihistamines, cimetidine was first introduced in 1976. It reduces the secretion of hydrochloric acid in the stomach and helps heal gastric and duodenal ulcers and heals inflammation of the esophagus.

Symptoms   On rare occasions, an overdose (or even a therapeutic dose) produces a toxic psychosis within a few hours of ingestion, with confusion, disorientation, agitation and hallucinations. Symptoms will usually clear within 24 hours.

Treatment   Treat symptoms of agitation with gastric lavage; barbiturates may be used cautiously to control central nervous system stimulation.

See also ANTIHISTAMINES.

cinchophen   A painkiller used to treat gout, it is available in both oral and injectable form. Cinchophen carries with it the risk of liver damage, which makes its use in the treatment of gout dangerous.

Symptoms   Appearing between six and 12 hours after ingestion, symptoms include gastrointestinal irritation, anorexia, diarrhea, vomiting, high fever, delirium, convulsions, coma and death.

Treatment   Treatment is the same as with salicylate poisoning (induce vomiting or perform gastric lavage followed by activated charcoal and a cathartic).

clematis   Many different species of this popular and quite beautiful flowering climber can be found throughout Canada and the north temperate United States.

Poisonous part   The whole plant is poisonous and contains the toxin protoanemonin, which irritates both the skin and the mucous membranes.

Symptoms   Ingestion causes intense pain, blistering and inflammation in the mouth and throat together with excess salivation, bloody diarrhea, abdominal cramps, dizziness and, in severe cases, convulsions and mental confusion.

Treatment   Usually, the immediate pain upon chewing leaves or flowers limits the amount of toxin ingested. In cases of large amounts of poisoning, gastric lavage should be performed and demulcents administered. Kidney function should be monitored.

climbing lily   *(Gloriosa rothschildiana; G. superba)*   Also called glory lilies, climbing lilies have striking bright crimson and yellow flowers with finger-like petals and lance-shaped leaves tipped with tendrils. They are primarily cultivated in the southern United States, the West Indies and Hawaii.

Poisonous part   The entire plant contains the toxin colchicine, especially the fleshy, tuberous roots.

Symptoms   Immediately after ingestion, the victim experiences burning pain in the mouth and throat with intense thirst followed by nausea and vomiting. Within two hours, abdominal pain and severe diarrhea develop, which may lead to shock. There is sometimes kidney damage. Because colchicine is not readily excreted, illness can last for some time.

Treatment   Give fluids, and monitor blood pressure and kidney function. Administer atropine and painkillers.

clove cigarettes   See PHENOL.

cobra   A large group of highly poisonous snakes of the family Elapidae, most of which expand the neck ribs to form a hood. Most species of cobras are found in warm regions of Africa and are favorites of snake charmers. Cobra bites are fatal between 10 and 50 percent of the time, depending on the species; if untreated, they can be fatal within minutes to several hours.

Cobras that are found in the East have fang openings facing forward, enabling the snake to spit. Snakes that spit their venom usually direct the poison at the victim's eyes at distances of up to more than seven feet; the venom can cause temporary or permanent blindness unless promptly washed out.

These snakes live in holes in the ground, and while they can climb into a shrub looking for food, they are usually seen underfoot. They are considered fairly placid, preferring to flee rather than fight. An angry cobra surprised in its hole will hiss loudly; if disturbed in the open, it will turn and face its victim, inflating its hood and looking very fierce. However, its striking range is limited, and it will often strike with its mouth closed in the hope of discouraging an attacker.

Included in the cobra family are the Indian or Asian cobra, the Egyptian or African cobra, the ringhals, the black-necked cobra and the tree cobra. Those of the cobra family without hoods include the blue krait, pama, black mamba, green mamba, taipan, death adder, tiger snake, Australian black snake, brown snake, eastern coral, Arizona coral, African coral, black-banded coral and the Brazilian giant coral.

Symptoms The venom of a cobra snake is a toxin chemically different from that of other snakes; some suggest it may contain a cardiotoxin. Within 15 to 30 minutes symptoms appear: pain, swelling, a drop in blood pressure, confusion, slurring of speech, dilation of the pupils, strabismus (deviation of the eye), drooping of the upper eyelid and muscle weakness. The respiratory muscles are affected last, and respiratory muscle paralysis is the most common cause of death. The venom from this snake family is twice as toxic as strychnine and nearly five times more toxic than the venom of a black widow spider.

Treatment The specific antiserum for the type of cobra involved should be used.

cobra, black-necked See COBRA, SPITTING.

cobra, Egyptian *(Naja haje)* Most likely the asp of ancient history and of Cleopatra's suicide, the Egyptian cobra is dark with a narrow hood ranging over much of Africa, in the savanna and sometimes near water. It has also been seen in a few small areas in Saudi Arabia. Also known as the African cobra, it is quiet but inquisitive and highly aggressive when restrained. It is considered small but can grow as long as six feet.

Cobras live in holes in the ground, and while they can climb into a shrub if they have to, it is unusual to see them anywhere but on the ground. These snakes will hiss if threatened in their holes, but if threatened in the open, they will pack their coils around themselves, spread their hoods and turn to face the enemy.

Symptoms Within 15 to 30 minutes symptoms appear: pain, swelling, a drop in blood pressure and confusion followed by death if the poison spreads to the respiratory muscles.

Treatment Antivenin is available, but only the specific antiserum for the type of cobra involved should be used; victims are often tested for sensitivity before being treated.

See also ANTIVENIN; SNAKES, POISONOUS.

cobra, Indian *(Naja naja)* Also known as the Asian cobra, this favorite of snake charmers kills many thousands of people each year. It is commonly found in paddy fields and urban areas of southern Asia, Indonesia, Taiwan and the Philippines. In India, the species has a black-and-white spectaclelike mark on a very wide hood; in other locations, the Indian cobra has a ring or bar on its hood. Growing up to six feet long, it is generally inoffensive but highly aggressive when restrained; it is active at dusk and during the night. When confronted by an aggressor, it rears up the front of its body and inflates its hood, standing its ground. Its venom is highly neurotoxic; it is fatal so often because it comes into populated areas to seek out rats.

Symptoms Pain radiating from the wound, swelling, numbness, drooping eyelids, difficulty in speaking, weakness, respiratory distress, blindness, convulsions and death.

Treatment Antivenin is available, but only the specific antiserum for the type of cobra involved should be used; victims are often tested for sensitivity before being treated.

See also ANTIVENIN; SNAKES, POISONOUS.

cobra, king (*Ophiophagus hannah* or *Naja hannah*)   The world's largest venomous snake, the king cobra (or hamadryad) is found in forests and areas of rural agriculture from southern China to the Philippines and Indonesia. This huge snake can grow as long as 18 feet; when angered, it raises its head and can stand as tall as a person. A normally quiet snake, the king cobra is highly dangerous when aroused; its bite is lethal about 10 percent of the time. It spreads a small hood, and while adult snakes have a dull color with no markings, young snakes sport a black skin with narrow chevrons of pale yellow on buff.

King cobras are often found in pairs, which may be the origin of the ancient belief that a person who kills a king cobra will be pursued and killed by its mate, intent on revenge.

King cobras are the most intelligent and curious of snakes and in captivity will watch any activity going on outside their cage. They are rarely kept in zoos outside of the tropics, however, because they are selective feeders, existing entirely on other species of snakes.

Symptoms Within 15 to 30 minutes symptoms appear: pain, swelling, a drop in blood pressure and confusion followed by death if the poison spreads to the respiratory muscles.

Treatment Antivenin is available, but only the specific antiserum for the type of cobra involved should be used; victims are often tested for sensitivity before being treated.

See also ANTIVENIN; SNAKES, POISONOUS.

cobra, spitting (*Naja nigricollis*)   This nervous and aggressive cobra is widely found throughout Africa, except in the extreme south and the Sahara. It is one of the cobras that can eject venom at a victim's eyes at distances of up to more than seven feet; the venom can cause temporary or permanent blindness unless promptly washed out. Also called the black-necked cobra, this snake prefers to spit and rarely bites. The sprayed venom is harmless to unbroken skin.

Symptoms The venom of a cobra snake is chemically different from the venom of other snakes. Within 15 to 30 minutes symptoms appear: pain, swelling, a drop in blood pressure and confusion followed by death if the poison spreads to the respiratory muscles.

Treatment The specific antiserum for the type of cobra involved should be used, and victims are often tested for sensitivity before being treated.

See also ANTIVENIN; SNAKES, POISONOUS.

cocaine One of the most popular of the abused drugs in America today, cocaine is an alkaloid of the coca plant grown on the slopes of the Andes, where it has been cultivated for thousands of years. The oval leaves that provide cocaine and 13 other alkaloids are picked four times a year, and the four-foot-high bushes continue to produce the leaves for up to 30 years. After the leaves are harvested, they are dried (sometimes in the sun or in a fire) and then packed for shipment. Cocaine has many uses as a medicine, and is especially valuable as a local anesthetic. As a solution of one of its acid salts, cocaine has long served as a topical anesthetic in the eye and on mucous membranes, but it is not commonly used in clinical medicine today. It is, however, still used in veterinary medicine.

Indians throughout the Andes chew coca leaves at an early age and continue the habit through their lifetime. Cocaine was first extracted from the leaves of the coca bush in Germany more than 100 years ago, and the kick obtained from sniffing the white powder was soon recognized. Indeed, cocaine was enthusiastically recommended by many medical authorities, including Sigmund Freud, who believed it could cure alcoholism and promote sexuality. Sir Arthur Conan Doyle, another cocaine adherent, popularized it further by making his character Sherlock Homes a sniffer and needle abuser of the white powder.

In the United States, a soft drink developed in 1886 by an Atlanta druggist contained a touch of cocaine and caffeine from the African cola nut, becoming famous as Coca-Cola; under pressure from the U.S. government in 1903, however, all cocaine was removed from the beverage. Coke's removal of the drug kicked off a federal crackdown on the use of cocaine, and beginning in 1906 a series of laws placed it under strict federal regulation.

Cocaine may be sniffed ("snorted"), smoked or injected; combined with heroin and injected, it is called a "speedball." Addicts prefer to inject it intravenously for the brief but intense elation that it induces. Similar to amphetamine in some of its action, cocaine even in a large oral dose dissipates quickly (usually within two to three hours).

"Crack" (the "freebase" form of cocaine) is made by dissolving cocaine salt in solution and extracting the freebase form with a solvent, such as ether. Heat is often applied to hasten solvent evaporation. Cocaine sold as a street drug may also contain caffeine, phenylpropanolamine, ephedrine or phencyclidine.

Cocaine is a local anesthetic and a central nervous system stimulant, with an intoxication resembling an amphetamine "high." It is well absorbed in the body, and smoking or injections can produce the maximum effects within a few minutes. Oral or nasal application may take up to 30 minutes. Its toxicity varies greatly from one individual to the next and is also affected by the presence of other drugs in the system. Still, the oral lethal dose is described as about one gram in adults, but some addicts are reported to have consumed as much as 10 grams in one day, reflecting an acquired tolerance. The method of use also affects toxicity; injecting or smoking cocaine may produce such rapid high levels in the brain or heart that convulsions or heart attack may occur, while the same dose ingested or snorted may produce only a feeling of euphoria.

Symptoms   Cocaine can be toxic to both the central nervous and the cardiovascular systems. Symptoms include anxiety, agitation, delirium, psychosis, muscle rigidity, hyperactivity, seizures and coma. Chronic cocaine use causes weight loss, insomnia and paranoid psychosis. In addition, symptoms may include fatal heart irregularities, severe hypertension, stroke, coronary artery spasm, heart attack, chronic heart disease, shock and kidney failure. Death is usually caused by a sudden fatal heart irregularity, seizure, brain hemorrhage or multiple organ failure. Other symptoms can occur from snorting or smoking cocaine, including chest pain, nasal septal perforation and skin ulcers ("coke burns").

Treatment   There is no specific antidote. Provide symptomatic treatment; after cocaine ingestion, perform gastric lavage but do not induce vomiting because of the risk of seizures. Administer activated charcoal and a cathartic. For those who have ingested large packets of cocaine in an attempt to smuggle or hide the drug, give repeated doses of activated charcoal and consider whole gut lavage (otherwise, laparotomy and surgical removal may be necessary).

codeine (methylmorphine) This narcotic painkiller is a naturally occurring alkaloid of opium (from the poppy plant) used in medicine as a cough suppressant and narcotic analgesic drug. It was first synthesized from morphine (an opium derivative) in 1832; although it can be extracted directly from opium, most of the codeine used in drugs is produced from morphine. When taken over a long period of time, codeine may be habit-forming.

Supertoxic, it is used to treat mild to moderate pain and can also be used as an antidiarrheal. It is found in combination with a wide range of other drugs, such as acetaminophen, aspirin, caffeine and cough suppressants. Because of its value as a cough suppressant, it had been included in a number of cough medicines in the past. But because they were available to those who experimented with drugs, codeine was removed from many of these products. However, more than 40 prescription cough medicines still contain codeine.

Nearly transparent, it has no odor and a bitter taste and is sold as either a powder or liquid. In some forms it is a Schedule II drug (a strictly controlled drug considered by law to have a high potential for abuse), and psychological dependence can develop fairly rapidly, but it is not a major drug of abuse.

Symptoms Within 20 minutes after ingestion, victims will begin to feel sleepy, giddy and clumsy, with a slow heartbeat; overdoses can lead to excitability, breathing problems, coma and death.

Treatment Naloxone is the antidote; other symptoms are treated as they appear.

See also ALKALOIDS; NALOXONE.

Cogentin See BENZTROPINE.

coliform bacteria The common microorganism *Escherichia coli* (or *E. coli*) that is found in the intestines of humans and other animals; in the gut the bacteria do not cause disease, but a high concentration of the bacteria in drinking water supplies or aquatic ecosystems is often an indicator of pollution.

See also FOOD POISONING.

colocynth *(Citrullus colocynthis)* Also known as bitter apple or bitter cucumber, this extremely toxic bitter fruit is native to the Mediterranean but can also be found in Central America.

Poisonous part The toxic fruit contains colocynthin, which is used as an insecticide, purgative and abortifacient.

Symptoms Within several hours of ingestion, symptoms of bloody diarrhea appear, followed by cramps, headache, kidney failure and death. Those who live more than two days will most likely recover.

Treatment Administer milk to relieve stomach irritation and atropine to minimize gastric secretions, plus medication for pain.

comfrey *(Symphytum officianale)* [Other names: gum plant, healing herb, knitbone, nipbone.] Once a popular tea herb found in every herbalist's garden and used to aid digestion and promote healing, comfrey has been shown to be poisonous by recent studies, although the findings are considered by some to be controversial.

Naturalized throughout North America and native to Europe and Asia, comfrey is a hardy perennial with a stout, brown-black root (from which the plant gets its nickname, "slippery root") and blue, yellow, white or red tubular flowers appearing in May and June. It grows to about three feet high and has coarse, hairy egg-shaped leaves; its fruit of black nuts can be seen in August. It is found along stream banks and in rich soils of moist meadows.

As early as 400 B.C. comfrey has been used to stop heavy bleeding and to treat bronchial problems. Its popularity as a treatment for broken bones gave the plant its name, a derivative from the Latin *conferta* ("to grow together"). In the 19th century during the Irish potato famines, the plant was seen as a solution to world hunger by Englishman Henry Doubleday, who founded an association still in existence today to promote the plant's use.

While remedies derived from the roots have been prescribed since the early 1500s for everything from tumors to burns and gangrene, in the early 1970s darker reports about this herb's character began to surface: a weed containing pyrrolizidine alkaloids fell into some wheat being harvested in Afghanistan. When the farmers and their families ate the bread made from the contaminated wheat, 25 percent of the 7,200 villagers developed liver ailments within two years.

Poisonous part   Recent studies show the roots and leaves of all varieties contain potentially dangerous compounds called pyrrolizidine alkaloids, which have caused liver tumors in animals. While comfrey leaves (from which tea is brewed) have only one-tenth the alkaloid concentration as the root, several teas on the market contain both root and leaves. In other comfrey products, such as comfrey-pepsin tablets (called "digestive aids"), comfrey root is a primary ingredient.

Symptoms   In 1976 and 1985 there were two cases of pyrrolizidine-alkaloid poisoning in humans, probably from drinking comfrey tea. One recent study found that rats fed a diet that was 8 percent comfrey developed liver cancers within six months; another showed that certain alkaloids in comfrey cause chronic liver problems in rats.

Treatment   Physicians suggest that since comfrey tea won't cure illness and may damage the liver, it is wise to avoid this herb until researchers perfect an accurate test for alkaloid levels in comfrey leaves.

See also HERBS, POISONOUS.

compound 1080   Also known as sodium fluoroacetate and used as a rat poison, this is one of the most toxic substances known; fluoroacetic acid is no longer sold in the United States because of its danger, but fluoroacetate is still available.

Fluoroacetate blocks cell metabolism, and as little as 1 mg is enough to cause serious symptoms. The effects of fluoroacetate poisoning are similar to those of cyanide and hydrogen sulfide, although they take longer to develop.

Symptoms   Within a few minutes to several hours after ingestion, symptoms appear, including nausea, vomiting, diarrhea, metabolic acidosis, agitation, confusion, seizures, coma, respiratory arrest and heartbeat irregularities. Death results from respiratory failure due to pulmonary edema or ventricular fibrillation.

Treatment There is no antidote. Perform gastric lavage but do not induce vomiting, since seizures may occur as early as 30 minutes after ingestion. Administer activated charcoal and a cathartic.

See also CYANIDE; HYDROGEN SULFIDE.

cone shell *(Conus)* These highly toxic stinging shells are found on or around coral reefs in warm waters, and although prized by collectors for their bright, spotted shells, they have caused several human deaths. Cone shells are tiny (only one to three inches long) members of the enormous mollusk family, with a cone-shaped shell with wavy stripes or an irregular pattern. The more than 70 different species in this family of toxic marine snails can fire a barbed harpoonlike device from a slit in their shell to obtain food and protect against predators.

There are three main types of cones—those that eat worms, mollusks or fish. Of all the cones, the fish-eating varieties are most dangerous to humans; they have teeth strong enough to pierce cloth.

Cones live in warm waters of barrier reefs in the Indo-Pacific, Australia and the Mediterranean, southern California and New Zealand. Some of the most common include the geography cone *(C. geographus)*, striated cone *(C. striatus)* and the tulip cone *(C. tulipa)*.

Poisonous part The cone shell uses its sting to secrete a neurotoxin that competes for acetylcholine in the body, and can be fatal within 15 minutes.

Symptoms Pain, swelling, numbness or tingling, dizziness, blurred vision, difficulty swallowing, weakness, ataxia, breathing problems, paralysis, coma and death.

Treatment There is no known antidote. Contact medical help immediately; flush the wound with fresh or salt water, and then soak the affected area in hot water or put hot compresses on it. The water should be very hot (122°F), so that the heat will deactivate the poison. Continue applying hot water for 30 minutes to an hour. Have the victim lie still with the stung part immobile and lower than the heart. Tie a flat strip of cloth around the stung arm or leg two to four inches above the sting. It should be snug but loose enough to allow a pulse farther out on the limb. Check periodically and loosen if necessary, but do not remove it. If swelling reaches the band, tie another band two to four inches higher up and remove the first one. Generally, victims recover within 48 hours.

coniine The most important of the six alkaloids found in all parts of *Conium maculatum* (poison hemlock), a plant widely found throughout the United States and Europe. The whole plant exudes a foul odor (similar to cat urine or mice) at least in part attributable to the volatile coniine.

Prolonged inhalation of the odors is said to cause a narcosis. The toxic potential of coniine has been known since earliest times and was presumably instrumental in the death of Socrates.

See also ALKALOIDS; HEMLOCK, POISON.

copperhead, Australian *(Denisonia superba)*   A poisonous snake of the cobra family found in Tasmania and along the coasts of southern Australia. About five feet long, this copperhead is usually copper or reddish brown. Although dangerous, it is unaggressive when not disturbed.

Symptoms   The venom of a cobra snake is a toxin chemically different from that of other snakes; some suggest it may contain a cardiotoxin. Within 15 to 30 minutes symptoms appear: pain, swelling, a drop in blood pressure, confusion, slurring of speech, dilation of the pupils, strabismus (abnormal deviation of one eye in relation to the other), drooping of the upper eyelid and muscle weakness. The respiratory muscles are affected last, and respiratory muscle paralysis is the most common cause of death.

Treatment   Antivenin is available, but only the specific antiserum for the type of cobra involved should be used; victims are often tested for sensitivity before being treated.

See also ANTIVENIN; SNAKES, POISONOUS.

copperhead snake *(Agkistrodon contortrix)*   Also called highland moccasin, this species of copperhead is a member of the Viperidae family and one of several unrelated snakes that get their name from the reddish color of the head. The *Agkistrodon* variety is the North American copperhead, a venomous species found in swampy, rocky and wooden regions of the eastern and central United States. It is considered a pit viper because of the characteristic small sensory pit between each eye and nostril.

Usually less than three feet long, the copperhead is a pink or red snake with a copper-colored head with reddish brown hourglass-shaped crossbands on its back. While many bites are reported, the venom of this snake is relatively weak and rarely fatal. The copperhead has retractable hollow fangs in the front of the upper jaw that can be folded back and then positioned forward as the mouth opens to strike.

Seriousness of the bite depends on a wide variety of variables, including the snake's size (usually the larger, the more venomous) and whether the snake is hungry or alert. The angle of the bite and its depth and length also affect the seriousness of the bite. In addition, the size of the victim can be important (children and infants are at greater risk), and the health of the victim at the time of the bite will also affect the outcome. People with diabetes, hypertension or blood coagulation problems and the elderly are particularly sensitive to snake venom, and menstruating women may bleed excessively following the bite of a pit viper. Several cases of miscarriage have been reported when pregnant women have been bitten.

Finally, the location of the bite itself is crucial to its seriousness; venomous snake bites on the head and trunk are twice as serious as those on the extremities, and bites on the arms are more serious than those on the legs.

Poisonous part   The venom is a mixture of proteins that acts on a victim's blood, and even snakes that appear to have been killed by the side of the road have been reported to bite. The size of the snake can give an idea of its potential dangerousness and can be judged by the distance between the fang marks. Fang marks less than 8 mm apart would be a small snake; between 8 to 12 indicates a medium-size snake and more than 12 mm suggests a large venomous snake. Even snakes that have been "de-fanged" can be dangerous, since all snakes grow new fangs from time to time.

Symptoms   Swelling, internal bleeding and changes in red blood cells; central nervous system symptoms include convulsions and sometimes psychotic behavior, muscle weakness and paralysis. In addition, there are general systemic symptoms of fever, nausea, vomiting, diarrhea, pain and restlessness. Tachycardia and bradycardia can develop, and kidney failure has been reported.

Treatment   Within the first 30 to 45 minutes after the bite, apply a venous tourniquet a few inches above the bite, loosening it every 15 to 30 minutes and reapplying it above the level of progressive swelling. Keep the victim quiet, lying down to decrease metabolic activity (which affects the spread of the venom). The wound area (especially if it is an arm or leg) should be kept lower than the heart. Within 30 minutes, trained individuals can incise the wound area and apply suction. Antivenin is available but should be administered within four hours; antivenin is rarely helpful if given more than 12 hours after the bite. Tetanus prophylaxis is advisable; other treatment might include blood transfusions, intravenous fluids, treatment for convulsions and antihistamines to control itching. In addition, broad-spectrum antibiotics may be administered, since snakebites are notorious for becoming infected. If antivenin has not been administered (or was given hours after the bite), sloughing of the skin around the bite is common.

See also ANTIVENIN; PIT VIPER; SNAKE, POISONOUS.

coprine   A water-soluble substance found in the wild mushroom *Coprinus atramentarius* and a few other less common species of the same genus. Its metabolites inhibit the liver enzyme acetaldehyde dehydrogenase. If even small amounts of ethanol (alcohol) are consumed within several days after eating the mushroom, acetaldehyde accumulates in the blood, causing illness. In the absence of alcohol, however, *C. atramentarius* is a safe, edible mushroom.

See also INKY CAP; MUSHROOM POISONING.

coral plant   (*Jatropha multifida*)   This plant is so poisonous that even a small amount—just one seed—can be toxic for a small child. This large, attractive plant is often kept as a houseplant despite its toxicity. It has large, deeply lobed circular leaves and coral-red flowers that bloom most of the year, and its yellow fruit has one seed in each of its three sides. It is a member of a large genus of shrubs or small trees with a three-sided seed capsule, found throughout the New World.

Poisonous part   Seeds and perhaps other parts of the plant contain the poison jatrophin, which interferes with protein synthesis in the intestinal wall. The coral plant also contains a plant lectin (toxalbumin) and cathartic oils that are toxic. Ingestion of just one seed can be serious. The plant lectin inhibits protein synthesis in cells of the intestinal wall and may cause serious or fatal poisoning.

Symptoms   The onset of symptoms (nausea, vomiting and diarrhea) occurs rapidly, unlike poisoning with other plants with toxic lectins.

Treatment   Give fluids and provide supportive treatment.

See also BARBADOS NUT; BELLYACHE BUSH.

coral poisoning   A cut from a coral reef may seem innocuous and is often ignored by visitors to the temperate waters where coral reefs are found. Because coral abrasions always contain pieces of animal protein and bits of coral material, even the slightest scratch may become infected, turning into a nasty ulcer that recurs for many years.

In addition to the true corals, there is also a "hydroid" coral, or stinging coral (also called fire coral), which is important to the formation of reefs. Its exoskeleton is made up of calcium carbonate, which is covered with tiny pores and is found off the Florida Keys and in the Caribbean.

Symptoms   Immediately after coming in contact with the coral, the victim exhibits welts, itching and burning at the wound site. The wound may weep and form wheals. Stinging coral causes burning pain on contact.

Treatment   Ideally, antiseptics should be applied as soon as a person gets the smallest coral cut. Cleanse with soap and water, dry and clean with alcohol, dry again, and rinse with hydrogen peroxide. In severe cases, the person should be put to bed with the wound elevated and given kaolin poultices, antibiotics and antihistamines.

Untreated, a coral cut—which looks innocuous enough at first—can within days become an ulcer that continuously sloughs off and is surrounded by a painful swelling. This ulcer can be incredibly painful—much more so than it looks—and can be quite disabling. If the wound is on the legs, the victim may be unable to walk for months. Generalized symptoms can include enlargement of local lymph glands, fever and malaise. Relapses are common and occur without warning.

Fire coral scrapes often result in bleeding that helps remove the toxin but may be severe enough to require direct pressure on the wound to control blood loss.

coral snake   There are about 65 species of this strongly patterned snake, a member of the cobra family—and all are dangerous. While true coral snakes are found primarily in the tropics, similar forms can also be found in Asia and Africa. In addition, there are two varieties of coral snakes found in the United States, the only species of Elapidae that are native here. They are the eastern coral snake *(Micrurus fulvius)* and the Arizona coral *(Micruroides euryxanthus euryxanthus)*.   Although coral snakes rarely bite when handled, the venom of some of them is capable of killing a person. The largest genus *(Micrurus)* ranges from the southern United States to Argentina. Other coral snakes include the African coral *(Aspidelaps lubricus);* the black-banded coral *(Micrurus nigrocinctus)* found in Central America; and the often-fatal Brazilian giant coral *(M. frontalis)*, found in southern South America.

Poisonous part   Strikingly colored, coral snakes have alternating red and black bands separated by narrow yellow or white rings. Their grooved fangs are fixed to the front part of the upper jaw and cannot be folded back, unlike the vipers and pit vipers. This is one of the snakes for which an old rhyme can sometimes be useful to differentiate poisonous from nonlethal varieties. Old folk rhymes hold that it is possible to tell the difference between harmless and deadly coral snakes by the stripes—deadly varieties have red stripes next to yellow ones. There are several versions of these rhymes: "Red on yellow, kill a fellow; red on black, okay Jack" or "Red touching yellow, dangerous fellow."

Symptoms   Numbness at bite, headache, facial swelling, sore throat, skin hypersensitivity, sore throat, drooping eyelids, photophobia, vomiting, rapid heartbeat, backache, irritability and death. Some species of coral snakes have a venom that breaks down the red blood cells and frees the hemoglobin, which then appears in urine.

Treatment   Antiserum is available for some species, but not for all. There is antivenin for the eastern coral snake; there is no antivenin for the Arizona coral snake.

See also ANTIVENIN; ANTIVENIN, CORAL SNAKE; SNAKES, POISONOUS.

coral snake, Arizona *(Micruroides euryxanthus euryxanthus)*   Also known as the Sonoran coral, this is one of two coral snake species found in the United States. A rare variety of coral snake, it has a potent bite but rarely strikes humans. Found in the southwestern United States deserts, it is quite small and rarely seen, coming out from its underground retreat only at night—usually after a warm rain. When disturbed, it buries its head in its coils and raises and exposes the bottom of its tail.

Several harmless snakes look very similar in color to the coral snakes, and it is important to be able to tell the difference. The Arizona coral has wide red and black bands separated by yellow rings, all almost the same width.

Poisonous part   The venom of the coral snakes contains a deadly neurotoxin that can be fatal and is believed to block the uptake of acetylcholine at the receptor sites. Their small, nonmovable fangs are not as efficient as those of vipers, and so this snake must hold on to its victim for a longer period of time in order to inject its venom.

Symptoms Symptoms appear within one to five hours, although occasionally it takes even longer. Early signs are systemic and include slurring of speech, dilation of the pupils, strabismus (eye movement), drooping of the upper eyelid and muscle weakness. The respiratory muscles are affected last, and respiratory muscle paralysis is the most common cause of death in coral snakebites.

Treatment Antivenin is available; should it be inaccessible, it may be possible to maintain life by intensive life support measures through the period of acute respiratory muscle paralysis. The poison is metabolized after about four days, symptoms fade and recovery is usually complete in those who survive.

coral snake, eastern *(Micrurus fulvius)* Also called a harlequin snake, this fairly small nonhooded member of the cobra family is found in North Carolina and Missouri to northeastern Mexico in moist, dense vegetation near ponds or streams and in hardwood forests, pine flats, rocky hillsides and canyons. While common, this nocturnal snake is rarely seen and prefers burrowing at night.

About 30 inches long, the eastern coral snake has wide bands of red and black separated by narrow yellow rings, and the head is completely black from the end of its blunt nose to just behind the eyes. The red rings are sometimes spotted with black. The eastern coral can be confused with the harmless scarlet snake and the scarlet king snake.

One of the few snakes that make a warning noise as they strike, the eastern coral has been heard to produce a succession of popping noises by drawing air at its vent and then expelling it.

Symptoms The bite of the eastern coral snake is unlikely to be fatal unless there is a prodigious amount of venom or the bite is in a particularly vulnerable place. Symptoms appear within one to five hours, although occasionally it takes longer. Early signs are systemic and include slurring of speech, dilation of the pupils, strabismus (abnormal deviation of one eye in relation to the other), drooping of the upper eyelid and muscle weakness. The respiratory muscles are affected last.

Treatment Antivenin is available.

See also ANTIVENIN; ANTIVENIN, CORAL SNAKE; SNAKES, POISONOUS.

corn cockle *(Agrostemma githago)* Native to Europe but introduced in America, the annual is tall and gray, with purple pin petals and pink flowers, and is occasionally grown as an ornamental. The milled seeds of this noxious weed may be found in flour.

Poisonous part The entire plant is poisonous (active ingredient is githagin and saponin glycosides), but the seeds are particularly deadly—especially if ground up with flour or cereal.

Symptoms Frequent ingestion of small amounts causes a chronic disease resulting in pain, prickling and burning of the lower extremities and increasing paralysis. Symptoms may appear within 30 minutes to an hour after ingestion and include dizziness, diarrhea, respiratory distress, vomiting, headache, sharp pain in the spine, coma and death.

Treatment Gastric lavage and treatment of symptoms.

corticosteroids Used principally as an anti-inflammatory agent, these drugs are used to treat arthritis, bursitis, certain skin diseases, adrenal gland insufficiency, thyroiditis, some cancers and other disorders.

See also ANTI-INFLAMMATORY DRUGS.

cortinarius mushrooms The members of the *Cortinarius* genus of mushrooms, once thought to be harmless, are deadly poison—almost as poisonous as the *Amanita* mushrooms. A little more than a cup of the cooked mushrooms can be fatal. Found in central Europe, the mushrooms have caps ranging from blue violet (which can be eaten) to those of brown or red (deadly); they get their name from the veil that sometimes covers the gills of young mushrooms.

Poisonous part The mushroom contains the poison orellanin, which damages the liver and kidneys.

Symptoms Symptoms do not appear until three days to two weeks after ingestion; by then, the victim develops excessive thirst and may drink several liters of fluid a day. By this time, the liver and kidneys usually have been irreversibly damaged. Other symptoms may include nausea, headache, muscular pains and chills.

Treatment Gastric lavage, if performed immediately after ingestion. In general, the only treatment once symptoms appear are kidney and liver transplants.

See also MUSHROOM POISONING; MUSHROOM TOXINS.

cottonmouth snake See WATER MOCCASIN.

crack cocaine See COCAINE.

creosote An oily wood preservative with a sharp, smoky smell, it is used to prevent or slow down decay and increase the life expectancy of wood, primarily on railroad ties and utility poles. It is also used extensively on construction lumber, fence posts, plywood and foundation materials. When used as a wood preservative, creosote is a mixture of chemicals produced by distilling wood or coal tar and may also include phenol, cresols (methyl phenol) and other benzene-based chemicals. It is also used as a waterproofing material, an animal dip, a constituent of fuel oil, a lubricant, and as an antiseptic and disinfectant.

No federal criteria have been set for creosote levels in water, and there are no air standards. In 1978, the Environmental Protection Agency (EPA) initiated a special review of creosote based on its cancer-causing reputation; as a result, it did not ban the substance but proposed a set of regulations intended to reduce exposure. Creosote is listed as a hazardous air pollutant in the 1990 Clean Air Act, requiring the EPA to set emission standards and is on the EPA community right- to-know list. Creosote is also a restricted-use pesticide, meaning that it may be applied only by certified applicators.

The Consumer Awareness Program recommends against using creosote-treated wood products in proximity to food, animal food and public drinking water. People are advised not to burn creosote-treated wood, and applicators must wear protective clothing, special face masks or goggles, respirators and gloves. If creosote is used on wood that will touch bare skin (such as in playground furniture or outdoor furniture), two coats of urethane or shellac sealer must be applied. A sealer should also be applied to treated wood used in areas where inhalation exposure may occur, such as in barns and stables.

Symptoms Ranked by the EPA as a possible human carcinogen, creosote causes both cancer and mutations in lab experiments. Both direct contact to the liquid and exposure to the vapors can cause burning, itching, discoloration and skin ulceration—followed ultimately by gangrene. It also causes eye injuries and can increase the skin's sensitivity to the sun. It may also cause skin cancer.

Acute poisoning causes systemic effects (throughout the body) including headache, vomiting, vertigo, low body temperature, convulsions, breathing problems and death.

Treatment If the victim is alert, give a slurry of activated charcoal and perform careful gastric lavage if there are no deep burns in the mouth or pharynx. AVOID ADMINISTRATION OF ALCOHOL. Remove contaminated clothing, and blot up liquid on skin (caregiver should wear gloves). Wash exposed areas of the skin, and give morphine for pain. Sodium bicarbonate may ease symptoms; give oxygen as needed and monitor electrocardiogram.

See also PHENOL.

crocus   See MEADOW SAFFRON.

croton *(Croton tiglium)* Also known as mayapple, this supertoxic plant is native to Southeast Asia and now also grows in the southwestern United States. Croton oil in alcohol is also known as a "Mickey Finn."

Poisonous part   Seeds and extracted oil from the plant are deadly.

Symptoms   Skin contact results in an immediate blistering and irritation, which can last up to three weeks. If the seeds or oil are ingested, symptoms appear within 10 to 15 minutes and include burning pain in the mouth and stomach, bloody diarrhea, kidney and liver damage, nausea, vomiting, fast heartbeat, coma and death.

Treatment   Vomiting and gastric lavage are ineffective. Give fluids orally along with intravenous infusion to correct electrolyte imbalance; treat symptoms.

cube jellies   See JELLYFISH.

curare   *(Strychnos)*   A centuries-old extract from the bark and juices of trees in Central America (*Strychnos toxifera*), it has been used as a poison for arrows and for blowgun darts in Central and South America. Curare is a skeletal-muscle relaxant drug, one of the alkaloid family of organic compounds.

It is used in medicine today as an auxiliary to general anesthesia (frequently with cyclopropane), especially in abdominal surgery. Curare acts as a neuromuscular blocking agent that produces flaccidity in striated muscle. Used by South American Indians against enemies and animals, curare is now widely available in the United States as a drug, where it is used to stop normal breathing and allow the patient to be placed on a respirator in order to treat the lungs.

Poisonous part   All parts of the *Strychnos toxifera* plant contain tubocurarine, a drug that interferes with muscle contractions by interfering with the action of the neurotransmitter acetylcholine. Curare is harmless if swallowed. Its poison is activated only if injected or administered intravenously.

Symptoms   Almost immediately, curare affects the muscles of the toes, ears and eyes, then those of the neck and limbs followed by muscles important for breathing. Death comes as a result of respiratory paralysis.

Treatment   There is no treatment or antidote, since curare works so quickly.

cyanide   [Other names: hydrogen cyanide (prussic acid), potassium cyanide, sodium cyanide.] The various forms of cyanide (gas, salts) can be swallowed, inhaled or absorbed through the skin, and it is one of the most rapidly acting poisons known. The inhalation of cyanide in its extremely volatile form called hydrocyanic acid (or prussic acid) can be fatal in just a few minutes. Hydrocyanic acid occurs naturally in a large variety of seeds and pits (such as peach, apricot, apple, plum, etc.) and has many industrial uses.

In addition, many other plants have cyanogenic glycosides that have a similar effect, although they take longer to act. These amygdalin-containing fruit seeds include choke cherries, cassava beans and bitter almonds.

Hydrogen cyanide is found in fumigants, insecticides, rat poisons, metal polish and electroplating solution and has also been used in gas chambers. Potassium cyanide and sodium cyanide are both white solids smelling faintly of bitter almonds. Certain of the cyanides irritate the eyes so powerfully that they have been used in some types of tear gas. In the household, cyanide can be found in many products from silver polish to rat poison.

Symptoms Cyanide prevents the body's red blood cells from absorbing oxygen by interfering with the body's enzymes. When the cells can't get oxygen, they produce a rapid progression of symptoms; a person who swallows or smells too much cyanide can lose consciousness, fall into convulsions and die within 15 minutes. Mortality from cyanide may be as high as 95 percent.

Treatment Call poison control before attempting any treatment, which must be rapid and efficient. The longer the patient can be kept alive, the better the prognosis, since the body can neutralize cyanide by combining it with sulfur compounds to form inactive sulfocyanates. An antidote kit (manufactured by Eli Lily Co.) is available; two antidotes currently in use in Europe have not yet been approved in the United States.

See also CYANOGENIC GLYCOSIDES; CHERRIES, WILD AND CULTIVATED; PRUNUS.

cyanogenic glycosides   A toxic glycoside (a compound found in plants that contains sugar) that gives off hydrocyanic acid and other cyanide compounds when exposed to acids and enzymes in the digestive tract. When this hydrogen cyanide is produced by cyanogenic glycosides, it interferes with the level of oxygen in the blood and causes the blue skin coloring common in cyanide poisoning. Cyanogenic glycosides are found in apricot, cherry and peach pits and apple seeds, but they are released only if the pits or seeds are ground and eaten; if swallowed whole, they cause no harm because of the hard outer shell covering.

See also, CHERRIES, WILD AND CULTIVATED; CYANIDE; PRUNUS.

cyclopropane   A flammable general anesthetic not widely used today because of its high cost and explosive nature. Cyclopropane works by depressing all functions of the central nervous system.

Symptoms When given in large amounts, this anesthetic will stop breathing with possible damage to heart, liver and kidneys. Symptoms include stupor, unconsciousness and respiratory paralysis. Convulsions may follow.

Treatment Symptoms will disappear once the anesthetic is removed. Keep warm, provide CPR if required. Stabilize blood pressure.

See also ANESTHETIC, GASEOUS/VOLATILE.

D

Dalmane (flurazepam) An anticonvulsant and a muscle relaxant used to relieve anxiety, Dalmane is not as strong as Valium (diazepam) but is still considered toxic. This is a drug often chosen for suicide, in combination with alcohol. It reacts negatively with other anticonvulsants, antidepressants, antihistamines, antihypertensives, oral contraceptives, disulfiram, erythromycins, monoamine oxidase (MAO) inhibitors, narcotics, sedatives, sleeping pills and tranquilizers.

Symptoms Within 10 to 20 minutes of ingestion, patients become groggy and fall into sleep, dropping further into unconsciousness if a large dose has been taken. Withdrawal psychosis is also possible.

Treatment Gastric lavage; increase oxygen while maintaining blood pressure.

See also DIAZEPAM.

dantrolene This drug is used in the treatment of the very high fevers common in anesthesia overdose. It is not, however, a substitute for other means of controlling temperature such as sponging and fanning. Dantrolene is a muscle relaxant that may cause diarrhea, muscle weakness and, sometimes, kidney damage.

daphne *(Daphne)* [Other names: bois joli, copse laurel, dwarf bay, February daphne, flax olive, lady laurel, spurge flax, spurge laurel, spurge olive, wild pepper, winter daphne, wood laurel.] One of the oldest plants recognized as a poison, daphne is found throughout the British Isles, the northeastern United States and eastern Canada. It is widely planted as an ornamental and is sometimes kept indoors as a flowering houseplant. This unusually fragrant rounded shrub has clusters of purple or white flowers that grow in the spring before the leathery leaves appear. Fruits are scarlet or yellow with a pit. Of all the daphne species, the *Daphne mezereum* variety is the most deadly, although all species are considered poisonous.

Poisonous part All parts of this plant are poisonous, especially the berries, bark and seeds; berries of *D. mezereum* are bright red; those of *D. laureola* are green, then blue and finally black when fully ripe. Poisonous substances are the glycoside daphnetoxin and mezerein, an irritating, blistering resin. This plant is considered particularly dangerous to children.

Symptoms Symptoms appear in 45 minutes to several hours and include swelling and blistering of the lips, salivation and problems in swallowing, burning and ulceration in the digestive tract, stomach pain, vomiting, bloody diarrhea, weakness, convulsions, shock, coma and death. Just a few berries can be fatal to a child. This plant may also cause systemic damage to the kidneys.

Treatment Gastric lavage—only with caution, since the mucous membranes may have been damaged as a result of this poison. Victims often go into shock after poisoning with daphne.

datura   See JIMSONWEED.

DDT (dichlorodiphenyltrichloroethane) One of a group of chlorinated hydrocarbons, this insect-fighting chemical was once widely used in agriculture and malarial control programs around the world. It was developed in Switzerland in the early 1940s and was found to be much more effective than previous insecticides and became an important weapon in fighting insect-transmitted diseases. Unfortunately, some insects have adapted to the poison and are resistant to its effects. However, because of its toxicity, it has been banned from commercial use because it does not disperse in the environment but accumulates in biological systems.

This broad-spectrum insecticide dissolves easily in oil and therefore builds up in fatty tissue; eating animals that have consumed DDT—or even that have eaten others that have consumed DDT—will poison anyone who eats the meat.

While it can be inhaled or absorbed through the skin, the most common means of human exposure is by eating DDT-contaminated food. In fact, inhaling the dust or coming in contact with the solution is rarely harmful to humans unless the person is wearing some sort of oily insect repellent that would aid absorption. However, toxic doses are possible if the skin contact area is large or the exposure lengthy.

Symptoms DDT affects the central nervous system, causing muscle weakness, excitability and convulsions, with tremor, confusion, headache, numbness of the tongue, lips and face and vomiting. Twitchings begin in the face and proceed in rising strength to involve all muscles. In fact, attacks resemble the convulsions of strychnine poisoning, since they can be set off by light or noise. Respiratory arrest and heart attack are followed by death.

Chronic poisoning causes weight loss, headache, loss of appetite, nausea, eye irritation, weakness and increasing tremors followed by convulsions, coma and death.

Contact with the eyes may cause a temporary blindness. People who work with DDT may also experience a gradual sensitization and allergic reactions to the chemical.

Treatment If convulsions continue for some time, recovery is not likely. Treat symptoms, and perform gastric lavage, but do not induce vomiting. Administer activated charcoal and a cathartic. Stimulants (such as epinephrine) may induce heart attack; administer anticonvulsants (such as Valium) to control convulsions.

See also CHLORINATED HYDROCARBON PESTICIDES.

deadly cort See GALERINA MUSHROOMS.

death camas *(Zigadenus venenosus)* [Other names: alkali grass, black snake root, hog's potato, myster grass, poison sego, sand corn, soap plant, squirrel food, water lily, wild onion.] One of the lily family and often mistaken for an onion, the death camas is found throughout North America (especially the extreme southeast) and Alaska and Canada.

Leaves are grassy and long and narrow—up to two feet tall—and at the top, the stem has a branched cluster of greeny white to yellow flowers. The plant's bulb looks like an onion, but does not have an oniony odor.

Poisonous part Fresh leaves, stems, bulbs and flowers are poisonous, but the seeds are particularly deadly. Poisons include zygacine, veratrine and zygadenine, protoveratridine, iso- and neogermidine. While cattle are usually poisoned by death camas, it is possible for humans to be poisoned as well.

Symptoms Symptoms appear within one hour and include burning of the mouth, vomiting, thirst, weakness, slow heartbeat, staggering, paralysis, convulsions, coma and death.

Treatment There is no antidote, but gastric lavage should be performed if the victim has not vomited. Fluids and the administration of atropine or ephedrine may also be required.

death cap/death cup *(Amanita phalloides)* One of the deadliest members of the *Amanita* genus of mushrooms, the death cap or death cup is found in woods or their borders and is responsible for most of the fatalities associated with mushroom poisoning. It has a green or brown cap and appears in summer or early fall. Some experts also include the destroying angel as part of the *Amanita phalloides* group.

Poisonous part This deadly mushroom contains peptide toxins, phalloidin and two amanitins that damage cells throughout the body within six to 12 hours after ingestion. The toxins are not affected by drying, cooking or boiling in water.

Symptoms First symptoms are caused by the action of the amatoxins on the intestine, but this is not responsible for the ultimate outcome. After about 12 hours following ingestion, symptoms include violent abdominal pain, vomiting, bloody diarrhea, loss of fluid and intense thirst. A latency period follows, up to five days, but by then the toxins have damaged the liver, kidneys and central nervous system. There is a decrease in urinary output and a drop in sugar levels in the blood, which leads to coma and—more than 50 percent of the time—death.

Treatment During the first phase, give fluids and monitor electrolytes; urine flow should be maintained, and repeat doses of activated charcoal may be given. If management is successful, the victim will recover within one week. Various strategies have been tried to treat this type of mushroom poisoning in Europe, including massive doses of vitamins, corticosteroids, sex hormones, high-dose glucose, penicillin G and thioctic acid. None of these has been proven effective.

See also AMANITA MUSHROOMS; MUSHROOM POISONING.

decongestants   A range of drugs used to relieve nasal congestion, they work by constricting blood vessels in the nose, which reduces swelling. They are used to treat sinusitis, allergies and acute upper respiratory infections.

Decongestants include phenylpropanolamine (PPA), phenylephrine (PHE), ephedrine (EPH) and pseudoephedrine (PEP), all available over the counter as nasal decongestants and cold preparations that usually contain antihistamines and cough suppressants as well. In addition, PPA is often used as an appetite suppressant. Combinations of these drugs with caffeine are sold on the street as amphetamine or cocaine substitutes.

Many of these drugs react negatively with other drugs. Patients sensitive to epinephrine, ephedrine, terbutaline or amphetamines may also be sensitive to drugs such as PPA.

Symptoms   Poisoning with products containing PPA, PHE and EPH may provoke symptoms after ingesting just two or three times the recommended dose. PEP is slightly less toxic (symptoms occur with four to five times recommended dose).

Patients taking monoamine oxidase (MAO) inhibitors may be extremely sensitive to these drugs, developing severe high blood pressure after ingesting even less-than-recommended doses.

The most serious symptom of these drugs is severe high blood pressure, together with hypertensive complications of headache, confusion, seizures and stroke. In fact, intracranial hemorrhage may occur in even normal, healthy young people after only a slight rise in blood pressure. The high blood pressure caused by PPA and PHE occurs together with slow heartbeat, while EPH and PEP usually cause high blood pressure with rapid heartbeat.

Using antihistamines or caffeine may increase the high blood pressure with PPA and PHE. PPA may also cause heart attack.

Treatment   There is no specific antidote. Give symptomatic treatment; monitor vital signs and electrocardiogram. Do not use beta blockers to treat high blood pressure without first giving a vasodilator (phentolamine or nitroprusside), for they will worsen the high blood pressure. Do not induce vomiting because of the danger of worsening the high blood pressure. Perform gastric lavage if the victim has ingested the drug within 30 to 60 minutes or has taken a large dose. Administer activated charcoal and a cathartic.

deferoxamine   This specific chelating agent is used in the treatment of iron overdose, particularly in the presence of shock, acidosis, severe gastroenteritis, leukocytosis and high blood sugar. It binds to the circulating free iron, and both are excreted in the urine, turning it an orange-pink color. Deferoxamine is also sometimes used to determine the presence of free iron in the body by administering the chelating agent and then looking for the characteristic pinkish rose color of the urine.

See also IRON SUPPLEMENTS.

Demerol   See NARCOTICS.

Depakene   (valproic acid) This anticonvulsant drug has been used since 1967 as a central nervous system depressant; it has a sweet odor and clear color.

Symptoms   Within a half hour after ingestion, Depakene causes stomach irritation, hair loss, psychosis and liver failure leading to death.

Treatment   Perform gastric lavage and treat symptoms.

derrin   See ROTENONE.

derris   The powdered root of various species of the botanical genus *Derris*, used as an insecticide. It is also used to kill fish without damaging the food supply, enabling game fish to be introduced into the same body of water. The toxic principles of derris include rotenone.

Symptoms   When absorbed through the skin, derris root may cause dermatitis. It is also more toxic than its rotenone and rotenoid content would suggest; it is believed this discrepancy may be due to the presence of other toxic agents in the derris powder. Absorption and toxicity are enhanced by olive oil.

Treatment   Symptomatic and supportive, including removal of the material from the skin and gastrointestinal tract. Oily cathartics should not be used, since absorption may be increased by their use.

See also ROTENONE.

destroying angel   (*Amanita bispongera* [smaller death angel], *A. ocreata*, *A. verna* [fool's angel] and *A. virosa* [destroying angel or death angel.]) A mushroom of the poisonous *Amanita* genus, the destroying angel (and its close relatives, named above) are extremely deadly, with a 90 percent fatality rate and no known antidote.

The fool's angel is the most common; it is relatively smaller than the others and chalky white. The destroying angels have a large white body and are found in forests during wet periods in summer and autumn. Experts disagree as to the classification of these related mushrooms, which is why they are listed together here. These amanitas are found in the mid-Atlantic states to Florida and west to Texas and are found in dry pine woods, although the smaller death angel can also be found in wooded lawns, especially near oak trees.

Poisonous part The main poisons found in these mushrooms are the slow-acting amanitin and the fast-acting phalloidin. Amanitin causes most of the symptoms, and phalloidin causes degeneration in kidney, liver and heart muscles. These mushrooms are deadly; one or two cooked mushrooms can be fatal, and there exists a report that one-third of one raw cap has killed a child.

Symptoms After these mushrooms are eaten, there are typically no symptoms for six to 15 hours—and sometimes as long as two days. Symptoms begin suddenly with severe abdominal pain, nausea, vomiting and diarrhea, followed by extreme abdominal pain, excessive thirst, violent vomiting, urinary problems, weakness, jaundice, convulsions, coma and death. Severe dehydration eventually results in cardiac arrest. Death occurs within two days of ingestion of a large amount of mushrooms, but more generally it may take up to three days of remissions followed by repeated, more acute attacks. Death occurs in between 50 and 90 percent of cases. Recovery can take up to one month.

Treatment There is no known antidote, although some victims survive if given a liver transplant. Gastric lavage is also instituted. Animal studies suggest that early treatment with penicillin silibinin or cimetidine may partially protect against liver injury. Treat fluid and electrolyte loss to head off massive circulatory collapse.

See also AMANITA MUSHROOMS; MUSHROOM POISONING.

dextromethorphan Found in many over-the-counter cough and cold medicines, dextromethorphan is frequently involved in poisonings with children, although fatalities are rare. Dextromethorphan is also frequently combined with antihistamines, decongestants or acetaminophen. It is a popular choice for cough suppressants because it works as well as codeine but is not addictive.

Symptoms Toxicity depends on other ingredients in the particular product that was ingested. Mild overdoses cause ataxia, clumsiness, restlessness and sometimes visual and auditory hallucinations. More serious overdoses produce stupor, coma and breathing problems, especially if alcohol has been ingested at the same time. In addition, persons taking monoamine oxidase inhibitors who ingest a normal dose of dextromethorphan may experience high blood pressure and severe hyperthermia (high fever).

Treatment Mild overdoses require only supervision; in more severe cases, the drug naloxone has reported to be an effective antidote in some cases, but not in others. Induce vomiting or perform gastric lavage; administer activated charcoal and a cathartic.

DFP See NARCOTICS.

diazepam (Valium) One of the group of benzodiazepines used in the treatment of anxiety or agitation caused by hallucinogenic drug overdose; to control seizures because of convulsant drug overdose; and to relax excessive muscle rigidity and contractions following strychnine poisoning or the bite of the black widow spider.

See also BENZODIAZEPINES; BLACK WIDOW SPIDER; STRYCHNINE.

dieffenbachia *(Dieffenbachia)* [Other names: dumb cane, dumb plant, mother-in-law's tongue, tuft root.] This extremely common plant has been used indoors as an attractive foliage houseplant for hundreds of years, but it can cause mouth pain if ingested and can be fatal in large amounts.

There are a number of dieffenbachia species, including *D. amoena, D. bausei, D. candida, D. exotica, D. maculata* and *D. seguine.* Dieffenbachia belongs to the family Araceae, which also includes other ornamental plants such as the jack-in-the-pulpit, philodendron, pothos and calla lilly.

These shade-loving plants have bright green oblong leaves and can grow quite tall, with fleshy stems as much as an inch thick. They may be found in outdoor gardens in southern Florida and Hawaii.

Dieffenbachia's toxic qualities have been known for a long time; in the past, slaves were punished by rubbing their mouths with dieffenbachia, and there are reports that the Nazis experimented with this plant in concentration camps during World War II.

Poisonous part All parts of this plant (including the sap) contain potent irritants including proteolytic enzymes, raphides of calcium oxalate and other, unknown toxins. The calcium oxalate raphides in this plant are really sharp crystals that puncture tissue; it is possible that the plant contains enzymes that attack cells through the punctures. The mechanisms behind its ability to cause systemic poisoning as well as localized irritation are not known.

Symptoms All varieties of dieffenbachia contain a range of potent irritants that can cause serious tissue damage to eyes, skin and mucous membranes. Chewing a leaf from this plant causes almost immediate, intense pain, blistering and burning of the mouth and tongue, excess salivation, swelling of the tongue and throat and difficulty in swallowing. Pain and swelling may persist for several days and leave damaged tissue behind. Because of the immediate pain upon ingestion, poisoning with large amounts of the plant is unlikely; however, in this event the toxins can swell the throat tissue, blocking the airway and leading to death. Some sources report that dumb cane can also cause systemic poisoning resulting in nausea, vomiting and diarrhea and damaging internal organs. The name "dumb cane" comes from its tendency to paralyze vocal cords.

Treatment Pain and swelling in the mouth will slowly fade even without treatment, although cool liquids (such as milk or Popsicles) and painkillers may help. Perform gastric lavage, and give antihistamines for local swelling.

See also PHILODENDRON.

dieldrin [Trade names: Compound 497, HEOD, Octalox.] A highly toxic chlorinated hydrocarbon pesticide used against potato beetles, corn pests and rape plant parasites. Its manufacture in the United States was banned in 1974 under the Environmental Protection Agency (EPA) Fungicide and Rodenticide Act, although it is still produced for use in Holland.

Dieldrin is highly soluble in fat, where it accumulates in humans or animals until a toxic level is reached. It can be inhaled, absorbed or ingested and is particularly dangerous when heated, as it can give off very toxic chloride fumes.

Symptoms Within 20 minutes to 12 hours dieldrin produces headache, dizziness, nausea, vomiting, sweating, excitability, irritability, convulsions, coma and death.

Treatment There is no specific antidote. Perform gastric lavage but do not induce vomiting because of the risk of sudden onset of seizures; administer activated charcoal and a cathartic. Irregular heartbeat may respond to propranolol.

See also CHLORINATED HYDROCARBON PESTICIDES.

digitalis A group of drugs used as a heart medicine that are purified from the seeds and leaves of the common foxglove plant *(Digitalis purpurea)*. Digitalis strengthens and slows contractions of the heart and restores circulation in persons with congestive heart failure. It also slows the rate of ventricular contraction in those with atrial fibrillation. In small doses, digitalis can strengthen a weak heart and slow down a rapid heartbeat; in large doses, however, it can be fatal by dangerously slowing down heart function. The most commonly used drugs in this group are digoxin and digitoxin.

The active principles in digitalis include a group of steroids called cardiac glycosides. Dosage must be measured with extreme care, since the lethal dose is only three times the effective dose.

Symptoms Overdose is evident with both gastrointestinal and neurologic problems, including anorexia, nausea, vomiting, diarrhea, depression, visual disturbances, fatigue, headache, delirium, confusion and hallucinations. A wide variety of cardiac problems are common and represent the most serious form of toxicity.

Treatment Management of mild overdose may require only stopping the drug. Acute poisoning requires gastric lavage or induced vomiting, followed by the administration of activated charcoal and a cathartic as soon as possible after ingestion.

See also CARDIAC GLYCOSIDES; DIGITOXIN; DIGOXIN; FOXGLOVE.

digitoxin   This cardiac glycoside is used to regulate the heart's rhythm after a congestive heart failure, increasing contractions and reducing fluid retention. While some physicians have prescribed digitoxin to treat obesity, its adverse affects can be fatal.

Symptoms   Almost immediately, overdose causes nausea, vomiting, diarrhea, blurred vision and heart problems such as premature contractions and atrial fibrillation.

Treatment   Wash the stomach with tannic acid (strong tea) and keep the victim lying down. Give stimulants such as caffeine, ammonia or atropine; if the pulse drops below 50 beats per minute, atropine is administered.

See also DIGITALIS; DIGOXIN; FOXGLOVE.

digoxin   (Lanoxin) This cardiac glycoside is used to regulate the heart's rhythm after a congestive heart failure, increasing contractions and reducing fluid retention.

Symptoms   Within six hours, overdose causes nausea, vomiting, diarrhea, blurred vision and heart problems such as premature contractions and atrial fibrillation.

Treatment   Discontinue administration; acute ingestion requires induced vomiting, gastric lavage and the administration of activated charcoal and a cathartic as soon as possible after ingestion.

See also CARDIAC GLYCOSIDES; DIGITALIS; DIGITOXIN.

digoxin-specific antibodies   The antidote for poisoning by digoxin and, to some degree, digitoxin and other cardiac glycosides. Digoxin-specific antibodies are produced in immunized sheep and can reverse the signs of digitalis poisoning within 30–60 minutes of administration with complete reversal within three hours.

See also CARDIAC GLYCOSIDES; DIGITOXIN; DIGOXIN.

Dilantin   See PHENYTOIN.

Dilaudid   See HYDROMORPHONE.

dimercaprol   This chelating agent is used to treat poisoning of arsenic, mercury, lead, antimony, bismuth, chromium, copper, nickel, tungsten, zinc or gold. It is not effective in the treatment of iron, selenium or cadmium poisoning.

dimethyl sulfate (sulfuric acid dimethyl ester, methyl sulfate) This color-less, odorless oily liquid is used to manufacture dyes, drugs, pesticides and perfumes; most poisonings occur when liquid or vapors leak from industrial machines. Its very mild oniony odor is barely perceptible and not useful as a warning. Dimethyl sulfate does not dissolve readily in water but does dissolve well in organic solvents.

Symptoms When absorbed through the skin or eyes, it is extremely irritating, although there is a latency period of up to five hours. Exposure to the vapors produces an immediate reaction of runny eyes and nose and swelling of the mouth, lips and throat, with hoarseness and sore throat. There may also be conjunctivitis (pink eye), perforation of the nasal septum similar to the side effects of cocaine and permanent vision problems. Liver and kidneys may also be damaged.

Upon ingestion, dimethyl sulfate hydrolyzes to sulfuric acid and methanol. Ingestion causes breathing problems and bronchitis within 12 hours, together with central nervous system side effects including drowsiness, temporary blindness, heart irregularities and irritation, followed by convulsions and death from pulmonary edema. Dimethyl sulfate is a carcinogen in animals.

Treatment Symptomatic treatment, including hydrocortisone to reduce injury.

dimethyl sulfoxide (DMSO) This clear liquid industrial cleaner, with its distinctive garlicky, oysterlike odor, is a powerful solvent and a by-product of the paper pulp industry. It is also used under medical supervision to treat skin inflammation or to improve absorption of drugs applied to the skin. It has also received sensational publicity regarding its miraculous pain-reliev-ing and anti-inflammatory characteristics when rubbed on the skin. Accord-ing to research, DMSO *is* mildly antifungal and antibacterial and is a promising treatment for ringworm. But (in 90 percent solution) it neither hindered nor helped experimental thermal burns, contact dermatitis and ultraviolet burns. It was not systematically harmful when applied to healthy subjects once a day for six months, but twice-daily treatments caused a mild scaling skin irritation in some subjects. The only DMSO product approved by the Food and Drug Administration is a 50 percent solution for the treatment of interstitial cystitis.

DMSO products currently available (for veterinary and industrial use) cannot be considered safe for human use, and the effects for human use have not been established, according to Jay Arena, M.D., *Poisoning: Toxicology, Symptoms, Treatment* (Springfield, Ill.: Charles C. Thomas, 1986).

dinoflagellate *(Gonyaulax catenella, G. tamarensis,* and others) The organ-isms responsible for "red tide," dinoflagellates are extremely toxic one-celled aquatic animals found on the Pacific coast of North America *(G. catenella)* and the east coast of North America *(G. tamarensis).* Dinoflagellates, some of which *(Noctiluca)* also produce part of the luminescence in the sea, have the characteristics of both plants and animals; most are microscopic and marine. A person becomes poisoned with dinoflagellates when eating contaminated shellfish; primarily, dinoflagellates cause paralytic shellfish poisoning, although at least one variety causes a type of poisoning more similar to ciguatera.

Under good conditions (warm climate, warm water), dinoflagellates may reach 60 million organisms per liter of water; these rapid growths (referred to as a "bloom") cause red tides that discolor the sea and poison fish and marine life. Usually, a person becomes poisoned with dinoflagellates when eating shellfish that have been feeding on the toxic protozoa. Bivalve shellfish (mussels, clams and oysters) are the primary shellfish at risk, and mussels are the most susceptible of all. Healthy bivalve shellfish filter large amounts of dinoflagellates, which form the primary ocean food from May through August. During these warm times, the dinoflagellates thrive by photosynthesis and can be so invasive that they kill birds and fish.

The first large epidemic of poisoning caused by dinoflagellate-contaminated shellfish occurred in San Francisco in 1927, when 102 people were sickened and six died. Today, largely because of the prohibition against eating certain shellfish during the summer months, such epidemics are rare.

Still, red tides and the resultant paralytic shellfish poisoning (PSP) and ciguatera are a problem in the warm months (May to November) on the Pacific coast between central California and the Aleutian Islands and on the Atlantic coast (St. Lawrence River estuary in Canada, the Bay of Fundy, and several northeastern states in the United States). Other countries have also experienced outbreaks of PSP, including England, Wales, France, Scotland, Germany, Norway, Ireland, Belgium, Denmark, Portugal, South Africa, Japan, New Guinea and New Zealand.

Not all dinoflagellate species are toxic to humans or marine creatures, and many varieties of phytoplankton bloom to large proportions without causing harm. Harmful dinoflagellates found in North America include *G. catenella*, *G. acatenella*, and *G. tamarensis*, all of which cause PSP; *G. breve*, found on the Florida Gulf coast, which causes a ciguatera-like poisoning; and *G. polyedra*, found on the southern California coast, causing a paralytic poison different from PSP. In Japan, the dinoflagellate *Exuviaella mariaelebouriae* causes "oyster poisoning," damaging the liver and kidneys. Several other dinoflagellates are injurious to fish and other marine creatures but do no harm to humans.

Symptoms Similar to curare poisoning and extremely fast acting (within 10 minutes), dinoflagellate poisoning causes a tingling and burning sensation and numbness of the lips, tongue and face, spreading elsewhere to the body; it can also cause weakness, dizziness, joint pain, intense thirst and difficulty in swallowing. As the illness progresses, breathing problems and muscular paralysis become more severe. Death is caused by respiratory paralysis within two to 12 hours, depending on the dose. Fatalities occur in 10 percent of poisoning cases. If the victim survives for 24 hours, prognosis is good and there do not seem to be lasting effects of poisoning.

Treatment   There is no antidote for shellfish poisoning caused by dinoflagellates. Gastric lavage and activated charcoal may be administered, since saxitoxin is readily absorbed by charcoal. It may be necessary to monitor blood pressure and the heart, and to provide respiratory support, since patients are often in critical condition.

See also CIGUATERA; PARALYTIC SHELL FISH POISONING.

dioxins   A group of highly toxic substances used in a variety of industrial and other applications. The herbicide Agent Orange used during combat in Vietnam contained small quantities of one type of dioxin. However, diagnosis of dioxin poisoning is difficult, since it is hard to detect dioxin in blood or tissue and there is no established correlation with symptoms.

According to research released by the Environmental Protection Agency, dioxin is a potent carcinogen with subtle immunological, developmental and neurological effects that may be even more of a public health threat than its carcinogenic problems.

Dioxin has spread well beyond its main industrial sources (paper processors, herbicide manufacturers and garbage incinerators) and can be found today in the bodies of anyone who eats fish, meat or dairy products. Research suggests dioxin may affect the body's hormonal messenger system; it may affect sex hormones and insulin and could create permanent health problems for children exposed in the womb— lowering sperm counts, interfering with sexual development and impairing brain development.

Symptoms   After exposure, victims experience skin, eye and mucous membrane irritation, nausea and vomiting. After a latency period of up to several weeks, additional symptoms appear, including chloracne, excessive hair growth, pigment abnormalities, motor weakness and sensory impairments. In animals, death occurs a few weeks after a lethal dose as the result of a wasting syndrome in which the animal stops eating and loses weight.

Treatment   There is no specific antidote. Symptomatic treatment, with induced vomiting or gastric lavage followed by the administration of activated charcoal and a cathartic. For eye or skin contamination, flush with water and soap; irrigate eyes with tepid water or saline. Anyone helping to wash the affected clothing or skin should wear protective clothing.

diphenhydramine   This antihistamine is used both as a treatment for the itchy skin rash from a wide variety of plants (such as poison ivy or sumac) and to partially prevent anaphylaxis caused by horse-serum–based antivenins or antitoxins.

See also ANTIVENIN.

dishwasher detergent   See ALKALINE CORROSIVES.

disulfiram   See ANTABUSE.

diuretics   These are the most commonly prescribed drugs for the treatment of high blood pressure. Overdoses are not generally harmful; more serious are the adverse effects from chronic use or misuse. Diuretics include acetazolamide, dichlorphenamide, methazolamide, bumetanide, ethacrynic acid, furosemide, mersalyl, amiloride, spironolactone, triamterene, bendroflumethiazide, benzthiadiazide, chlorthalidone, chlorothiazide, cyclothiazide, flumethiazide, hydrochlorothiazide, hydroflumethiazide, indapamide, methyclothiazide, metolazone, polythiazide, quinethazone and trichlormethiazide.

Symptoms   Lethargy, weakness and dehydration, which may be delayed for two to four hours until the diuretic action begins. The diuretic spironolactone may not produce symptoms until the third day; thiazide diuretics may cause hyperglycemia.

Treatment   There are no specific antidotes; treatment is symptomatic. Replace fluid loss and correct electrolyte abnormalities; monitor potassium levels. Induce vomiting or perform gastric lavage followed by activated charcoal and a cathartic (unless the patient is dehydrated).

See also MEDICATIONS AS POISONS.

DMSA   (2,3-dimercaptosuccinic acid) This chelating agent is being tested for possible use in the treatment of heavy metal poisoning such as lead, arsenic and mercury (especially methyl mercury).

DMSO   See DIMETHYL SULFOXIDE.

dog hobble   *(Leucothoe)*   [Other names: dog laurel, fetterbush, pepper bush, sweet bells, switch ivy, white osier.] This deciduous or evergreen shrub grows from Virginia to Florida, Tennessee, Louisiana and California. Its white or pink flowers grow in clusters.

Poisonous part   The leaves and nectar (in honey) are toxic and contain the toxin grayanotoxin (andromedotoxin).

Symptoms   Burning in the mouth, followed gradually by increased salivation, diarrhea and prickly skin; headache, vision problems, bradycardia, severe hypotension and possibly convulsions and coma.

Treatment   Fluid replacement, atropine for bradycardia; ephedrine for hypotension that does not respond to fluid replacement.

drain cleaners   See ALKALINE CORROSIVES.

dwale   An ancient name for deadly nightshade, popular in the time of Chaucer, meaning "to sleep."
See also NIGHTSHADE, DEADLY.

dyphylline (7-dihydroxypropyltheophylline) One of the group of bronchial tube relaxers given to control asthma, bronchitis and emphysema, dyphylline was introduced in 1946 and is available in time-release tablets or syrup.
Symptoms   Within one hour, overdose produces headache, nervousness, insomnia, nausea, vomiting, rapid heartbeat, low blood pressure, convulsions and circulatory failure.
Treatment   Perform gastric lavage, followed by symptomatic treatment.
See also BRONCHIAL TUBE RELAXERS; MEDICATIONS AS POISONS.

E

edrophonium chloride   Antidote used in the treatment of curare poisoning reversing the neuromuscular blockade produced by curare, tubocurarine or gallamine. It also treats the respiratory depression caused by curare overdose. It must be used with caution, however, among patients with chronic lung disease and heart problems.

See also CURARE.

elderberry, black and scarlet elders   *(Sambucus canadensis* and *S. pubens)* [Other names: American elder, sweet elder.] Often cultivated for its ornamental foliage, this indigenous shrub is found throughout the United States and Canada in low, damp ground and waste places. The elderberry grows from five to 12 feet with a rough gray bark and a faintly sweet odor. It flowers in June and July with white, star-shaped clusters; its black berries mature in September and October. Sometimes, flower and fruit appear at the same time. The European elder is larger than its American cousin but is otherwise quite similar.

Poisonous part   The entire plant is toxic, although the ripe fruit is edible when cooked, and in limited amounts it may not cause symptoms even if eaten raw. According to some sources, the flowers are probably nontoxic and the berries cause nausea only if eaten raw in large numbers. The poison is cyanogenic glycosides found mostly in the roots, stems and leaves and an unidentified cathartic mostly in the bark and roots of some species. Proper cooking destroys the toxic principle. Children have been poisoned by eating the roots or using the pithy stems as blowguns.

Symptoms   Eating leaves, bark, root or immature berries may cause serious diarrhea. Juice from the berries of *S. mexicana* has caused nausea, vomiting and cramps within 15 minutes, dizziness, numbness and stupor. There have been no cases of cyanide poisoning in humans from this plant in toxocological literature.

Treatment   Administration of fluids.

See also CYANOGENIC GLYCOSIDES.

endrin   [Trade names: Compound 269, Experimental Insecticide 269.] A highly toxic chlorinated hydrocarbon insecticide and rat poison, endrin has been responsible for numerous fatalities. This white crystalline solid can be inhaled, ingested or absorbed through the skin.

Symptoms   Between 30 minutes and 10 hours after ingestion, symptoms appear including giddiness, weakness, nausea, confusion, insomnia, lethargy, repeated convulsions and loss of consciousness followed by respiratory failure and death.

Treatment   There is no specific antidote. Perform gastric lavage but do not induce vomiting because of the risk of sudden onset of seizures; administer activated charcoal and a cathartic. Irregular heartbeat may respond to propranolol.

See also CHLORINATED HYDROCARBON PESTICIDES.

ephedrine   A potent central nervous system stimulant used to treat low blood pressure following overdose with antihypertensive drugs such as beta blockers, calcium channel blockers (verapamil, nifedipine), vasodilators (minoxidil, prazosin), etc.

See also BETA ADRENERGIC BLOCKERS.

epinephrine   This catecholamine produced naturally in the body is used to treat anaphylaxis or cardiac arrest. It may also be helpful in raising low blood pressure resulting from an overdose of beta adrenergic blockers and other heart-depressant drugs.

See also BETA ADRENERGIC BLOCKERS.

ergot *(Claviceps purpurea)*   This parasitic fungus is found primarily in rye grain, which can also contaminate flour made from the grain. Ergot poisoning can occur after eating rye meal or bread that has been prepared from the contaminated grain. Originating in Europe, ergot is now found throughout the world.

Ergot poisoning was epidemic during the Middle Ages, when 40,000 Frenchmen died from "St. Anthony's Fire." It is no longer a danger today because of widespread screening programs used to check cereal grains for the fungus.

Ergot was used in earlier times as an abortifacient because of its ability to contract the uterus; however, doses necessary to expel the uterine contents also tended to be fatal. In the 17th century, midwives used ergot to help the uterus contract after childbirth, and today it is still found in hospitals, where it is used for the same purpose.

Symptoms   Drowsiness, headache, giddiness, nausea, vomiting, cramps, itching and respiratory and cardiac arrest. In severe poisoning cases, gangrene involving the fingers, toes, ears and nose may occur. Ingestion can also cause painful convulsions, permanent damage to the central nervous system and psychosis.

Treatment   Gastric lavage followed by activated charcoal, together with symptomatic and supportive treatment. Amyl nitrate is sometimes used to ease spasms.

ethanol   The alcohol in alcoholic drinks; ethanol is administered either intravenously or orally to treat methanol or glycol poisonings.

See also ISOPROPYL ALCOHOL; METHANOL.

ether (diethyl ether) The first general anesthetic, ether was first demonstrated successfully in Boston in 1846, when a tooth was extracted without pain while the patient was breathing ether. Soon after, the anesthetic properties of chloroform and nitrous oxide were added to the anesthesiologist's arsenal.

A colorless liquid, ether is administered on a gauze mask over a patient's nose and mouth and produces unconsciousness when inhaled. It is so flammable that even static electricity can cause an explosion. For this reason, ether was abandoned after the 1930s when it was replaced by other, safer anesthetic agents.

Symptoms Excessive use depresses the central nervous system and stops breathing.

Treatment Remove the gas and force ventilation, maintain breathing and keep warm to avoid shock. If a high fever develops, pack the body in wet towels or administer dantrolene sodium and procainamide.

See also ANESTHETICS, GASEOUS/VOLATILE; CHLOROFORM; NITROUS OXIDE.

ethyl alcohol Another name for ethanol, the alcohol in alcoholic drinks. It is used as an antidote to antifreeze poisoning.

See also ANTIFREEZE; ISOPROPYL ALCOHOL.

ethylene chlorohydrin This colorless, odorless liquid is used as an industrial solvent and to facilitate seed germination. It evaporates quickly at room temperature. Because it has no smell and does not irritate the mouth or nose, it is possible to become exposed before danger is realized.

Symptoms In the wake of continued exposure, ethylene chlorohydrin is a central nervous system depressant and damages the heart, lungs, liver and kidneys. It is not yet certain whether it causes cancer or fetal damage. Symptoms appear soon after exposure, including nausea, vomiting, headache, vertigo, delirium, low blood pressure, slow breathing, cyanosis and coma. Death occurs from respiratory and circulatory failure. In addition, there have been reports of impaired DNA and possible birth defects.

Treatment Move the victim into fresh air and remove all contaminated clothing. Perform artificial respiration or administer oxygen as needed. For ingestion, perform gastric lavage followed by a saline cathartic. Do not administer epinephrine or other stimulants.

ethylene dibromide (EDB) This volatile liquid is found in leaded gasoline and is used as a pesticide and fumigant for soil, fruits and vegetables. It can cause chemical burns or (if inhaled) respiratory tract irritation and pulmonary edema. Its use as a pesticide has been restricted since 1984 because of its suspected carcinogenic role. In cases of inhalation poisoning, rescuers must wear breathing apparatus and protective clothing to avoid exposure. Once absorbed in the body, EDB can disrupt cell metabolism and initiate a multisystem failure throughout the body.

Symptoms   If inhaled, EDB can irritate the eyes and upper respiratory tract; pulmonary edema is found within six hours but may take as long as two days to develop. Ingestion causes vomiting, diarrhea, central nervous system depression, seizures and metabolic acidosis. In fatal cases, there is acute kidney failure, liver damage and muscle necrosis. Ingestion of 4.5 ml of liquid EDB can be fatal.

Treatment   There is no specific antidote. Treat symptoms, and provide oxygen if needed. For skin/eye contamination, remove clothes and wash with soap and water; irrigate eyes with saline or tepid water. For ingestion, do not induce vomiting because of corrosive effects and danger of rapid onset of coma or seizure. Perform gastric lavage followed by the administration of activated charcoal and a cathartic.

See also PESTICIDES.

ethylene glycol   See ANTIFREEZE.

eucalyptus   (*Eucalyptus globulus*   Labill.) Also known as a gum tree, this genus includes more than 600 species (both trees and shrubs) in the myrtle family. It is the essential oils of this tree that can be toxic. The eucalyptus is native to Australia, New Zealand, Tasmania and nearby islands and is cultivated throughout the temperate regions of the world as shade trees or in forestry plantations. About 90 species are grown in California, and a few are found in Florida.

The bark of the eucalyptus tree is distinctive, peeling off in long strips exposing the inner layer. Leaves are leathery and smooth, and the flower petals (white, yellow or red) form a cap when the flower expands and attract honeybees. The fruit is surrounded by a woody, cup-shaped receptacle and contains many tiny seeds.

Poisonous part   The leaf glands of many species contain a volatile aromatic oil known as eucalyptus oil, and is an active ingredient in expectorants and inhalants. It contains 70 percent eucalyptol; the toxic dose is 5 ml.

Symptoms   Following an acute overdose by mouth, symptoms may appear within five to 30 minutes and include burning in the mouth and throat followed by nausea and vomiting. Drowsiness, confusion, restlessness, delirium, muscle twitching and coma may follow. Death may occur as a result of depression of the central nervous system and respiratory arrest.

Treatment   Treat seizures and coma if they occur. There is no specific antidote. Perform gastric lavage but do not induce vomiting because of the risk of inducing seizures. Administer activated charcoal.

exotoxin   Exotoxins include some of the most poisonous substances known, which are released by some types of bacteria into the bloodstream. Tetanus and diphtheria bacilli produce some of the best-known exotoxins; the former affects the nervous system and causes muscle spasms and paralysis, and the latter damages the heart and nervous system. Vaccinations for some of the potentially fatal bacterial diseases use detoxified exotoxins to prevent the disease. Once infection has occurred, however, treatment includes antibiotics and an antitoxin to neutralize the exotoxin.

See also TOXOID.

F

false Jerusalem cherry *(Solanum pseudocapsicum)* This decorative pot plant has spread through cultivation from its native Gulf Coast region and Hawaii. It is a member of a very large genus with 1,700 species, most of which have not been evaluated toxicologically.

Poisonous part Human poisoning is usually attributed to immature fruit, which contains the toxin solanine glycoalkaloid.

Symptoms While there is little danger of fatal poisoning in adults, children may ingest a fatal amount of this plant. Symptoms appear several hours after ingestion and include gastric irritation, scratchy throat, fever and diarrhea (solanine poisoning is often confused with bacterial gastroenteritis).

Treatment Provide the same general supportive care that would be given in gastroenteritis cases; fluid replacement may be required.

false morel See TURBANTOP.

fenoprofen See NONSTEROIDAL ANTI-INFLAMMATORY DRUGS.

fentanyl See NARCOTICS.

fer-de-lance This extremely venomous pit viper lives in cultivated lands and tropical forests of central Mexico into South America. A member of the viper family, it is considered a pit viper because of its sensory pit between each eye and nostril.

The fer-de-lance is gray or brown with black-edged diamonds on a lighter border and is found in tropical America ranging from farms to tropical forests. Its name (French for "lancehead") is sometimes used to refer collectively to all snakes of the Central and South American genus *Bothrops* and the Asian genus *Trimeresurus*, and it is called *barba amarillo* ("yellow chin") in Spanish. Other pit viper relatives include the dangerous South American wutu *(Bothrops alternatus)*, the jumping viper or tommygoff *(B. nummifera)* of Central America, the Okinawa habu *(Trimeresurus flavoviridis)* found in the Ryukyu Islands and Wagler's pit viper *(T. Wagleri)*.

Symptoms With a bite from this viper, blood cannot coagulate and hemorrhages into muscles and nervous system. There is local pain, bleeding from the bite, gums, nose, mouth and rectum. Shock and respiratory arrest are followed by death.

Treatment Antivenin is available.

See also ANTIVENIN; PIT VIPERS; SNAKES, POISONOUS.

fertilizers   Plant foods that contain one of three ingredients necessary for plants to grow: potassium, nitrogen or phosphorous. They are not generally considered particularly toxic even if ingested by children, *unless the fertilizer also contains herbicides or insecticides.* If a child ingests products containing only these three ingredients, usually the only symptoms that occur will be vomiting or diarrhea. However, many fertilizers also contain additives that could produce toxicity.

See also HERBICIDES; INSECTICIDES.

fire ant   *(Solenopsis)*   Several species of these small, aggressive ants, also known as thief ants, are found in North America. These red or yellow ants live in loose mounds with open ventilation craters and long tunnels, usually located in meadows of clover and Bermuda grass and in row crops; they occasionally invade homes.

Poisonous part   The release of histamine causes the painful symptoms common in fire ant stings.

Symptoms   A sting from the fire ant can cause severe pain, swelling, itching, reddening, warmth and burning.

Treatment   Ice, compresses and cleansing of the wound to prevent infection. Neither antihistamines, corticosteroids nor antibacterial ointments significantly ease symptoms.

fireworks   According to federal regulations, all fireworks must be sealed to prevent leakage of gunpowder during shipment and handling and must be constructed to prevent burnout through the sides or blowout through the bottom of the device after ignition. Still, each year fireworks injure many thousands of Americans, usually children and teenagers. These products are also toxic if ingested.

Gold sparklers may contain barium nitrate, paste, chalk, dextrin, iron and aluminum; green sparklers contain barium nitrate, potassium perchlorate, wheat pastes, gum, dextrin and aluminum powder. Red sparklers contain strontium carbonate, nitrate and potassium perchlorate, plus gums, wheat pastes, dextrin and aluminum powder.

Symptoms   The soluble barium salts contained in these products can cause vomiting, abdominal pain, bloody diarrhea, shallow breathing, convulsions, coma and death from respiratory or cardiac failure. Strontium may cause vomiting, abdominal pain, bloody stools and methemoglobinemia; perchlorates may cause vomiting, abdominal pain and methemoglobinemia.

Treatment   When a sparkler has been eaten, induce vomiting or perform gastric lavage; in the case of nitrate-induced methemoglobinemia, intravenous solution of 1 percent methylene blue is recommended.

fish contamination   High in protein, low in calories, fat and cholesterol—

and widely suspected to fight against heart disease and cancer—this highly praised health food can also be a site of contamination and spoilage.

The problem is that fish readily soak up poisons and contaminants in water; tiny fish pick up contaminants from the plankton they feed on in polluted water, concentrating heavy metals (such as methyl mercury) in their organs. These fish are eaten by larger fish, further concentrating the toxins, and in big fish, such as swordfish and tuna, the contaminants may reach levels harmful to humans.

Fatty fish like salmon, bluefish and herring are vulnerable to chlorinated compounds such as PCBs, dioxins and DDT, which linger in the body for years. Very minute quantities of these substances in the water will produce very high concentrations in fish.

Indeed, one of the more insidious types of mercury poisoning occurs through the contamination of fish in lakes and streams throughout the United States as a result of extensive agricultural fungicide and pesticide use and the industrial by-products of chlorine production. Current estimates suggest up to 10,000 tons of mercury infiltrates the sea each year; once in the water, it enters the food chain where it is converted into organic methyl mercury, one of the most toxic substances known. The presence of sewage in the water facilitates this deadly conversion by bacteria living in the mud; once it occurs, the contaminated bacteria are then eaten by plankton, which are in turn eaten by pike, pickerel, perch, walleye, muskie and white bass.

Unlike inorganic mercury compounds, methyl mercury is hard to detect in the blood; it does not readily break down in the body and can take months to be excreted. In addition, it can pass easily through the blood-brain barrier, irreversibly damaging brain cells; it also crosses the placenta and builds up in the fetal brain and blood. Methyl mercury seems to affect women more than men, and children and infants most of all.

The first cases of contaminated fish poisoning occurred in Japan in 1953 and 1970, when more than 121 cases—and 46 deaths—were reported. At that time, methyl mercury chloride flowed directly into a bay and river near a manufacturing plant.

According to research conducted in the 1970s, fish in the Great Lakes were also contaminated with methyl mercury (2.8 parts per million). Today, the Food and Drug Administration mandates that tuna must contain less than 0.5 mg/kg, but scientists estimate that to be safe, humans should ingest no more than 0.1 mg of mercury per day; if a fish contains 1 parts per billion of mercury, then the safe weekly limit would be about three portions of fish a week (1 1/2 lb.). Still, no methyl mercury fish poisonings have been reported since Japan's incidences.

Studies suggest that there is greater danger in blood levels of mercury in infants. Very little is known about the effects of methyl mercury on genetics, except that it is 1,000 times more genetically toxic than the next most dangerous substance, colchicine.

FISH AND SHELLFISH POISONING

Type	Onset	Fish/shellfish	Effects
Ciguatera	1–6 hrs	Barracuda, grouper, red snapper	Gastroenteritis, hot and cold reversal, weakness, myalgia
Scombroid	Immediate to delayed	Tuna, mahi mahi, mackerel, bonita	Gastroenteritis, flush, wheezing, rash
Neurotoxic shellfish	Up to 3 hrs	Mussels	Gastroenteritis, ataxia, paresthesias
Paralytic shellfish	Within 30 min.	Mussels, clams, "red tide"	Gastroenteritis, ataxia, respiratory paralysis
Tetrodotoxin	30–40 min.	Pufferfish, sun fish, porcupine fish, California newt	Vomiting, twitches, weakness, respiratory paralysis

In addition, there is very little known about ways to remove the methyl mercury pollutants from contaminated water, which may remain poisoned for between 10 and 100 years.

Fish spoilage   The danger of fish contamination is not just with the contaminants they ingest. Because bacteria that live on fish are adapted to withstand the cool and cold waters of lakes and oceans, they can thrive in temperatures cold enough to preserve other food. These microbes will quickly spoil the fish, unless it is kept at temperatures close to freezing. Even under the best conditions, fish lasts only seven to 12 days; but it often takes seven days for fish to get from the water to the supermarket, where it may sit for several more days.

How to protect against contamination   Seafood should look and smell fresh, with vivid skin and bright eyes and no fishy or ammonia odor. It should be displayed on ice in the store; otherwise, fish is best selected from the bottom of the refrigerator case where it is coldest. Once home, it should be kept very cold and eaten within one or two days. Cook thoroughly, but no amount of cooking will destroy contaminants. Scrape off the fatty skin before cooking. Pregnant women, nursing mothers and young children should limit consumption of fish that might have high levels of mercury and PCBs.

floor polish and wax See PETROLEUM DISTILLATES.

Flumazenil   This nontoxic drug is used to rapidly reverse a coma brought on by benzodiazepine overdose. After intravenous administration, the reversal takes effect within two minutes.
See also BENZODIAZEPINES.

fluoride   Fluoride poisoning is usually caused by the accidental ingestion of roach powder insecticides, although it can also occur in children who ingest large amounts of vitamin-fluoride tablets or eat too much fluoride toothpaste. The recommended dose of fluoride for children under age two is 0.25 mg/day; vitamin-fluoride tablets contain 1 mg, as does the average amount of toothpaste on a toothbrush. If too much toothpaste is swallowed by a child in one day, it could result in fluoride poisoning and severe mottling of the tooth enamel. For this reason, new research suggests children under age two should brush without toothpaste; those between ages two and five should be given toothpaste no larger than a pea and required to rinse their mouths thoroughly after brushing.
In addition, the American Dental Association Council of Dental Therapeutics suggests that fluoride supplements prescribed by pediatricians should be limited to those children whose drinking water has a fluoride concentration less than 70 percent of the 1-part-per-million level recommended for community water. Still, fluoride is an effective weapon against the development of dental cavities and should not be abandoned because of potential problems.
The most famous case of fluoride poisoning occurred at the Oregon State Hospital in 1943, when workers accidentally mixed 11 pounds of flouride sodium salt with 10 gallons of scrambled eggs, killing 47 of the 263 patients who ate the tainted breakfast.
Symptoms   Following ingestion, symptoms include pain, salivation, nausea, vomiting and diarrhea. Vomiting and diarrhea usually get rid of most of the poison in the stomach, although the gastrointestinal tract readily absorbs fluoride salts. In the event of ingesting large amounts of fluoride, death from respiratory paralysis can result within a few minutes. Death may also be caused by shock as a result of the effects of fluid loss from violent vomiting and the effects of the fluoride on the heart muscle, causing arrhythmias and heart failure.
Although the lethal dose of sodium fluoride in adults is fairly large (5 grams), a fatal dose as low as 2 grams has been recorded.
Treatment   Intravenous glucose in isotonic saline in order to increase the amount of water in the urine secreted from the body is the most effective way of removing fluoride from the body. Administer limewater, calcium chloride solution or milk in order to bind as much fluoride ion as possible, followed by gastric lavage with any of the above fluids. This is followed by

administration of calcium gluconate or calcium chloride to head off muscular spasms; calcium solution should also be used to wipe away corrosive materials after being vomited or excreted. For hydrofluoric skin burns, wash with cold water and administer magnesium oxide. Treat shock as it occurs.

fluoroacetate   See COMPOUND 1080.

fly agaric (yellow or red)   *(Amanita muscaria)* Sometimes confused with its close relative, the panther mushroom *(Amanita pantherina)*, this is a member of the poisonous *Amanita* mushroom genus that has been used for at least 3,000 years as an intoxicant in the rituals of many Asian and Indian tribes. Some mycologists believe it is the source of Soma, the mystical drug of the ancients. It gets its common name from its ancient use as a fly poison, since it attracts—and kills—any fly that lands on it.

This mushroom is found in pastures and fields in summer throughout Europe and the United States in wooded areas and conifer forests, and sometimes in open pastureland. It generally appears at the beginning and end of the summer months and in many places is more abundant than common edible mushrooms.

Similar in appearance to the *Amanita phalloides*, the fly mushroom cap ranges in color from yellow, red, orange to deep brown, all with white warty patches on the caps that disappear as the mushrooms age. Because of its color variations, the panther mushroom is sometimes confused with the fly agaric. Both varieties have the unattached, white gills with white spores that are typical of the *Amanita* genus. While both varieties are poisonous, the panther mushroom is the more deadly of the two. The taste is bitter and unpleasant.

In most cases, people who have been poisoned by eating this mushroom have done so deliberately to experience hallucinations.

Poisonous part   The fly agaric and *A. pantherina* mushrooms contain the strong hallucinogen muscimol and the potent insecticide ibotenic acid. Despite its name, *A. muscaria* usually contains insignificant quantities of muscarine.

Symptoms   While poisoning is rarely fatal, severe symptoms appear quickly, between 30 minutes and three hours, and include severe gastrointestinal distress, drowsiness, lowered blood pressure, slow heartbeat, blurred vision, watery diarrhea and intoxication featuring euphoria and hallucinations. There may be intermittent drowsiness and manic behavior. In more severe cases, psychosis, convulsions and coma can follow.

Deaths have been reported in those whose immune systems were already compromised or in those who ate large amounts of the mushroom. Although deaths are rare in adults, they must be protected against injury during the manic phase of the intoxication. In preadolescents, however, ingestion of these mushrooms may cause convulsions and coma.

Treatment   Vomiting soon after ingestion will lessen the severity of symptoms. While some scientists have advocated the administration of atropine as a specific antidote, many others prefer to counteract delirium and coma with the use of physostigmine.

See also AMANITA MUSHROOMS; MUSHROOM POISONING; PANTHER MUSHROOM.

fly mushroom   See FLY AGARIC.

folic acid   A B-complex vitamin that is very helpful in the treatment for methanol and ethylene glycol poisoning. Folic acid is essential for the synthesis of protein in the body and is believed to help eliminate the toxic metabolite formic acid from the body.

See also METHANOL; VITAMINS.

food poisoning   An illness that appears suddenly and within 48 hours of eating contaminated food and causes stomach pain, vomiting and diarrhea. Most cases of food poisoning are caused by the presence of bacteria or viruses in food.

The greatest danger from food poisoning is loss of fluids from vomiting and diarrhea, which are the body's natural responses to poison. If dehydration becomes serious, the victim should be hospitalized and given fluids intravenously.

Botulism is an exception, however. Unlike other food poisoning, botulism affects the nervous system and only occasionally causes vomiting or diarrhea. Botulism is life threatening, and any suspected case should be immediately referred for medical help, since there is an antitoxin available.

BACTERIAL CAUSES

Bacterial gastroenteritis   This is caused by the *Yersinia enterocolitica* bacterium found in meat, water, raw vegetables and unpasteurized milk; it multiples rapidly at room temperature. Between two to five days after eating, the victim experiences fever, headache, nausea, and diarrhea—sickness often mistaken for the flu. It is common in children but also appears in adults.

Botulism   This is the most deadly type of food poisoning, caused by a bacterial toxin associated with home canning. Fortunately, it is rare today because of modern canning techniques. It occurs when sealed foods are not processed at high enough temperatures to kill the organism. Cooking the canned food after removal from the container will not destroy this toxin. Before opening a canned food, check the can to see if it is swollen or if the safety button in the center of the lid has popped up. If either occurs, the food must be thrown away.

Campylobacterosis Caused by the *Campylobacter jejujni* bacterium found in raw poultry, meat and unpasteurized milk. From two to five days after eating, symptoms appear and last between two and seven days, including diarrhea, stomach cramps, fever and bloody stool.

Cereus Caused by the *Bacillus cereus* bacterium, this type of food poisoning multiplies in raw foods at room temperature. Onset of symptoms is between one and 18 hours after eating. It may cause stomach pain and diarrhea or nausea and vomiting but rarely lasts longer than 24 hours.

Cholera This disease is caused by the *Vibrio cholera* bacterium found in fish and shellfish harvested from contaminated water; main sources are fish and shellfish eaten raw. Symptoms begin from one to three days after eating and can range from mild diarrhea to a life-threatening dehydration from intense diarrhea. Hospitalization is recommended for severe cases.

Clostridium perfringens A form of infectious diarrhea caused by *C. perfringens* resulting from allowing cooked meat to cool slowly to room temperature over a period of 12 to 24 hours. It can also be caused by unsanitary food handling practices. Symptoms of abdominal pain and diarrhea begin within six to 12 hours after ingestion of contaminated meat and last about 24 hours.

Listeriosis This rare (but potentially lethal) illness can strike pregnant women, the elderly and people with damaged immune systems who eat food contaminated with the *Listeria monocytogenes* bacterium. Symptoms include chills, nausea, blood poisoning, complications of pregnancy and stillbirths. In severe cases, this illness can lead to meningitis (an infection of the membrane surrounding the brain and spinal cord).

Salmonellosis The *Salmonella* bacteria—one of the most common causes of food poisoning—are most often found in poultry. If poultry is not properly cooked and prepared, the bacteria can cause salmonellosis in those who eat the birds. Salmonella can also be transferred to food from the excrement of infected animals or people. Contaminated food left at room temperature can also contribute to the multiplication of large colonies of bacteria that cannot be detected by the naked eye. Still, proper handling and cooking of even contaminated food will kill the *Salmonella* bacteria.

Shigellosis (bacillary dysentery) This is caused by the *Shigella* bacterium, found in milk and dairy products, poultry and mixed salads but which can develop in any moist food that is not thoroughly cooked. The bacteria multiply rapidly at or above room temperature. Symptoms usually appear eight hours to eight days after ingestion and begin with nausea, vomiting, diarrhea, stomach cramps, weakness, vision problems, headache, difficulty in swallowing, slurred speech, dilated pupils and progressive paralysis. Shigellosis usually runs its course in between three and six days, but it can be fatal.

Staphylococcus aureus Other bacteria are not so easy to kill, even by heating at high temperatures. Toxin-forming strains of staphylococcal

PROPER FOOD HANDLING
TO PREVENT FOOD POISONING

The foods that are most vulnerable to contamination during storage, preparation, cooking and serving are meat, poultry and eggs. Here are the principles of proper food handling and kitchen safety:

- *Refrigeration*   Temperature in the refrigerator must be 40°F or below; 0°F in the freezer. Cooling doesn't kill bacteria, but it stops their growth. Allow air to circulate around refrigerated items. Always wrap food in refrigerator to keep off bacteria in the air.
- *Wash hands*   To avoid contamination by *Salmonella* bacteria or other organisms when preparing food, wash hands thoroughly with soap and water *before* and *after* handling the food.
- *Wash utensils*   Wash cutting board and utensils with hot soapy water before touching any other food with them. An acrylic cutting board is best, since it can be washed in the dishwasher where the high temperatures kill bacteria. Unlike wood, acrylic also resists pits and grooves where bacteria can hide. To disinfect a wooden cutting board, wash with a solution of 2 teaspoons of household bleach mixed with 1 quart of water; flush board thoroughly after applying bleach. It's best to reserve a separate cutting board for poultry and meat.
- *Thawing meat*   Don't thaw meat at room temperature; thaw meat or poultry in a microwave oven or in the refrigerator and then cook immediately.
- *Marinades*   If you marinate meat or poultry, don't serve the marinade unless it has been cooked at a rolling boil for several minutes.
- *Serving*   Serve meat and poultry on a clean plate with a clean utensil to avoid contaminating the cooked food with its raw juices.
- *Cook thoroughly*   Use a meat thermometer in the thickest portion of the meat, not touching bone. The thermometer should register 180°F to 185°F for poultry and 160°F for pork. Juices should run clear when meat is pierced. Do not cook poultry at a low temperature for a long period of time
- *Leftovers*   Cool poultry and meat quickly when refrigerating leftovers; do not let stuffed poultry stand for long periods. Remove the stuffing after cooking and promptly refrigerate it.
- *Eggs*   Never use cracked eggs, because they may contain *Salmonella* bacteria; it's best to check eggs for cracks before you use them. However, even an uncracked egg may contain bacteria; since *Salmonella* is killed by heat, it's best to cook eggs thoroughly. Raw eggs should be avoided (such as in Caesar salad dressing, homemade eggnog, hollandaise sauce, etc.). Eggs keep longer when refrigerated in their cartons—but don't keep on the refrigerator door. Eggs must be kept in the coldest part of the refrigerator to stop bacteria from multiplying.

- *Mold* In general, throw out any food with mold (except for cheese, which may be eaten after the mold is trimmed off).
- *Microwave* A turntable should be used to rotate dishes as they cook; because microwave ovens heat food unevenly, cold spots in a food may harbor dangerous bacteria and hot spots can cause burns.
- *Cleaning cues* Don't season wooden salad bowls with oil; it can become rancid. Keep can opener and blender free from food particles. Always scrub down the sink after working with poultry or meat. Sponges in the kitchen used to wipe dishes or countertops should be discarded after one week, and never left to sit in water (it encourages bacterial growth). Clean sink and counters with detergent containing bleach, which kills harmful bacteria.

For more information about food safety, call the U.S. Department of Agriculture's Meat and Poultry Hotline at (800) 535-4555. In Washington, D.C. call (202) 477-3333 between 10 A.M. and 4 P.M.

For questions about storing or handling fish, call the helpline of the Rhode Island Seafood Council at (800) EAT-FISH between 8 A.M. and 5 P.M. ET.

bacteria may contaminate food from a cook's septic abscess. Outbreaks of this type of food poisoning, called a "staph infection," can occur among large numbers of people. Foods with mayonnaise or cream bases are especially good environments for these bacteria. Within three to six hours after eating, people will experience nausea, vomiting and diarrhea that last for 12 hours.

Traveler's diarrhea This is still another type of common bacterial food hazard, caused by eating strains of the intestinal bacterium *Escherichia coli* (known as *E. coli*). The *E. coli* bacterium produces toxins that cause a severe diarrhea lasting for several days. This is most often found while traveling to foreign countries, where it is common in the water supply and on foods prepared in unhygienic conditions.

To protect against this type of food poison, travelers should not consume untreated water and ice, salads, raw fruits and vegetables that can't be peeled and uncooked milk products. Contamination from *E. coli* can also occur from eating raw or partially cooked ground meat.

VIRAL CAUSES

Norwalk virus The most common cause of viral contamination is the Norwalk virus, which often contaminates shellfish. These can cause food poisoning when raw or improperly cooked food has been in contact with water contaminated by human excrement.

Hepatitis A It's possible to contract hepatitis A from eating raw shellfish with the hepatitis A virus, harvested from sewage-contaminated waters. Vegetables can also harbor the virus, especially if they are handled a lot and are

---

KEEPING HOT FOODS SAFE

To keep hot foods safe, follow these guidelines from the U.S. Department of Agriculture:

- Use a meat thermometer to make sure meats and poultry are cooked completely. Put the thermometer into the thickest part (avoiding fat and bone). Bacteria are killed at 160°F (poultry at 180°F or higher).
- Don't partially heat food, then finish cooking later; half-cooked food may be warm enough to encourage bacterial growth but not hot enough to kill it. Subsequent cooking might not kill the bacteria.
- Allow at least one and a half times longer than usual to cook frozen foods that have not been prethawed.
- Keep hot foods at 140° to 160° until serving time, especially those served in chafing dishes or warmers. Food should never be kept between 40° and 140° for more than two hours, as this encourages bacterial growth.
- Thoroughly reheat leftovers, and make sure food is evenly heated. Gravies should be brought to a rolling boil.

---

eaten raw. Even though federal regulations and posting of contaminated waters offer some protection, there is still a risk of eating raw shellfish. Symptoms begin from two to six weeks after eating: fever, weakness, anorexia and jaundice. Severe cases may damage liver and can be fatal.

PROTOZOA

Giardiasis This type of food poisoning is caused by the *Giardia lamblia* protozoan, which is found in the human intestinal tract and in feces. It can be introduced to food when sewage is used as fertilizer, or when food handlers don't wash their hands. Symptoms include diarrhea, stomach pains, gas, loss of appetite, nausea and vomiting.

Amebiasis Also known as amebic dysentery, it is caused by *Entamoeba histolytica* found in the human intestinal tract and feces. The protozoa can be introduced to food when sewage is used as fertilizer or when food handlers don't wash their hands. Symptoms include tenderness over the colon area or liver, loose morning stools, diarrhea, nervousness, weight loss and fatigue.

CONTAMINATED FISH

Tainted fish Fish sometimes ingest a particular type of toxic one-cell organism (for example, snapper, sea bass, barracuda and amberjack caught off Florida or the West Indies). The contaminated fish cause symptoms similar to those of other food poisoning, plus a rash, numbness in the hands and feet, headache, muscle ache, tingling of the lips and tongue and face pain. Sometimes symptoms can last for months.

Decomposition Eating certain kinds of fish that aren't fresh can also be toxic. Bacterial decomposition of tuna, mackerel, bonito, mahi mahi, bluefish or albacore can cause immediate gastrointestinal problems, rash and abdominal pain. Symptoms subside after a day or two.

Sushi Sushi, the Japanese dish made of raw fish, can cause a type of food poisoning from a parasitic worm, anisakiasis, which infests small crustaceans on which many kinds of fish feed. This causes gastrointestinal distress, nausea and vomiting.

OTHER CAUSES

Food poisoning can also be caused by eating poisonous mushrooms or fruit and vegetables contaminated with high doses of insecticides. Certain other types of more exotic food, such as the Japanese pufferfish or cassava, can also cause poisoning from mild to fatal if improperly prepared and cooked. In addition, even the common potato can develop a toxin (present in green areas in the potato, in the sprouts or eyes). Peanuts can develop a toxic mold when not properly stored; never eat a moldy or shriveled peanut.

Symptoms While the time between ingestion and the onset of symptoms varies according to the cause of poisoning, symptoms usually develop within 30 minutes in the case of chemical poisoning, between one and 12 hours for bacterial toxins, and between 12 and 48 hours for virus and salmonella infections. Symptoms also vary depending on how badly the food was contaminated, but they often include nausea, vomiting, diarrhea, stomach pain, and—in severe cases—shock and collapse. Diagnosis of food poisoning can be made from a culture or sample of vomited material or fecal matter.

Treatment Medical assistance should be obtained if severe vomiting or diarrhea appears suddenly, if the victim collapses *or if the victim is a child, an elderly person or someone with a chronic illness.* In cases of severe poisoning with chemical or bacterial toxins, gastric lavage is indicated. In all cases, rehydration (drinking liquids such as water, tea, bouillon and ginger ale to replace fluid loss) is important. Mild cases may be treated at home, with a soft diet and plenty of fluids, including some salt and sugar.

Symptoms can be treated much the way one would treat a bout of flu. Most cases of food poisoning are not serious (except for botulism and some types of mushroom poisoning), and recovery is usually within three days. Samples of any food left from recent meals should be saved for testing, if possible. According to the U.S. Department of Agriculture's Safety and Inspection Service, consumers should report possible food poisoning in three situations:

SAFE FOOD STORAGE *

Food	Where	How Long
Poultry		
Raw	Refrigerator	1–2 days
	Freezer	9 months
Cooked	Refrigerator	3–4 days
	Freezer	4–6 months
Seafood		
Lean fish, raw	Refrigerator	1–2 days
	Freezer	6–8 months
Fatty fish, raw	Refrigerator	1–2 days
	Freezer	4 months
Raw shrimp	Refrigerator	1–2 days
	Freezer	9 months
Cooked seafood	Refrigerator	3 days
	Freezer	2 months
Meat		
Ground meat	Refrigerator	1–2 days
	Freezer	3–4 months
Chops (all)	Refrigerator	3–5 days
Frozen lamb chops	Freezer	6–9 months
Frozen pork chops	Freezer	4–6 months
Roasts	Refrigerator	3–5 days
Frozen beef roasts	Freezer	6–12 months
Frozen veal/pork roast	Freezer	4–6 months
Frozen lamb roast	Freezer	6–9 months
Steak	Refrigerator	3–5 days
		6-12 months
Cooked leftovers	Refrigerator	3–4 days
	Freezer	2–3 months
Luncheon meats,		
(unopened)	Refrigerator	2 weeks
(opened)	Refrigerator	3–5 days
	Freezer	1–2 months
Dairy		
Raw eggs in shell	Refrigerator	3 weeks
Hard-boiled (in shell)	Refrigerator	1 week
Milk	Refrigerator	5 days
	Freezer	1 month
Mayonnaise (opened)	Refrigerator	2 months

*Guidelines provided by the USDA and the Food Marketing Institute

- If the food was eaten at a large gathering.
- If the food was from a restaurant, deli, sidewalk vendor or other kitchen that serves more than a few people.
- If the food is a commercial product (such as canned goods or frozen food), since contaminants may have affected an entire batch.

When making a report, officials need to know your name, address, telephone number, a detailed explanation of the problem, when and where the food was eaten, who ate it and the name and address of the restaurant or establishment where the food was obtained. If the food is a commercial product, you should provide the manufacturer's name and address and the product's lot or batch number. These codes reveal which factory shift prepared the food and on which day—vital information in tracing the source of the contamination. If the tainted food is meat or poultry, look for the USDA inspection stamp on the wrapper, which will identify the plant where the food was made or packaged.

See also BOTULIN; BOTULIN ANTITOXIN; BOTULISM; BOTULISM, IN-FANT; CIGUATERA; DINOFLAGELLATE; ERGOT; FISH CONTAMINATION; GROUPER, SPOTTED; PARALYTIC SHELLFISH POISONING; PTOMAINE POI-SONING; PUFFERFISH; SALMONELLA; SALMONELLOSIS; SAXITOXIN; SCOM-BROID POISONING; SHELLFISH POISONING; STAPHYLOCOCCUS ENTEROTOXIN; SUPERANTIGENS; SUSHI.

formaldehyde   This colorless, pungent irritant gas has an unpleasant odor and is considered to be supertoxic. It is most commonly found as formalin, a solution of 40 percent formaldehyde, water and methanol used in medicine to preserve tissue specimens. It is also found in many everyday products: the glue and resin odor in new automobiles and furniture is formaldehyde; it is also contained in antiseptics, disinfectants, fabric sizing, some explosives and adhesives.

In fact, formaldehyde is the most common chemical irritant in modern buildings—found in plywood, particleboard, stain-resistant carpets, insulation and adhesives in flooring. However, the amount of formaldehyde emitted by these products fades in time. Workers and homeowners are exposed to low levels of formaldehyde from cloth, foam insulation and plywood (especially in mobile homes). Formaldehyde is a suspected carcinogen.

Symptoms   Most dangerous when inhaled or ingested, formaldehyde is less toxic when absorbed through the skin. It attacks the respiratory system, and, if it is ingested, victims experience immediate severe abdominal pain, with vomiting, pain in the throat and diarrhea, corrosive gastritis and collapse within a few minutes, loss of consciousness and liver failure, with death from circulatory failure. Shock may cause death within a few hours up to two days. If the patient does not die, recovery may be rapid.

Inhalation of fumes irritates the eyes, nose and respiratory tract; chronic inhalation causes pulmonary edema and death. Skin contact (especially with paper and cloth containing formaldehyde) causes discoloration and may result in sloughing and allergic dermatitis, and the higher the concentration of formaldehyde in a product, the greater the danger of explosion.

Treatment Gastric lavage immediately after ingestion, followed by large amounts of water and then a saline cathartic. In the event of skin contamination, wash thoroughly. Otherwise, treatment is supportive; dialysis may be effective.

formalin See FORMALDEHYDE.

foxglove *(Digitalis)* [Other names: dead man's thimbles, fairy bells, fairy cap, fairy finger, fairy glove, fairy thimbles, folks gloves, foxes glofa.]

Named for the resemblance of its flowers to fingers of the fairy "folks gloves," the foxglove has been considered medically useful since the first century A.D. and was first written about as a drug in the year 1200. The name refers to any of about 30 species of plant's including the common foxglove *(D. purpurea)*, which is a powerful poison and plant source of the heart drug digitalis.

Together with paintbrush, speedwell, snapdragon and monkeyflower, foxglove is a biennial member of the figwort family (Scrophulariaceae). During its first year, the plant produces a soft rosette of full, tapering, finely toothed leaves covered with white down, and on the second year it produces a beautiful, tall flower stalk column of three to five feet, with bell-shaped hanging flowers of yellow, white, pink, and purple. The stalk has a few small leaves and a long succession of flowers that open from the bottom to the top; each flower droops over the one below it on the stalk, and the flowers bloom in midsummer.

Native to Europe, the Mediterranean region and the Canary Islands, foxglove is grown as an ornamental in the United States and is often seen in foundation plantings of older homes. It is also naturalized on the Pacific coast from northern California to British Columbia.

Its name originates in Britain, where residents called it "folks gloves" (the gloves of the little people, or fairies) and believed that the small spots on the lower lip of the foxglove flower were tiny fairy fingerprints. It was also called "dead man's thimbles" because of its shape and toxicity, and its Latin genus—Digitalis—also refers to a finger, or thimble.

In fact, it was in Britain that its usefulness as a heart medication was first discovered in 1775, when the physician to Benjamin Franklin discovered that a cold infusion made from the dried, powdered leaf of the foxglove acts as a heart stimulant and also a diuretic. The strengthened heart pumps more blood through the kidneys, carrying off water that has accumulated in the tissues.

Foxglove is considered by some to be a magical plant, ruled by the planet Venus, and has, since ancient times, been considered to be an herb of protection.

Welsh housewives rubbed foxglove leaves into the stone cracks in their floors and painted crossed lines on the floor with foxglove dye to prevent evil from entering their homes.

Digitalis works by slowing the heartbeat and making it stronger, thereby increasing the efficiency of the heart. It reduces congestion in the veins and causes the kidneys to produce more urine. In the past, digitalis was administered by using the entire leaf, until digitoxin was isolated in 1869. Digoxin was isolated in 1930, which allowed physicians to refine the dosage and control the drug's action on the heart. No synthetic drug has been discovered that can take the place of *Digitalis purpurea*.

Recent research also suggests digitalis may be beneficial against glaucoma and as a component in a drug program in the treatment of muscular dystrophy.

Poisonous part   All parts of this plant—particularly the leaves—are poisonous and contain several glycosides that affect the heart and kidneys as well as irritant saponins. Ingestion of the dried or fresh leaves, which are not rendered harmless by cooking, will cause a severe case of poisoning. Most cases of foxglove poisoning have resulted from therapeutic overdose or by drinking foxglove herbal teas, not from accidental ingestion. Children have been poisoned after sucking on flowers or swallowing the seeds.

Symptoms   Eating even small amounts of foxglove leaves, flowers or other parts can dangerously disrupt heartbeat rhythm. In large amounts it can depress heart function or stop it completely. Symptoms appear within 20 to 30 minutes after ingestion and include nausea, vomiting, diarrhea, stomach pain, severe headache, blurred vision, loss of appetite, irregular heartbeat and pulse, delirium, tremors, convulsions and death from paralysis of the heart muscle. In excess amounts, foxglove increases the force of the heart's contractions to the point where it causes irritation and stimulates the central nervous system. Some sensitive individuals experience headache, rash and nausea from handling the plant.

Treatment   Gastric lavage followed by the administration of activated charcoal, together with potassium chloride every hour (unless urination stops). Victims must have their heart and potassium levels constantly monitored.

See also DIGITALIS; DIGITOXIN; DIGOXIN; GLYCOSIDES; SAPONIN.

free base cocaine   The cocaine alkaloid (or base) that results when the hydrochloride is removed from cocaine hydrochloride, a common form of the drug.

See also COCAINE; NARCOTICS.

fungicide   Fungicides are inorganic and organic compounds used to protect against rot and eliminate fungi. While some are fairly nontoxic to humans, others are extremely poisonous. Among the most common substances used as fungicides are mercury and copper compounds, pentachlorophenol, dithiocarbamates, tetramethylthiuram disulfide, hexachlorobenzene and iodine.

G

galerina mushroom *(Cortinarius speciosissimus, C. gentilis, G. venenata, G. autumnalis* and *C. orellanus)* Members of the *Cortinarius* genus, they cause some of the same symptoms. The brown-capped galerinas are also known as deadly cort, deadly galerina and deadly lawn galerina; all are supertoxic.

C. orellanus is found primarily in Europe; *C. gentilis, G. venenata, G. autumnalis* (deadly galerina) and *C. speciosissimus* are found throughout the United States, particularly in the Northeast.

Poisonous part The poison orellanin found in these mushrooms is toxic to the kidneys, but experts believe the mushrooms contain other as-yet-unidentified poisons.

Symptoms Latency period following ingestion is longer than 10 hours and may last as long as two weeks; when symptoms appear, they include acute stomach pain, headaches, pain in back or joints, kidney failure, damage to the intestines, genital organs, liver, heart and nervous system. The victim's course may seem to improve, only to worsen and improve again until death finally occurs several months later.

Treatment There is no antidote or successful treatment known. Vomiting soon after ingestion may expel the poison, and medical treatment may save some victims.

See also CORT MUSHROOMS; MUSHROOM POISONING; MUSHROOM TOXINS.

gasoline See PETROLEUM DISTILLATES.

gelsemine A plant alkaloid found in yellow jessamine, gelsemine depresses and eventually paralyzes motor nerve endings, with contractions or spasms and—in severe cases—convulsions and respiratory arrest.

See also ALKALOIDS; JESSAMINE, YELLOW.

giant milkweed *(Calotropis procera, C. gigantea)* This tree is found in the tropical Americas and Africa; its sap is used as an arrow poison in Africa. The treelike shrubs have rubbery leaves and clusters of white or lilac flowers with a sweet scent. The seeds have silky attachments, similar to other types of milkweed seeds, which are shaken from the pods as they dry. The two species are different heights (*C. procera* is less than six feet; *C. gigantea* may grow to 15 feet).

Poisonous part The latex sap contains a mixture of cardiac glycosides with digitalis-like action, and unidentified allergens.

126

Symptoms   Ingestion results in irritation, burning and swelling of the mucous membranes, but because of the bad taste ingestion of large amounts is not normally a problem. In addition, skin contact may cause an allergic reaction. Exposure to the eyes (cornea) may cause a severe keratoconjunctivitis.

Treatment   The ingestion of a large amount of this plant may produce heart irregularities, which are managed by monitoring an electrocardiogram.

See also CARDIAC GLYCOSIDES; DIGITALIS.

giardiasis   An infection of the small intestine caused by the protozoan *Giardia lamblia*, which is found in the intestinal tract and feces. Contamination occurs when sewage is used as a fertilizer or when food handlers don't wash their hands. Although giardiasis is generally found commonly in tropical countries and travelers to those areas, in recent years outbreaks have been common in the United States among people in institutions, preschool children and in catered affairs and large public picnic areas. It is most common in this country where large numbers of young children gather. It is spread by contaminated food or water or by direct personal hand-to-mouth contact. Infection can be prevented by thoroughly washing hands before handling food.

Symptoms   Giardiasis is not fatal and will eventually pass, and about two-thirds of infected people have no symptoms. When they do occur, symptoms appear about one to three days after infection and are uncomfortable. They include explosive diarrhea, foul-smelling and greasy feces, stomach pains, gas, loss of appetite, nausea and vomiting. In some cases, the infection can become chronic. Giardiasis is diagnosed by examining a fecal sample for the presence of the parasites.

Treatment   Acute giardiasis usually runs its course and then clears up, but antibiotic metronidazole or quinacrine will help relieve symptoms and prevent the spread of infection.

See also FOOD POISONING.

Gila monster   *(Heloderma suspectum)*   The Gila monster is one of only two poisonous lizards in the world; both are similar in appearance and habits. This sluggish, shy little fellow grows to about 20 inches, with a stout body, black and pink spots and bands extending onto a blunt tail and beadlike scales. It has a black face, with large toes and strong claws, and is smaller than its poisonous relative, the Mexican beaded lizard.

Named after the Gila River Basin, the Gila monster lives in the gravelly and sandy soils found in the deserts of the Southwest, particularly in Arizona, southern Utah and New Mexico. It prefers rocks and other animals' burrows; it may also dig its own holes. Gila monsters mate during summer and lay between three and five eggs in autumn and winter, and more than 95 percent of their time is spent underground.

Poisonous part   The venom of this lizard, used principally to immobilize prey, is extremely dangerous for humans as well. It is produced in eight glands in the lower jaw; venom is secreted into the mouth and then flows through the grooves of the teeth into the bite wound as the lizard chews; it is not injected as is snake venom. The whole system is not particularly efficient, requiring the Gila monster to hang on to its prey for some time and chew its tissues, enabling the poison to flow. The bite is extremely painful but rarely fatal (no deaths have been reported in modern times), but the Gila monster is extremely tenacious; often the victim must be cut away.

Symptoms   Severe pain at the wound site, swelling, weakness, tinnitus (ringing in the ears), nausea, breathing problems, cardiac failure and sometimes death. Symptoms occur within one to three hours after the bite; their severity depends on the amount of venom injected, where the wound is located and the victim's health.

Treatment   There is no known antivenin. Treatment is supportive, with tetanus prophylaxis and pain relief.

See also MEXICAN BEADED LIZARD.

glue   See SOLVENT ABUSE.

glycoside   Also known as glucosides, the glycosides are more common in the plant kingdom than alkaloids. Glycosides are a group of compounds containing at least one type of sugar that are released when the plant is eaten. ("Glyco" comes from the root word meaning "sugar.") The amount of glycoside in a plant depends on genetics, the part of the plant, its age and, to a large degree, environmental factors such as climate, moisture supply and fertility of the soil. While many glycosides are not poisonous, a number of them are, including cardiac glycosides, cyanogenic glycosides and saponins.

Glycosides that yield hydrocyanic acid after hydrolysis are called cyanogenetic; one of the most common is the glycoside amygdalin, found in many members of Rosaceae plants that have cyanogenetic compounds, including hydrangea, flax, cassava, lima bean, cherries, apple, white clover, and vetch seed.

See also ALKALOIDS; CARDIAC GLYCOSIDES; CYANOGENIC GLYCOSIDES; SAPONIN.

golden dewdrop (*Duranta repens* L.) [Other names: pigeon berry, sky-flower.] This large shrub usually cultivated as a hedge is native to Key West and is also found in southern Texas, the West Indies, Hawaii, Guam and Australia. It produces small, light blue or white flowers and masses of poisonous orange berries.

Poisonous part   The berry contains toxic saponins, but reports of poisoning with them have occurred only in Australia.

Symptoms   Sleepiness, fever, tachycardia, swelling of the lips and eyelids, convulsions and gastrointestinal irritation.

Treatment   Gastric lavage, control of convulsions with diazepam and maintenance of fluid and electrolyte balance.

See also SAPONIN.

gout stalk   *(Jatropha podagrica)*   This plant is a member of a large genus of shrubs or small trees with a three-sided seed capsule, found throughout the New World.

Poisonous part   The seeds are poisonous and contain jatrophin (curcin), a plant lectin (toxalbumin) and cathartic oils. Ingestion of just one seed can be serious. The plant lectin inhibits protein synthesis in cells of the intestinal wall and may cause serious or fatal poisoning.

Symptoms   The onset of symptoms (nausea, vomiting and diarrhea) occurs rapidly, unlike poisoning with other plants with toxic lectins.

Treatment   Treat symptoms; give fluids.

ground cherry   *(Physalis)*   There are about 17 species of this plant growing in the United States, most with an attractive fruit resembling a Chinese lantern; inside the papery pod is a berry filled with tiny seeds.

Poisonous part   The unripe berries are poisonous and contain toxic solanine glycoalkaloids.

Symptoms   While solanine rarely is toxic to adults, children can be fatally poisoned. Symptoms include stomach irritation, a harsh, scratchy feeling in the throat, diarrhea and fever.

Treatment   Replace fluids, treat symptoms and give supportive care.

grouper, spotted   Any of a number of species of fish in the family Serranidae (including yellowfin) widely found in warm seas with large mouths and heavy bodies; they can grow to be more than six feet long. Many carry a toxic substance in the flesh that can cause ciguatera, a form of poisoning, when eaten. Ciguatera is caused by blue-green algae, which is eaten by reef herbivores, which are in turn eaten by larger fish.

Poisonous part   The toxin believed to be involved in ciguatera is fat soluble, odorless and tasteless and is not destroyed by heat.

Symptoms   After eating, symptoms may develop quickly or slowly and involve tingling sensations in the lips and mouth followed by numbness, nausea, vomiting, abdominal cramps, weakness, paralysis, convulsions, skin rash, coma and death in about 12 percent of cases.

Treatment   Recent research suggests that pralidoxime chloride (a cholinesterase reactivator) is an effective antidote.

See also CIGUATERA; FISH CONTAMINATION; FOOD POISONING.

grouper, yellowfin   See GROUPER, SPOTTED.

Gyromitra   This species of mushroom, also known as the false morel, contains a toxin usually removed during cooking, although a few individuals are sensitive to it even when cooked completely. The species has no gills, and its spores develop in microscopic sacs on the surfaces of the fruiting bodies. The appearance of the body of the fungus gives this mushroom its nickname, brain fungi. While many species of *Gyromitra* are edible, it usually takes an expert to tell the difference.

   Poisonous part   While the chemical ingredient in this species is not known, many varieties contain gyromitrin, which is hydrolyzed to form the active toxin monomethylhydrazine, a substance that affects the central nervous system and is also used as rocket fuel. This toxin is volatile and dissolves readily in water; therefore, the mushroom may be made edible by air drying or extracting the toxin with boiling water.

   Symptoms   Between six and 24 hours after ingestion or inhalation of the vapor while cooking, symptoms suddenly appear: The victim begins to vomit and develops dizziness, fatigue and muscle cramps. In severe cases, this may be followed by delirium, coma and convulsions and can sometimes be fatal. In nonfatal cases, victims recover within two to six days.

   Treatment   Supportive, which may include blood transfusions and correction of acidosis. Intravenous pyridoxine is the specific antidote.

   See also MONOMETHYLHYDRAZINE; MUSHROOM POISONING; MUSHROOM TOXINS.

H

habu, Okinawa *(Trimeresurus flavoviridis)*   The most dangerous pit viper in Asia, this large, aggressive snake, known as one of the collective group called fer-de-lance, is found on the Amami and Okinawa groups in the Ryukyu Islands—often in houses. Marked with a wavy band of dark green splotches, it sometimes grows to be five feet long and can cause disability or death. Its smaller relative, the kufah *(Trimeresurus okinavesis)*, is also dangerous. Both are happy to live in trees, along with the other genus of this group, *Agkistrodon*.

Symptoms   Because the venom interferes with the coagulation of the blood, it hemorrhages into muscles and the nervous system and results in bleeding from the gums, nose, mouth and rectum. Shock and respiratory distress is followed by death if untreated.

Treatment   Antivenin is available.

See also ANTIVENIN; FER-DE-LANCE; PIT VIPERS; SNAKES, POISONOUS.

Halcion   See BENZODIAZEPINES; SLEEPING PILLS.

Haldol   See ANTIPSYCHOTIC/PSYCHOMETRIC DRUGS.

hallucinogenic mushrooms   A group of mushrooms, important to the sacred ceremonies of the American Indian religions (and also to drug abusers), that produce hallucinations when eaten. These mushrooms include three main groups: the psilocybes *(Psilocybe caerulescens, P. mexicana, P. pelliculosa, P. cyanescens, P. baeocystis, P. cubensis)*, conocybes *(Conocybe cyanopus, C. smithii)* and stropharias, all of which produce visual and auditory hallucinations about 15 minutes after eating.

The *Conocybe* and *Psilocybe* mushrooms contain psilocybin and psilocin as active constituents.

Symptoms   The onset of effects for all varieties usually occurs with three hours of ingestion, and symptoms include drowsiness, loss of ability to concentrate, dizziness and sometimes muscle weakness. The hallucinogenic effects are dose dependent and may vary according to the personality of the person; both space and time distortion are reported, together with visual and auditory imagery. The hallucinations are usually described as pleasant.

Treatment   Recovery following ingestion of such a mushroom is normally uneventful. The period of intoxication is not long, usually between three and six hours, after which all symptoms disappear. However, there is a danger that patients may become destructive during the hallucinatory period, and therefore their movements should be restricted. Phenothiazine drugs may be used to end the psychosis if extreme agitation is experienced.

See also MEXICAN HALLUCINOGENIC MUSHROOM; MUSHROOM POISONING.

harlequin snake   See CORAL SNAKE, EASTERN.

hemlock, deadly   See HEMLOCK, POISON.

hemlock, ground   See YEW.

hemlock, lesser   See HEMLOCK, POISON.

hemlock, poison *(Conium maculatum)* [Other names: California fern, deadly hemlock, herb bonnett, kill cow, lesser hemlock, muskrat weed bunk, Nebraska fern, poison parsley, poison root, snake weed, spotted hemlock, spotted parsley, wode whistle.] The ancient poison drink of Socrates, poison hemlock is rapidly fatal. The plant (which resembles a carrot) has large lacy leaves as much as four feet long that produce a disagreeable garlicky odor when crushed, and a white root. It is found in South America, northern Africa and Asia, and in the United States and Canada where it has been naturalized. In Europe, it is called "fool's parsley."

Poisonous part   Leaves are most toxic when the plant is flowering, but all parts of the hemlock are deadly. Its root resembles the wild carrot, and its seeds have been mistaken for anise. Hemlock contains coniine, a muscle relaxant similar to curare, and related alkaloids. In addition, quail may eat poison hemlock seeds and pass on the poison to a human who consumes the flesh. This type of secondary hemlock poisoning can cause diarrhea, vomiting and paralysis in humans within three hours of eating the affected quail.

Symptoms   Responsible for many human fatalities, hemlock poisoning can begin within 30 minutes after ingestion. Symptoms include gradual muscular weakness and increasing muscular pain, paralysis, blindness, respiratory problems, and death within several hours, which comes from paralysis of the lungs.

Treatment   Gastric lavage must be performed immediately after ingestion of the poison or it is ineffective; give diazepan to relieve convulsions.

See also ALKALOIDS; CONIINE.

hemlock, water *(Cicuta maculata, C. californica, C. douglasii, C. vagans, C. bolanderi, C. bulbifera, C. curtissii, C. occidentalis)*   One of the most poisonous plants and the most violent poison contained in plants in the United States, the several species of water hemlock are found in waste places, pastures and swamps of the northern temperate regions. Water hemlock is a perennial herb and member of the carrot family, growing up to eight feet tall with purple spots and small, white, heavily scented flowers. Underground, there is a bundle of roots that, when cut, smell very much like parsnips. Water hemlock *(C. maculata)* is found in eastern North America to the Great Plains; California water hemlock *(C. californica, C. bolanderi)* in midwestern California; Douglas water hemlock *(C. douglasii)* along the Pacific coast and British Columbia; tuber water hemlock or Oregon water hemlock *(C. vagans)* in the Pacific Northwest; western water hemlock *(C. occidentalis)* in the Rocky Mountain states to the Pacific coast; bulbous water hemlock *(C. bulbifera)* in the northern United States.

Poisonous part The entire water hemlock contains the poison cicutoxin, although the root has the most. Many people have been poisoned by mistaking water hemlock for parsnips or artichokes, and children have been poisoned by using water hemlock to make peashooters and whistles. One mouthful of the root may kill an adult, and many Americans (especially children) have died after eating this plant; 30 percent of water hemlock poisonings are fatal. The powerful nerve toxin causes excruciating spasms and convulsions so powerful that people have been known to bite through their own tongue and break their teeth.

Symptoms This is a fairly fast acting toxic plant, with symptoms beginning 15 minutes after ingestion, including restlessness, abdominal pain, nausea, vomiting, diarrhea, respiratory problems, hypersalivation, weak and rapid pulse, delirium, violent convulsions and—within one hour—death.

Treatment Both emetics and cathartics are used to get the poison out of the body, and morphine and barbiturates can control convulsions. Once seizures appear imminent or have already occurred, gastric lavage should not be attempted without an anesthesiologist. Prolonged problems in mental function and abnormal electroencephalograms have been reported.

henbane *(Hyoscyamus niger)* [Other names: black henbane, devil's eye, fetid nightshade, henbell, hog's bean, insane root, Jupiter's bean, poison tobacco, stinking nightshade.] This powerful plant is the most common species of the nightshade/potato family Solanaceae, comprising 11 biennials or perennials. Naturalized in the eastern United States, it is grown commercially in North America and is found wild in garbage dumps and in isolated spots in Great Britain, central and southern Europe and western Asia.

The annual form of the plant grows to one to two feet tall and then flowers and sets seed; the biennial produces only a tuft of basal leaves that disappear in winter leaving a root. In the spring, a branched flowering stem grows from this root that is usually much taller and more vigorous than the flowering stems of the annual plants. The whole henbane plant has a strong, unpleasant odor, and its leaves, if bruised when fresh, emit a strong narcotic smell similar to that of tobacco. Its root is a long, tapering brown tuber with a bad odor and could be mistaken for parsnips and eaten, with fatal results.

Three drugs are made from the dried leaves of the henbane plant: Atropine, hyoscyamine and scopolamine. In addition, the leaves are smoked as a narcotic and are prepared as a beverage in India.

Poisonous part   All parts of the plant are poisonous, especially the seeds, pods and leaves, which contain varying amounts of the belladonna alkaloids atropine, hyoscyamine and scopolamine. The seeds have the highest amount of scopolamine, which depresses the central nervous system.

Symptoms   A fast-acting toxin (within 15 minutes), henbane produces symptoms similar to those caused by deadly nightshade or atropine poisoning. Children are poisoned by eating seeds and pods. Poisoning causes dry mouth, tachycardia, fever, blurred vision, excitement, delirium and confusion; hallucinations are frequently reported in children.

Treatment   If poisoning is severe, a slow intravenous administration of physostigmine is given until symptoms subside.

herbicides   Chemicals used to kill weeds. They can be divided into two groups: those that are poisonous to anything with which they come in contact, including animals and humans in addition to weeds; and those that are poisonous only to a selected group of weeds and will not harm humans or animals. Contact weed killers commonly used include sodium chlorate, dinitrophenol derivatives, potassium cyanate, sodium arsenite, caustic acids and alkalis, petroleum distillates, trifluralin, diquat and paraquat.

See also PARAQUAT; PETROLEUM DISTILLATES.

herbs, unsafe   Long before the beginnings of modern medicine, the earliest health care practitioners—the shamans, the medicine men and the healers—prescribed herbs and herb extracts to treat disease. Many of these herbal medicines were beneficial (for example, digitalis heart drugs are extracted from foxglove). But many of the early remedies have been discovered to be quite dangerous—even toxic—inducing violent episodes of vomiting or seizures and causing serious liver, kidney or other organ damage. Some cause abortions, and others are simply of no value at all.

According to the Food and Drug Administration, there are three categories of herbs: unsafe herbs, herbs of undefined safety for food use and safe herbs (GRAS—generally recognized as safe). For its own purposes, however, the FDA considers herbs as foods, not as medicine. Still, the FDA notes that even the GRAS herbs can cause problems if used to excess. "Too much of any herb is toxic," the FDA warns in one of its reports. In particular, eating too much red pepper, sorrel or nutmeg can be decidedly toxic.

While plant ingestions are second only to drugs as the most common poisoning emergency in children, serious poisoning or death from ingesting herbs is rare because the amount of toxin is usually quite small. However, there has been an increase over the past 20 years in the public use of herbal remedies and traditional herbal healing products.

In fact, brewing or mixing some herbal remedies can be dangerous, not only because of the toxic makeup of the plants, but because the content of various toxins varies considerably with the soil and climate conditions in which the plant was grown. Beneficial and harmful components in any herb can vary tremendously from one garden to another, from one year to another and even from one plant to another in the same garden grown at the same time.

Unfortunately, in addition to natural toxicity in some plants, "herbal" or "traditional" preparations may sometimes actually contain drugs such as phenylbutazone, corticosteroids, salicylates, ephedrine or toxic metal salts (mercury or lead).

Herbal mail-order suppliers and health food stores do a brisk business in health food products, and there are almost 400 different herbs available in the form of commercial teas; there are almost 200 herbs blended into a variety of commercial cigarettes or smoking mixtures. But some teas contain plants that can be very dangerous—nutmeg, mandrake or jimsonweed (identified as "thorn apple," its other name).

See also COMFREY; DIGITALIS; FOXGLOVE; JIMSONWEED; MANDRAKE, AMERICAN; NUTMEG.

heroin (diacetylmorphine) A narcotic drug derived from morphine, the principal alkaloid of opium, which is extracted from the pods of the opium poppy and often processed in Turkey. Currently, the Middle East is the world's primary morphine/heroin source.

Heroin was created in an attempt to find a safer type of morphine, and the resulting product was a would-be cough medicine called Heroin, named for the drug's presumably "heroic" ability to mimic the effects of morphine without causing addiction. Developers hoped the new drug would be used to cure morphine addiction. Unfortunately, heroin is in fact highly addictive.

Heroin is a white or brown powder (depending on where it has been processed) that can be smoked, sniffed or dissolved in water and injected. It can be smoked when the end of a cigarette is dipped in heroin powder and lighted (this is called ack-ack); "chasing the dragon" or "playing the organ" involves mixing heroin with barbiturates. The drug is lighted and the smoke inhaled. Subcutaneous injection is called skin popping; intravenous injection is mainlining.

In addition to its painkilling properties, heroin produces sensations of warmth, calmness, drowsiness and a loss of concern for outside events. Long-term use causes tolerance, which means the user needs more and more of the drug to maintain the same level of intoxication. It also produces both psychological and physical addiction. Sudden withdrawal of the drug causes shivering, abdominal cramps, diarrhea, vomiting, sleeplessness and restlessness.

It was originally invented to cure morphine addiction, but in fact heroin is more toxic than morphine or codeine, since it acts primarily on the respiratory system. Heroin is also four times more addictive than morphine.

As yet, there is no legal medical use for heroin in the United States, although a few researchers are investigating its ability to control cancer pain. Heroin is an accepted cancer painkiller in Britain; because it is stronger than morphine, it is a better and longer-lasting pain reliever.

Symptoms Heroin is a central nervous system depressant. An overdose frequently results in death. Following an injection, the user feels an immediate rush; if an overdose, death occurs within a few minutes unless the drug was sniffed or injected under the skin (then death may take up to four hours). Symptoms include pinpoint pupils, slow and shallow breathing, vision problems, restlessness, cramps, cyanosis, weak pulse, low blood pressure, coma and death from respiratory paralysis.

Treatment The antidote is naloxone; treat symptoms.

See also MORPHINE; OPIUM, NARCOTICS.

holly *(Ilex)* There are about 400 species of red- or black-berried plants, including the popular Christmas hollies, American holly *(Ilex opaca)* and English holly *(I. aquifolium)*. The hollies have alternate, glossy and thick-spined leaves (either single or clustered) with small, green flowers and bright red or black berries. Male and female flowers are usually on separate plants.

American holly is native from Massachusetts to Florida, west to Missouri and Texas; English holly is cultivated from Virginia to Texas, the Pacific coast states and British Columbia. Yaupon *(Ilex vomitoria)*, also known as Carolina tea and emetic holly, is native to the Atlantic and Gulf coast states and North Carolina to Texas and Arkansas.

Poisonous part Berries (and in some reports, leaves) of this plant are poisonous and contain alkaloids, glycosides, saponins and terpenoids, caffeine and theobromine (a caffeinelike alkaloid). In some species, the leaves are brewed for their caffeine and other xanthines.

Symptoms In small doses, holly may be a nervous system stimulant. In large doses, it can cause nausea, vomiting, diarrhea, inflamed and numb sensations in the mouth, drowsiness and altered state of consciousness. The berries are particularly poisonous and can be fatal to children if enough are eaten and the symptoms are not treated. Some estimate that 20 berries are poisonous, but a fatal dose may be less in children.

Treatment Treatment for gastroenteritis—administer fluids to prevent dehydration.

See also ALKALOIDS; GLYCOSIDE; SAPONIN.

honey Honey of any type can contain *Clostridium botulinum* spores, which are harmless to everyone *except infants under one year of age.* For this reason, infants should never be fed raw honey of any type, since botulism spores can be fatal to this group.

See also BOTULISM; BOTULISM, INFANT; FOOD POISONING.

horse nettle See CAROLINA HORSE NETTLE.

hyacinth *(Hyacinthus orientalis)* A plant widely cultivated throughout the United States for its fragrant bell-shaped flowers.

Poisonous part The bulb of this plant is poisonous.

Symptoms Ingestion of the bulb of the hyacinth causes severe stomach problems, which, while not fatal, can be very painful.

Treatment Perform gastric lavage or induce vomiting; treat symptoms.

hydrangea *(Hydrangea)* The hydrangea is considered to be one of the most poisonous plants. About 80 species of this common flowering shrub are found throughout the entire Western Hemisphere; *H. macrophylla* is the most popular.

This deciduous mounded shrub can grow to be 15 feet, with large oval leaves with toothed edges up to six inches long, and white, pink or blue flowers in a showy cluster. Flower color usually depends on the acidity of the soil, and the color grows brown as the flowers age.

Poisonous part All parts of the plant (but especially the flower buds) are toxic and contain the poison hydrangin, which is believed to produce toxic cyanide compounds activated by stomach acids.

Symptoms Several hours after ingestion, the glycosides decompose in the gastrointestinal tract and release the poison, which causes gastroenteritis and other cyanide poisoning symptoms. Cyanosis may develop, and in cases of large doses, convulsions, coma and death.

Treatment Gastric lavage followed by a 25 percent solution of sodium thiosulfate. In unconscious victims, acidosis should be corrected and shock treated together with the administration of oxygen to aid breathing. Cyanide antidote should be administered.

hydrocarbon An organic compound that contains primarily hydrogen and carbon atoms, usually of biological origin. Hydrocarbons include ethylene, acetic acid (vinegar), methylene chloride, formaldehyde, benzene, DDT, PCB, propylene, butylene, toluene and xylene.

hydrochloric acid (hydrogen chloride) Hydrochloric acid is usually marketed as a solution containing 28 to 35 percent by weight hydrogen chloride, commonly known as concentrated hydrochloric acid. It is also found in the stomach lining, forming part of the stomach juices and important in the digestion of proteins.

A fatal dose of hydrochloric acid is almost impossible to swallow, since the highly corrosive nature of the acid would close up the throat. Skin absorption or breathing in the vapors can cause fatalities, however. The acid produces burns, ulcers and scarring, destroying any tissue it touches.

Symptoms   Eye contact will cause blindness; skin contact will result in redness, peeling, burns and scarring. Inhalation will inflame the throat, tongue and lungs and cause coughing, choking, headaches, dizziness and weakness followed some hours later by chest constriction, foaming at the mouth and cyanosis. Blood pressure falls while pulse races, as pulmonary edema is followed by death.

When ingested, hydrochloric acid can cause burning pain, vomiting, bloody diarrhea, low blood pressure, swelling of the throat (causing suffocation) and a usually fatal peritonitis.

Treatment   Administer a mild alkali (such as milk) to neutralize acid; treat symptoms as they appear.

hydrogen peroxide   This popular antiseptic found in most home medicine cabinets is used as a mouthwash, to treat infections and to bleach hair and is usually sold in concentrations of 3 percent. Toddlers frequently ingest hydrogen peroxide, but it is considered to be of low toxicity. It generally breaks down in the gastrointestinal tract before it can be absorbed in the body; as it decomposes, however, it may release large amounts of oxygen, causing stomach distention and nausea.

hydrogen sulfide   This is an irritant gas that occurs in the presence of decomposing vegetables or animals, such as in liquid manure pits, sewers, tanneries, fishing boats or coal mines; its presence is announced by the distinctive smell of rotten eggs. Hydrogen sulfide is also an industrial by-product of petroleum refineries and blast furnaces.

Symptoms   Poisoning with this gas resembles that of cyanide and interferes with the body's oxygen supply. In mild exposure, it causes painful and reddened eyes, blurred vision and seeing colored halos around lights. In higher amounts, it can cause cyanosis, confusion and pulmonary edema; at very high levels, it can cause an almost immediate fatal coma. In the case of serious poisoning, the fatality rate is 6 percent.

Treatment   Remove the victim from exposure; give oxygen and intravenous nitrite therapy. There is no antidote to hydrogen sulfide poisoning. If the victim lives for four days, recovery is likely, although there are lingering side effects for months (including lethargy, headache, fatigue, memory loss and lack of initiative).

hydromorphone   The chemical name for Dilaudid, this is a potent analgesic used for moderate to severe pain available in a wide variety of forms (tablet, injection, rectal suppositories and oral solution). It has become a highly abused drug because of its euphoric effects. Clinical effects of this drug are quite similar to those of morphine at similar doses.

Symptoms Chronic use may result in both physical and psychological addiction, but an overdose—even in those who have been chronic abusers—may cause breathing problems and death. Acute overdose causes depression of the central nervous system, convulsions, shock, cardiopulmonary arrest, low body temperature, pneumonia, low blood pressure and slow heart rate.

Treatment Induced vomiting is not recommended; however, gastric lavage may be performed even several hours after ingestion, followed by the administration of activated charcoal and a saline cathartic. Seizures may be controlled with intravenous diazepam. Naloxone may be administered.

See also MORPHINE; NARCOTICS; MEDICATIONS AS POISONS.

hypochlorite   See ALKALINE CORROSIVES.

I

ibuprofen   (Trade names: Motrin, Nuprin, Motrin IB, etc.) See NONSTE-
ROIDAL ANTI-INFLAMMATORY DRUGS.

indane derivatives   These insecticides are chemicals that dissolve readily
in fat and include aldrin, dieldrin, endrin, kepone, chlordane, and heptachlor, although chlordane, heptachlor, aldrin and dieldrin have all been
banned. Of these, aldrin is the most toxic; recent cancer studies in rodents
have suggested that heptachlor (contained in chlordane) is a carcinogen.
Food and Drug Administration studies suggest that 70 percent of all meat,
fish, dairy products and poultry in the United States contain residues of these
pesticides. And the EPA found that 97 percent of Americans tested in a 1973
study had heptachlor and chlordane present in fatty tissues.
   Symptoms   After ingestion or skin contamination, acute poisoning
causes excitability, tremors, restlessness and convulsions. In animals, lower
doses are associated with liver problems; humans with liver disease may be
more sensitive to indane exposure.
   Treatment   Gastric lavage followed by saline cathartics. Avoid all fats
and oils (including milk), since they increase the rate of absorption.
Administer phenobarbital sodium for tremors and barbiturates for
convulsions, and provide oxygen if necessary. If the skin has been
contaminated, wash with soap and water immediately to head off skin
problems and systemic absorption. Remove contaminated clothing.
   See also ALDRIN; CHLORDANE; DIELDRIN; ENDRIN; INSECTICIDES.

Indian tobacco *(Lobelia inflata)*   [Other names: asthma weed, bladderpod,
eyebright, lobelia.] This deadly poisonous plant with its attractive red, white
and blue flowers is found in waste areas, along roadsides and in woodland
throughout eastern North America, westward to Nebraska and Arkansas.
Used homeopathically to treat laryngitis and asthma, it was also dried and
smoked by Native Americans. It gets its name from the Flemish botanist
Matthais de L'Obel.
   Indian tobacco is an annual or biennial relative of the bellflowers, with its
flowers appearing in July and August as loose spikes and alternate, toothed
leaves. Similar in many respects to nicotine, Indian tobacco has been
advertised as a substitute for tobacco and as a weight-reducing aid.
   Poisonous part   The entire plant is poisonous and contains alkaloids
of lobeline and lobelamine. These toxins act by exciting, and then
depressing, the central nervous system. In limited amounts Indian tobacco

can open the bronchioles, but in larger amounts it can slow breathing and cause a drop in blood pressure. In addition, leaves, stems and fruit cause a skin rash.

Symptoms   Quite similar to nicotine poisoning, ingesting Indian tobacco causes symptoms within one hour, including nausea, vomiting, weakness, tremors, convulsions, coma and death. As little as 50 mg of the dried plant, or one ml of tincture of Indian tobacco, can cause these reactions.

Treatment   Gastric lavage, artificial respiration and the administration of atropine and Valium.

See also NICOTINE.

indomethacin   (Indocin) See NONSTEROIDAL ANTI-INFLAMMATORY DRUGS.

inky cap   *(Coprinus)*   The inky cap is the common name for the 100 different types of mushroom species of the genus *Coprinus*, which get their name from the fact that after the mushrooms discharge their spores, the cap disintegrates into an inklike liquid that has been used for writing. The mushrooms are found growing on dung or buried wood, and the caps of *C. atramentarius* and *C. comatus* (shaggy mane or shaggy cap) are edible if picked young, before the gills turn black.

Symptoms   While these mushrooms are edible, the coprine in the mushrooms is similar to disulfiram (Antabuse) and interferes with the metabolism of ethanol, causing intoxication when alcohol is drunk within 72 hours of eating the mushroom. The alcohol is believed to increase the solubility and absorption of the poison and causes giddiness, nausea, vomiting, sweating, breathing problems and even tachycardia. Many victims recover within a few hours, but eating a large amount of mushrooms with alcohol can result in low blood pressure and cardiovascular collapse. The reaction persists for several hours.

Treatment   Supportive, including the administration of intravenous fluids. There is no antidote, and once they appear, the symptoms usually fade within several hours.

See also ANTABUSE; COPRINE; MUSHROOM POISONING; MUSHROOM TOXINS.

***Inocybe* mushroom**   These members of the cort family range in toxicity from mild to fairly poisonous, but none are as toxic as the *Amanita* mushrooms; the most dangerous are the *I. napipes* and *I. fastigiata*. They are found in pine forests throughout the United States, with graey-brown spores and small, brown caps.

Poisonous part   These mushrooms contain the parasympathetic stimulant muscarine, which is not affected by cooking and affects the autonomic nervous system and the liver.

Symptoms   Ingesting small concentrations of muscarine is associated with sweating and sometimes abdominal pain; other symptoms develop rapidly and include salivation, cyanosis, weak muscles, twitching, weak pulse, delirium, hallucinations and convulsions, but rarely death. Heart attacks occur only 4 percent of the time, since treatment is generally started in time to prevent this. Intoxication usually subsides within two hours.

   Treatment   Induce vomiting or perform gastric lavage, since it is possible to get rid of the poison this way and recover quickly. Atropine is the antidote for muscarine poisoning and may be given to those who experience severe discomfort or anxiety.

   See also AMANITA MUSHROOMS; CORT MUSHROOMS; MUSCARINE; MUSHROOM POISONING; MUSHROOM TOXINS.

inorganic chemical insecticides   One of four major groups of insecticides, the inorganic chemical insecticides include arsenic compounds, fluorides, thallium, selenium, metaldehyde, mercury, phosphorus, sodium borate, hydrocyanic acid (cyanide), pyrethroid and antimony.

   See also ANTIMONY; ARSENIC; CYANIDE; INSECTICIDES; MERCURY; METALDEHYDE; PHOSPHORUS; SELENIUM; THALLIUM.

insecticides   There are many wide-spectrum or all-purpose products to kill insects, and in the past most were synthetic chemical compounds created in laboratories to mimic nature. These products were convenient and effective; however, gardeners came to recognize that such panaceas carry certain penalties—they poisoned more than the insects they were designed to attack.

   Today, insecticides fall into two groups: those that coat the outside of a plant, and those that are absorbed by the roots, stems or leaves into the plant itself. There are six major types: minerals, such as kerosene or borax; botanicals or natural organic compounds (nicotine, pyrethrin and orotenone); chlorinated hydrocarbons (DDT, lindane, chlordane); organophosphates (malathion and diazinon); carbamates (carbaryl and propoxur); fumigants (such as naphthalene) and benzene (mothballs, etc.).

   Newer insecticides include insect-growth regulators and natural predators (such as beetle-eating wasps, or insect-killing bacteria).

   While all insecticides are toxic, most fatal poisonings occur only when large quantities are accidentally or intentionally ingested or inhaled.

   See also BENZENE; BOTANIC INSECTICIDES; CARBAMATE; CHLORDANE; CHLORINATED HYDROCARBON PESTICIDES; DDT; LINDANE; MALATHION; NAPHTHALENE; ORGANOPHOSPHATE INSECTICIDES.

insect repellents   Substances that, when applied or sprayed on the skin, repel mosquitoes, gnats and other insects. Because these products are designed for human use, they are generally considered nontoxic, although they are not recommended for use on small children. While poisoning from insect repellents is rare, there have been a few cases of toxicity with DEET (diethyltoluamide).

insulin   Insulin is a hormone produced by the pancreas. Supplements of insulin have been used to treat diabetes mellitus since 1922; today, they are used in all cases of insulin-dependent diabetes mellitus, and sometimes for non–insulin-dependent diabetes when oral hypoglycemic drugs don't work. These supplements are produced from pig or ox pancreas and by genetic engineering; there are a variety of short-, medium- and long-acting insulins available. Insulin may either be injected by the patient before meals or introduced with an insulin pump to deliver the hormone over a 24- hour period. Oral doses of insulin are not absorbed and are not toxic.

Symptoms   An overdose can cause hypoglycemia (low sugar level) with dizziness, sweating, irritability and weakness; severe hypoglycemia coma and permanent brain damage have occurred following injections of 800–3,200 units of insulin.

Treatment   Administer concentrated glucose as soon as possible after drawing blood samples; treat symptoms.

See also MEDICATIONS AS POISONS.

iodine   This element is one of the oldest antiseptics used in medicine, found most often in compound form as an antiseptic and cough remedy. Discovered in 1811, tincture of iodine was first used in 1839 by a French surgeon and put to work again on the battlefields of the American Civil War. It remains a popular choice for home medicine cabinets today as an inexpensive skin antiseptic. It is also used in contrast dyes for X rays and fluoroscopy, and in making dyes, photo film, water treatment and medicinal soap.

The brownish element is not soluble in water but dissolves readily in alcohol; it is available in solid and tincture preparations. While earning a deadly reputation as a serious poison, iodine does not often cause toxic poisonings in the amounts normally found in the household. Iodoform, iodochlorhydroxyquin and sodium and potassium iodides are all powders or crystals with similar solubility.

Symptoms   Oral ingestion of iodine produces toxic symptoms similar to those of acid corrosives; absorbed through the skin, it is toxic because of its ability to be well absorbed through the skin of burn patients or neonates. Iodine is a central nervous system depressant and also interferes with cellular activity. Following ingestion, symptoms include vomiting, diarrhea, abdominal pain, thirst, shock, fever, delirium, stupor and death. A fatal dose of iodine and iodoform is about 2 g. However, food in the stomach inactivates iodine by converting it to harmless iodide. Fatalities from iodochlorhydroxyquin and iodide salts are rare. Accidental ingestion of the tincture is rarely fatal, since it is not rapidly absorbed.

When iodine is applied to the skin, it can cause hypersensitivity in some people, including a fever and generalized skin reaction. Because of this sensitivity in some individuals, iodophors have generally replaced the use of iodine tinctures; one of the most widely used iodophors is a complex of povidone and iodine (Betadine). These iodophors are compounds of iodine linked to a carrier agent.

Treatment   After acute ingestion, give milk immediately followed by a starch solution (such as 15 mg of cornstarch or flour to 500 ml of water). Vomiting is not advisable if there is any esophageal injury, and milk should be repeatedly given every 15 minutes to ease stomach irritation. Antidote is sodium thiosulfate, which reduces iodine to iodide. In the event of an allergic reaction, administer epinephrine and intravenous hydrocortisone.

ipecacuanha *(Cephaelis ipecacuanha)*   Ipecacuanha is a poisonous plant found throughout Europe and South and Central America and is the plant source for ipecac syrup, which is used, ironically, as an emetic to rid the stomach of poisons. (When used incorrectly, however, this syrup can be fatal.) *The fluid extract from the plant is 14 times more toxic than the commercially available ipecac syrup and should never be used as a substitute.*

Poisonous part   The berries and juice are most toxic and contain the alkaloid emetine, which weakens the heart.

Symptoms   Vomiting occurs immediately after ingestion but may not be fatal until 24 hours to a week later. Recovery can take up to a year.

Treatment   Gastric lavage, morphine and bed rest.

See also IPECAC SYRUP.

ipecac syrup   A substance that makes people vomit (an emetic), ipecac syrup (also called ipecacuanha) comes from the dried roots of a poisonous shrub *(Cephaelis ipecacuanha)* found in Europe and Central and South America. The commercially available syrup is used in the treatment of accidental poison to remove the toxic substance from the stomach before it is absorbed into the blood.

It is a thick, amber liquid that will stay fresh for several years in a tightly closed container stored at room temperature. It is available over the counter in syrup form but should be kept out of the hands of youngsters, as ipecac is poisonous.

Ipecac syrup should never be given to a suspected poisoning victim unless instructed to do so by a health care specialist. Not all poisons require the removal of the poison, and sometimes vomiting can be dangerous—especially if the toxic substance is caustic or petroleum based. Syrup of ipecac should not be given to anyone not fully conscious or to a child under age one without careful supervision. While ipecac syrup saves lives, it is itself poisonous and should never be given in more than two doses. More may be toxic.

In a recent study (the first ever done in an emergency room on pediatric poisonings), researchers at Children's Hospital of Buffalo tested whether giving ipecac in addition to charcoal would help remove poison from the body even better. In that study, 32 of 70 children less than six years old at the hospital took syrup of ipecac before taking activated charcoal; the rest of the group received charcoal alone. The children treated with both took an average of 39 minutes *longer* to recover than the group treated with charcoal alone. Doctors had to wait from 30 minutes to two hours until the ipecac's work was done and the children stopped vomiting so they could administer the charcoal. Even then, the queasy feeling caused by the ipecac made it more difficult for the children to keep from vomiting the gritty charcoal solution, while most of the children who took the charcoal alone had no problems.

Because time is so important in the treatment of poisoning cases, many scientists now believe that activated charcoal alone may be the better emergency room treatment. Ipecac only empties the stomach of its toxic contents, but by the time a child sees a physician in the emergency room, it has usually been at least an hour since the poison was ingested and chances are the poison has already traveled into the small intestine.

Ipecac taken within five minutes of ingestion will remove about 50 or 60 percent of the poison, which can reduce a substance like aspirin to a safe level. But after an hour, only 20 percent of the poison will come back up. At that point, activated charcoal does a better job, since it can pass through the intestine, bind with the poison and move it out of the body through the stool.

Charcoal, then, may well replace ipecac in hospitals. At home, however, charcoal is more difficult to administer because children don't like the tasteless, gritty solution. According to Allan Kornberg, M.D., head of the emergency medicine department at the Children's Hospital of Buffalo and author of the above study, ipecac should continue to be used at home for emergencies—but always with the guidance of a poison control center.

While the correct dosage should be prescribed by a physician or poison control center, a normal dose for a person over age one is 2 tbsp. followed by at least two to three glasses of water, *not milk*. If the victim hasn't vomited within 20 minutes, the dose may be repeated. If the victim doesn't vomit after the second dose, call the poison control center for further instructions. If possible, the victim should vomit into a container so the material can be identified by medical experts at the hospital. Vomiting is effective only if it occurs within four hours of ingestion of a solid substance, or within two hours after ingestion of a liquid.

See also CHARCOAL ACTIVATED; IPECACUANHA.

iron supplements   Dietary supplements that contain iron (ferrous sulfate, ferrous gluconate, ferrous fumarate) are common—but overlooked—potential poisons in children. An acute overdose of iron can damage the stomach and small intestine, affect blood circulation and damage the liver and other organs, causing shock and even death. Young children have been seriously injured by swallowing doses of 200–400 mg of iron, equivalent to 14–27 children's vitamin-and-mineral supplements with iron or 4–7 tablets of a typical adult iron supplement. More than 2,000 people are poisoned each year with iron, and a large number of these poisonings are fatal; mortality may be as great as 50 percent.

Iron is used by the body to produce the red blood cells that transport oxygen, and it helps the cells in the muscles and other parts of the body turn oxygen into energy. But recent research by a team of Finnish researchers links excess iron stored in the body to heart disease. Men who ate iron-rich food (such as red meat) faced a higher likelihood of heart attack. The findings could help force public health experts to rethink dietary recommendations for iron ingestion, since even normal levels of stored iron may prove damaging. Over-the-counter vitamin supplements often contain iron, as do some enriched foods such as cereals.

Up until the late 1800s, iron therapy was used to treat anemia, but it later fell out of favor. Recently, however, ferrous sulfate has been widely prescribed to treat iron deficiency anemia, and its popularity has greatly increased the risk of poisoning. There are about 120 iron products currently marketed in the United States.

The exact mechanism behind iron poisoning is not known, nor is it understood how death results—whether from shock, from systemic effects due to the passage of large amounts of iron into the blood or from the metabolic effects of absorbed iron, which cause respiratory collapse.

Symptoms Within 30 minutes of overdose, the first symptoms appear: lethargy, vomiting, fast and weak pulse, low blood pressure, shock, pallor, cyanosis, acidosis, clotting problems and coma. Then, symptoms may disappear, and the victim may seemingly begin to improve. One or two days later, the victim goes into shock, with pulmonary edema, vasomotor collapse, coma and death within 12 to 48 hours.

Treatment Control shock; perform gastric lavage with sodium bicarbonate and administer a chelating agent. Peritoneal dialysis or hemodialysis, or early exchange transfusion, may be needed. Give supportive and symptomatic therapy as required, including multiple vitamins and antibiotics.

See also VITAMINS.

irritant oils Some glycosidal oils in high concentrations can irritate the digestive tract. While in small quantities they are harmless (such as the oils in plants of the mustard family, horseradish and radishes), in large amounts they are more upsetting and cause the irritations found with some plants of the buttercup family and anemone species.

See also VOLATILE OILS.

isopropanol See ISOPROPYL ALCOHOL.

isopropyl alcohol Widely used as a solvent, antiseptic and disinfectant, isopropyl alcohol (also known as isopropanol) is found in products such as shave lotion and window cleaners and is twice as toxic as its relative ethyl alcohol. It is also found in the home as a 70 percent solution (rubbing alcohol), which is commonly drunk by alcoholics as a substitute for liquor. But unlike other common alcohol substitutes (methanol and ethylene glycol), isopropyl alcohol is not metabolized to highly toxic organic acids.

While the effects of isopropyl poisoning resemble drunkenness, they may last up to four times longer than those induced by alcoholic drinks. Rubbing alcohol can be swallowed, inhaled (as a vapor) or absorbed. In fact, alcohol sponge baths were once prescribed as a way to reduce fever, until it was discovered that the alcohol sometimes produced a nonfatal coma.

Isopropyl alcohol is a potent central nervous system depressant, and ingestion or inhalation of it can cause coma and respiratory arrest. It is metabolized to acetone, which may contribute to and prolong the central nervous system depression.

Symptoms Within 10 to 30 minutes after ingestion (depending on how much food is in the stomach), overdose symptoms appear: nausea, vomiting, stomach pain, depressed respiration, vomiting blood, excessive sweating, hemorrhage in the trachea and bronchial tubes, pneumonia, swelling, and coma.

Treatment There is no specific antidote. Ethanol is not given as an antidote, and if the victim has only drunk a few swallows or more than 30 minutes has passed, there is no point to emptying the stomach, since the alcohol is rapidly absorbed after ingestion.

However, for large ingestions, perform gastric lavage (do NOT induce vomiting) and administer activated charcoal and a cathartic, although charcoal will not absorb isopropyl alcohol very well. Hemodialysis removes isopropyl alcohol and acetone, but it is usually not necessary because the majority of victims can be managed with supportive care alone. Dialysis is indicated when levels are very high, or if low blood pressure does not respond to fluids.

See also ETHANOL; ETHYL ALCOHOL; METHANOL.

isoproterenol This drug, similar to catecholamines, is useful in the treatment of excessively slow heartbeat following an overdose of beta blockers.

ivy *(Hedera)* Of the five species in the genus *Hedera*, *H. helix* (English ivy) is the most common. This form is poisonous if eaten because of the presence of saponins; in small amounts it can cause stomach upset and a tingling sensation around the mouth, but large amounts can lead to labored breathing, convulsions and coma. While no fatal cases have been reported in the United States, European children have been poisoned with this plant.

English ivy is a climbing evergreen plant with three- or five-lobed leaves and a woody stem and prefers shade and damp, moist ground. Occasionally, it produces black berries. There are more than 200 cultivars, and ivy has been a known toxicant since early Greek times.

Poisonous part   All parts of the ivy plant are poisonous if eaten and contain the saponin hederin.

Symptoms   Burning sensation in the throat, nausea, vomiting, diarrhea, excitement, difficulty in breathing, abdominal pain, excess salivation and skin irritation; rarely, it causes coma.

Treatment   Traditional treatment of gastroenteritis and fluid replacement, especially in young children.

See also SAPONIN.

J

jack -o'- lantern fungus *(Clitocybe illudens)* This cousin of the *Inocybe* mushroom also contains muscarine and induces sweating. An orange fungus found growing on wood, it can induce severe vomiting but is not fatal.

Symptoms This fungus can cause gastrointestinal upset. Ingestions of small amounts of the parasympathetic stimulant muscarine contained in these mushrooms also cause vomiting and blurred vision.

Treatment Intoxication usually subsides after two hours; when the victim experiences severe discomfort or anxiety, atropine may be given. Other treatment is symptomatic.

See also INOCYBE MUSHROOM; MUSHROOM POISONING; MUSHROOM TOXINS.

jellyfish Although the term is used to refer to any marine member of a group of invertebrates, the true jellyfish family includes about 200 species, all of which are disk-shaped animals with four, eight or more dangling tentacles, found drifting along the shoreline. Jellyfish, together with corals, sea anemones and Portuguese men-of-war all belong to the group of marine animals called coelenterates, which have tentacles with capsules that sting when touched.

Most common in tropical waters, jellyfish float on the surface of the water, trailing tentacles that can penetrate human skin and inject venom. Most live for only a few weeks, but some live as long as a year, and the deep-sea species may live longer. Jellyfish are by far the most common of the coelenterates and cause a significant number of injuries in the United States coastal areas.

Produced in a wide variety of sizes, colors and shapes, jellyfish often are almost transparent with brilliant tentacles, ranging from a few millimeters to more than two meters across the top. Because some varieties have such long tentacles, it is possible to be stung without ever seeing the top of the jellyfish floating on the surface. Jellyfish are also dangerous after storms have broken them up and sprinkled them across the sandy beaches, where they can still sting—even when dry.

One of the most poisonous of the jellyfish is the sea wasp, which swims from Queensland north to the central Atlantic coast of the United States; a moderate sting from a sea wasp can cause death within a few minutes. While most stings from poisonous fish and jellyfish may not cause much harm, some jellyfish and Portuguese men-of-war can inflict severe stings, and the victim may panic and drown. The lion's mane jellyfish *(Cyanea capillata)* is the giant of all the species of jellyfish, its sac reportedly measuring eight feet or more across. Its tangle of poisonous tentacles arranged in groups of eight (each group with 150 tentacles) may reach over 100 feet long. The lion's mane ranges in the Atlantic and Pacific oceans, and although it is not believed to be fatal to humans, its sting is very painful. The most common jellyfish is the moon jellyfish, only slightly venomous and found in all warm and temperate waters.

Symptoms Stings from a jellyfish cause severe burning pain and a red welt—or a row of lesions—at the site of the sting. Some victims also suffer from headache, nausea, vomiting, muscle cramps, diarrhea, convulsions and breathing problems. In the water, the initial shock of the sting may cause a swimmer to jerk away, which stimulates the tentacles to release more poison. On shore, more poison is released if the victim tries to rip off the sticky threads. On those who have been stung by jellyfish but survive, the wounds from the jellyfish stings become red blisters that can leave permanent scars. One or two weeks after the sting, the victim may experience a recurrence of the lesions at the site, which can be treated with antihistamines.

In the United States, it is not particularly important to identify the type of coelenterate, but in Australia (where many lethal varieties exist) it is crucial.

Treatment Alcohol, ammonia or vinegar and salt water (*do not use fresh water*) poured over the site of the sting will deactivate the tentacles, which should then be scraped off with a towel or with sand held by a bath towel—*not the hand*. Pull off—do not rub—the tentacles. The tentacles will continue to discharge their stinging cells (nematocysts) as long as they remain on the skin. Watch carefully for signs of shock or breathing problems.

Baking soda in a paste with water should be applied to the sting to relieve pain; after an hour, moisten again and scrape off the baking soda with an object to remove any remaining nematocysts. Calamine lotion also will help ease the burning sensation, and painkillers may help with the stinging pain. (Other local remedies for pain include meat tenderizer, sugar, ammonia and lemon juice.)

Jellyfish often cause allergic reactions, which can be eased by the administration of Benadryl or a steroid. A severe reaction to the sting requires hospitalization and perhaps CPR. Antivenin, effective against more dangerous species, may be available but must be administered immediately together with a tourniquet. Another type of jellyfish, the Portuguese man-of-war, is rarely fatal but causes hives, numbness and severe chest, abdominal and extremity pain. If given early, the calcium blocker verapamil may be effective.

See also PORTUGUESE MAN-OF-WAR.

Jerusalem cherry *(Solanum pseudocapsicum)* One of the nightshade family, this popular houseplant has luscious orange or red berries that are deadly poison. It is a decorative pot plant and has escaped from cultivation in Hawaii and the Gulf Coast states.

Poisonous part   Human poisoning is usually attributed to immature fruit, which contains the toxin solanine glycoalkaloid, the poison of the true nightshades.

Symptoms   While there is little danger of fatal poisoning in adults, children may ingest a fatal amount of this plant. Symptoms appear several hours after ingestion and include gastric irritation, scratchy throat, fever and diarrhea (solanine poisoning is often confused with bacterial gastroenteritis).

Treatment   Provide the same general supportive care that would be given in gastroenteritis cases; fluid replacement may be required.

See also NIGHTSHADE, DEADLY.

jessamine, yellow   *(Gelsemium sempervirens)*   Also known as Carolina jessamine, this plant is a highly toxic member of the olive family which has about 300 tropical and subtropical species of fragrant, flowering shrubs. The plants are found in woodlands and are native to all continents except North America. Still, it is found today from eastern Virginia to Tennessee, and Arkansas south to Florida and west to Texas; it is also grown in parts of California.

A perennial evergreen with lance-shaped leaves and fragrant, bright yellow flower clusters, the plant has a small fruit capsule with winged seeds. It is not a member of the jasmine species *(Jasminum)*, which causes only a mild skin rash.

Poisonous part   All parts of this plant contain the poisons gelsemine, gelsemicine and other related alkaloids, which cause strychninelike effects. There are cases of children who were poisoned after sucking on the flowers; honey made from the nectar of this plant has been implicated in three deaths.

Symptoms   At high doses, poisoning can be fatal in 10 minutes, but it may take several hours in lower doses. Symptoms include frontal headache, dizziness, drooping eyelids, sweating, weakness, convulsions, anxiety, difficulty in breathing, depression and death through respiratory failure.

Treatment   Immediate gastric lavage with instillation of a slurry of activated charcoal, intravenous fluids and respiratory support.

See also GELSEMINE.

jimsonweed   *(Datura stramonium)*   [Other names: apple of Peru, devil's trumpet, Jamestown weed, mad apple, stinkweed, thornapple.] Responsible for more poisonings than any other plant, jimsonweed is an extremely deadly member of the potato family. Originally called "Jamestown weed," it got its name in 1666 following a mass poisoning in the town when starving soldiers ate the berries of the plant. Jimsonweed is found throughout much of the Northern Hemisphere in roadside and waste places but never in mountains or woods.

An annual, jimsonweed grows to about six feet with ovate, unevenly toothed, strong-scented leaves; large, white or violet trumpet-shaped flowers; and a large, spiny fruit (often called a thornapple). Seeds are small and dark brown or black when ripe and yield what is called "datura." Jimsonweed is the source for the alkaloidal drug hyoscyamine. There are about 15 species of *Datura*, and while all are poisonous, their fragrance can be sweet or unpleasant depending on the season.

Poisonous part All parts of this plant are poisonous and harbor belladonna alkaloids (the poisons hyoscyamine, hyoscine and atropine). The juices, seeds and wilted leaves are especially deadly. Four to five grams of crude leaf or seed will be a fatal dose for a child. Poisonings have occurred from sucking nectar from the flower tube or eating fruits containing the poisonous seeds.

Symptoms Within several hours after ingestion, the first symptoms appear: excessive thirst and dry mouth, dilated pupils, dry, hot and flushed skin, headache, vertigo, weak pulse, visual difficulty, fever, hallucinations, disorientation, urinary retention, decreased bowel activity, high blood pressure, delirium, convulsions, coma and death. Handling the leaves and rubbing the eyes can dilate the pupils.

Treatment Sedatives are effective for convulsions, and a purgative may also be used. If intoxication is severe, slow intravenous administration of physostigmine is usually advised until symptoms diminish.

K

kerosene See PETROLEUM DISTILLATES.

kokoi frog One of the "arrow poison" frogs, this frog has a venom in its skin that has been used for centuries as an arrow poison by the Cholo Indians of Colombia. Ten times more deadly than the toxin found in the Japanese pufferfish, it is the most active venom known. The molecular structure of the toxin found in the kokoi frog is related to that of steroid hormones secreted by the adrenal gland.

Symptoms The toxin in the kokoi frog blocks the transmission of nerve impulses to the musculoskeletal system, causing death within minutes.

Treatment There is no known antidote.

See also ARROW POISON FROGS.

krait, blue *(Bunguras coeruleus)* This is one of the nonhooded members of the cobra family; it has powerful venom but seldom bites humans. Still, of those who *are* bitten, nearly half die if untreated. The krait is generally passive and has shiny scales and bands of yellow and black, or white and black.

Similar to the blue krait is the banded krait, or pama (*B. fasciatus*), also a member of the cobra family. This variety is almost harmless, although larger than its blue krait cousin. While the venom is lethal, bites are very rarely reported.

The kraits are fairly small and are mainly nocturnal; when disturbed, they tend to roll up into a loose ball and only bite under great provocation. They are found throughout most of southern Asia and range from four to seven feet long with light and dark bands and short fangs.

Symptoms The venom of snakes in the cobra family contains a neurotoxin chemically different from that of other snakes. While there is little local reaction, within 15 to 30 minutes more generalized symptoms appear: pain, swelling, a drop in blood pressure and confusion followed by death if the poison spreads to the respiratory muscles. The venom from this snake family is twice as toxic as strychnine and nearly five times more toxic than that of a black widow spider.

Treatment Immediate administration of specific antivenin — only the specific antiserum for the type of cobra involved should be used. Many types of antivenins are available for the krait bite in southern Asia; other antivenins are produced in Bangkok for both the blue krait and the pama.

See also ANTIVENIN; COBRA; SNAKES, POISONOUS.

L

labetalol This drug is used in the treatment of high blood pressure and racing heartbeat associated with stimulant drug overdose (such as cocaine or amphetamines).

laudanoisine See MORPHINE.

laudanum A solution of opium once used as a sedative and painkiller and to treat diarrhea. It was created in the 16th century by the Swiss physician Paracelsus, and it was a popular medication during Victorian times, when physicians would prescribe it for women suffering from "the vapors." Elizabeth Barrett Browning, Charles Baudelaire, Theophile Gautier, Alexandre Dumas, Edgar Allan Poe and Samuel Taylor Coleridge were all users of laudanum; in fact, Coleridge wrote his poem "Kubla Khan" while in an opium reverie. Unfortunately, the pleasurable effects that laudanum brought came at a cost: long, dry spells in their creativity and occasional loss of ambition. In order to achieve the euphoric effects, they had to risk overdose and addiction.

See also MORPHINE; NARCOTICS; HEROIN; OPIUM.

laurel, mountain *(Kalmia latifolia)* [Other names: Alpine laurel, calfkill, calico bush, hook heller, ivy bush, lambkill, mountain ivy, narrow-leaved laurel, pale laurel, poison laurel, sheep laurel, spoonwood, swamp laurel.] Like its cousin the rhododendron, the evergreen mountain laurel is a deadly narcotic poison found in moist areas and rocky hills throughout North America. Ancient Greek legends reported that these two plants poisoned Xenophon's army by honey made from the flowers' nectar. Closer to home, the Delaware Indians used wild laurel for suicide.

The ornamental bush grows to heights from four to eight feet, with three-inch-long leaves and white, pink or purple flowers appearing in June and July. The leaves may also be poisonous to animals, which in turn can poison any other human or animal who eats the meat. Native to North America, the plant is not a true laurel but a member of the heath family.

K. latifolia grows in the northeastern United States but not in Canada; *K. angustifolia* grows in eastern North America from Ontario to Labrador east to Nova Scotia, and south to Michigan, Virginia and Georgia; *K. microphylla* is found from Alaska to central California.

Poisonous part All parts of the plant are poisonous, especially the leaves and nectar (in honey), and contain carbohydrate andromedotoxin—the same poison as rhododendron. A tea made from two ounces of the leaves of the laurel has caused poisoning.

Symptoms Usually beginning within six hours, they include severe gastrointestinal distress, watery eyes and mouth, respiratory problems and bradycardia followed by depression, convulsions, paralysis, coma and death. Death from mountain laurel poisoning may occur anywhere from several hours to days after ingestion. Children can be poisoned by eating leaves.

Treatment Gastric lavage, fluid replacement and respiratory support; atropine for bradycardia and ephedrine for hypotension that does not respond to fluid replacement.

See also RHODODENDRON.

laxatives A group of drugs used to treat constipation. There are a variety of types of laxatives, each causing different symptoms in overdoses. They include bulk forming, stimulant, lubricant and saline. In addition, chronic overuse can produce bowel function dependency.

Symptoms Stimulant laxatives may cause abdominal cramps and flatulence; prolonged use of saline laxatives is likely to cause a chemical imbalance in the blood. Lubricant laxatives may coat the intestine and prevent vitamin absorption. Resulting diarrhea from laxative overdose causes fluid and electrolyte imbalance.

Treatment Since systemic absorption is not really a problem, laxative overdose is simply treated by reestablishing the fluid and electrolyte imbalance caused by diarrhea. In cases where the patient is at risk for dehydration, perform gastric lavage or induce vomiting followed by the administration of activated charcoal.

See also MEDICATIONS AS POISONS.

lead poisoning Lead poisoning in adults is rare, but unfortunately it is one of the most common and preventable childhood health problems today. It can be a problem for those who lick or eat flakes of old paint containing lead. Lead can also contaminate water flowing through old lead pipes, slowly poisoning those who drink it. Lead poisoning causes the most damage to the brain, nerves, red blood cells and digestive system and is considered to be a cumulative poison, since it remains in the bones for as long as 32 years and in the kidneys for seven. Several recent studies have also shown that high levels of lead in the blood can hinder a child's growth, and this may occur early in the chemical chain of events regulating bone growth—perhaps in the brain.

Lead poisoning in children is particularly serious because it doesn't take much lead to harm a child and the potential damage to the child's developing neurological system is much more serious. Furthermore, the danger of lead poisoning is especially great with young children, who tend to put everything into their mouths—which is how lead dust and flecks from old lead paint get into children in the first place.

In 1991, the Centers for Disease Control lowered the amount of lead it considers dangerous in children, from 25 microliters to 10 microliters per deciliter of blood.

Although lead is found in many different products, it is most often associated with paint; until about 40 years ago, all house paint contained some amount of lead. Lead was added to paint because it helped the paint dry more quickly and gave it a shinier and harder finish. In fact, the more lead in a can of paint, the better and more expensive the product; some paints were as much as 50 percent lead.

By the late 1970s, laws were passed to regulate the amount of lead in paint, but they did nothing about the lead-filled paint already on the walls in millions of older homes throughout the United States. It is this lead-based paint—often found in inner-city homes—that causes most of the lead poisoning in children. Children suck and chew on toys and furniture, pick at peeling paint and eat the chips they pull off and even chew on windowsills. Today, 57 million American homes still contain lead paint; 14 million housing units have high levels of lead in dust or chipping paint, and 3.8 million of these housing units have young children living there. If a house was built before 1950, chances are very high that its paint contains the toxic substance; if it was built between 1950 and 1978, there is still a 50 percent chance that it has lead paint.

Lead poisoning is usually a chronic problem, building up in the body over a period of time. When a child eats lead, the body absorbs about 10 to 15 percent of the metal, slowly excreting the rest. Most of the absorbed lead is stored in the child's bones, with smaller amounts in the bone marrow, soft tissues and red blood cells. If the child continues to ingest lead, large amounts will accumulate and eventually reach a toxic level. If the lead poisoning is not noticed and corrected, the toxic lead levels in the child's body can lead to serious complications, including mental retardation.

According to the Centers for Disease Control, the usual source of lead poisoning among adults is contamination in the workplace. It is also possible to get lead poisoning from drinking liquor from illegal stills with lead piping, or inhaling fumes from burning battery casings. Eating or drinking anything contained in lead-glazed or lead-soldered containers can also contribute to lead poisoning; even storing—and then drinking—wine in lead crystal decanters may contribute to the problem. And almost everyone is exposed to lead from cars' exhaust fumes, although atmospheric lead levels have recently decreased thanks to legislation requiring autos manufactured after 1975 to use only unleaded gasoline.

According to the Food and Drug Administration, the lead-foil wraps around wine bottles are another potential source of lead poisoning among adults. When drinking from these bottles (which will be found in home wine

---

LEAD REMOVAL

- To temporarily reduce lead paint and dust, clean floors, windowsills and window wells at least twice a week with a trisodium phosphate detergent available at hardware stores. Sponges used for this purpose should not be used for anything else.
- Move cribs and playpens away from chipped or peeling paint.
- Wash the child's hands, face and toys often.
- Children and pregnant women should not be in the area while removing lead paint.
- Never sand, scrape or burn off lead paint; this disperses toxic particles onto other surfaces and into the air. Dry scrape, cover the contaminated area or hire a professional.
- Before beginning work, protect all food, clothing, appliances, utensils, bedding, toys and clothing from dust by either removing them or bagging them in plastic and sealing tightly.
- Never attempt a large lead-removal project yourself; working with lead can be very risky for the untrained.
- If hiring a lead abatement contractor, ask specific questions about credentials. Where was he trained? How much experience does he have in lead abatement? How does he protect his workers? How does he dispose of the toxic material?
- All members of the family should be checked for lead poisoning once renovations are complete.

---

cellars, restaurants and hotels for many years to come), it is important to be sure the lead is twisted off below the lip of the bottle, and to wipe the lip before pouring. Other sources of lead include juice or food contained in an improperly fired ceramic dish coated with lead- based glaze; painted furniture; and color-tinted newspapers.

"Lead" pencils, however, are not made of lead, but of nontoxic graphite. In any event, one should not encourage a child to eat or chew on them.

While lead poisoning is almost always a chronic problem, it is possible—albeit extremely rare—to suffer from an acute case of lead poisoning, when a large amount of lead is taken in by the body over a short period of time.

Home test kits for testing lead paint are sold in hardware stores throughout the country.

Symptoms Lead is excreted very slowly from the body, so it builds up in tissues and bones and may not even produce detectable physical effects, although it can still cause mental impairment. If they do appear, early symptoms include listlessness, irritability, loss of appetite and weight, constipation and a bluish line in the gums followed by clumsiness, vomiting, stomach cramps and a general "wasting." Acute poisoning symptoms include a metallic taste in the mouth, abdominal pain, vomiting, diarrhea, collapse and coma. Large amounts directly affect the nervous system and cause headache, convulsions, coma and, sometimes, death.

Treatment Individuals with suspected lead poisoning should be given a simple blood test, which can determine the level of lead in the blood. A person with enough absorbed lead in the body to show symptoms will probably require hospitalization. Treatment usually includes the administration of medicines (called chelating agents) to help the body rid itself of lead. In mild cases, the chelating agent penicillamine may be used alone; otherwise, it may be used in combination with edetate calcium disodium and dimercaprol. In acute cases, perform gastric lavage.

Lepiota **mushrooms** *(Lepiota josserandii, L. brunneoincarnata, L. helveola, L. subincarnata)* The poisonous mushroom *L. josserandii* contains the deadly poison amatoxin, and the others in the *Lepiota* genus are assumed to contain amatoxins as well. Amatoxins prevent protein synthesis and cause cell death, sometimes affecting the kidneys as well. These mushrooms are not made less toxic by drying, cooking or boiling in water.

Symptoms Initial symptoms are caused by amatoxin on the intestine. After about 12 hours following ingestion, the victim experiences persistent nausea and vomiting, intestinal pain and watery diarrhea. This is followed by a period of remission of up to five days, followed by liver problems similar to those caused by acute viral hepatitis.

Treatment Give fluids and monitor electrolytes; maintain urine flow, since amatoxins are partially excreted by the kidneys. Give repeat doses of activated charcoal with water. If the victim will recover, it will occur within one week. European physicians suggest a wide range of additional therapy, including high-dose vitamins, corticosteroids, sex hormones, glucose, penicillin G. and thioctic acid; their value has not been established.

See also AMATOXINS; MUSHROOM POISONING; MUSHROOM TOXINS.

Librium See BENZODIAZEPINES.

lidocaine A local anesthetic related to cocaine, this is a synthetic version of the coca bush alkaloids. It is used to control possible irregular heartbeat following poisoning by a variety of cardioactive drugs and toxins (such as digoxin, cyclic antidepressants, stimulants and theophylline. It is also used to relieve pain and irritation caused by sunburn or hemorrhoids, to numb tissues before minor surgery and as a nerve block. It is used topically to relieve pain when inserting needles, and it is given intravenously as an antiarrhythmic agent following a heart attack to reduce the danger of ventricular arrhythmias (irregular heartbeat).

Although lidocaine is used to treat poisoning by other drugs, it is also toxic itself if used excessively.

Symptoms Immediately upon ingestion, lidocaine causes giddiness followed by dizziness, blue color, low blood pressure, tremors, irregular and weak breathing, collapse, coma, convulsions and respiratory arrest.

Treatment Efforts to remove the drug after 30 minutes are useless. The ingested drug must be removed, and absorption from the injection site limited by tourniquet and wet cloths. Give oxygen and artificial respiration until the nervous system depression lifts. If the victim survives for one hour, recovery outlook is good.

See also ANTIDEPRESSANTS; DIGOXIN; MEDICATIONS AS POISONS; THEOPHYLLINE.

lighter fluid See PETROLEUM DISTILLATES.

lily of the valley *(Convallaria majalis)* Often mistaken for wild garlic, the beautiful white-flowered plant is deadly—*even the water in which the flowers are kept is toxic.* Found throughout western North America through the Midwest and into Canada and Britain, the plant also occasionally bears orange-red berries. It is a hardy perennial, with hanging, bell-shaped white flowers and smooth, dark green leaves, and spreads by underground roots to form thick beds.

Poisonous part All parts of this plant are poisonous, especially the leaves. The poison, which is similar to digitalis, is a glycoside called convallatoxin; the plant also contains irritant saponins.

Symptoms Immediately after ingestion, the following symptoms appear: nausea, rash, headache and hallucinations. If large amounts are eaten, dizziness and vomiting may occur one or two hours later; slow heartbeat can lead to coma and death from heart failure.

Treatment Gastric lavage together with cardiac depressants to control cardiac rhythm. Activated charcoal may be given and repeated later, and saline cathartics may also be used.

See also GLYCOSIDE; SAPONIN.

lindane The common name for cyclohexane hexachloride, this is a synthetic organic insecticide used to control insects resistant to DDT and those that attack cotton. A cancer-causing agent, lindane was formerly used as a general-purpose insecticide against indoor pests. The Environmental Protection Agency canceled the registration of all indoor fumigating devices containing lindane in 1986.

Symptoms Less serious poisoning incidents will result in nausea, dizziness, headache, tremor and weakness. Acute cases of ingestion or skin contamination cause vomiting and diarrhea, excitability, loss of a balance and convulsions. If the insecticide also contains an organic solvent, symptoms may also include breathing problems and cyanosis followed rapidly by circulatory failure. Exposure to the fumes from a thermal insecticide vaporizer can cause eye, ear, nose or throat irritation in addition to the above symptoms. While symptoms will fade after exposure ends, there have been reports of the development of aplastic anemia.

Treatment Gastric lavage followed by saline cathartics. Avoid all fats and oils (including milk), since they increase the rate of absorption. Administer phenobarbital sodium for tremors and barbiturates for convulsions, and provide oxygen if necessary. If the skin has come in contact with these insecticides, wash with soap and water immediately to head off skin problems and systemic absorption. Remove contaminated clothing.

See also DDT; INSECTICIDES; PESTICIDES; SYNTHETIC ORGANIC INSECTICIDES.

lionfish *(Pterois)* [Other names: butterfly cod, firefish, rock perch, turkeyfish.] The lionfish includes any of several species of the scorpionfish family often found off the beaches in Barbados, where it hides in coral and stings unwary swimmers. Lionfish are famous for their poisonous fin spines, which can produce a painful sting that is not usually fatal but extremely uncomfortable.

While these fish would normally not cause a problem, their beautiful coloring makes them desirable aquarium species. The fish have 18 spines along their back, which sometimes break off in the wound, leading to secondary infections and sometimes gangrene. Unaggressive fish, they drift peacefully along the coral reefs in which they live.

Symptoms Perspiration, tachycardia, vomiting, diarrhea and intense abdominal pain. The wound site is swollen, inflamed and painful, with the pain radiating outward.

Treatment Supportive; local anesthetic can ease pain around the wound site.

See also SCORPIONFISH.

listeriosis A rare but potentially fatal illness caused by eating toxic food contaminated by the *Listeria monocytogenes* bacterium. The illness is common among cattle, pigs and poultry but is rarely found in humans; however, it is more likely to strike those with compromised immune systems, the elderly and pregnant women.

In the past 10 years, there have been several outbreaks that seem to have been linked to the ingestion of soft cheeses (such as feta and some types of Mexican cheeses) and deli-type lunchmeats. While most people don't have to worry about the disease, scientists at the Atlanta-based Centers for Disease Control warn that pregnant women, the elderly and those with damaged immune systems might want to avoid deli-counter foods and soft cheeses.

Symptoms Ingesting the bacteria can cause blood poisoning, flu-like symptoms, complications of pregnancy and stillbirths. In severe cases, it can lead to meningitis (an infection of the membranes covering the brain and spinal cord).

Treatment   Administration of antibiotics clears the infection in most cases.

See also FOOD POISONING.

lithium   Appearing either as a pill (lithium carbonate) or liquid (lithium citrate), this is the treatment of choice for manic-depression, for which it is given orally. It is also used to treat alcohol toxicity and addiction and schizoid personality disorders, and sometimes to boost the white blood cell count in persons with leukopenia.

However, toxic levels can be quickly reached, causing fatal acidosis or alkalosis, particularly in chronic overmedication for long-term treatment. For this reason, patients given lithium treatment should have frequent blood checks to make sure a toxic level has not been reached. Lithium is not recommended for those who have kidney or heart disease or for women in early or late pregnancy.

It should not be taken with alcohol (combination can result in lithium poisoning); combination with caffeine reduces lithium's effect, and combination with cocaine can cause psychosis. In addition, lithium in combination with a wide range of drugs can cause a variety of problems, including increased toxicity, hypothermia, major seizures and excessive sedation.

Poisonous part   It is not clear how lithium produces toxic effects, but it seems to focus primarily on the kidneys. Lithium is thought to stabilize cell metabolism; in large amounts it depresses neural function, but entry into the brain is slow. This explains the delay between peak blood levels and central nervous system effects after acute overdose.

Symptoms   Within 15 minutes to an hour after ingestion of an excessive dose, tremors appear followed by twitching, apathy, difficulty in speaking, anorexia, hair loss, sodium retention, dry mouth, seizures, blurred vision, confusion, and coma and death. After acute ingestion, victims experience mild nausea and vomiting, but these are delayed for several hours. Patients with chronic intoxication have more serious symptoms, and toxicity may be severe with levels only slightly above recommended doses.

Treatment   There is no specific antidote. Stop administering lithium and give sodium chloride intravenously. In the ingestion of acute large doses, perform gastric lavage and administer activated charcoal followed by a saline cathartic. Drink plenty of fluids; dialysis may be required. Potassium may be given as well.

See also MEDICATIONS AS POISONS.

loquat *(Eriobotrya japonica)* [Other names: Japanese medlar, Japanese plum.] This small evergreen tree is cultivated in California, Florida, the Gulf coast states, Hawaii and the West Indies. It has large, stiff leaves and fragrant white flower clusters; the fruit is yellow and shaped like a pear.

Poisonous part   While the unbroken seed is harmless, the pit kernel is toxic and contains cyanogenic glycosides that release hydrocyanic acid upon interaction with water in the gastrointestinal tract.

Symptoms   Since the glycosides must be hydrolyzed before the hydrocyanic acid is released, some hours may pass before symptoms appear. When they do, they include abdominal pain, vomiting, sweating and lethargy—cyanosis may or may not occur. In severe poisoning cases, convulsions and coma may result.

Treatment   If conscious, victims may be given gastric lavage followed by a 25 percent solution of sodium thiosulfate distilled into the stomach; activated charcoal absorbs cyanide but releases it slowly during passage through the intestine. In those who are losing consciousness, treat shock, correct acidosis and give respiratory assistance with oxygen, together with the administration of a cyanide antidote.

See also CYANOGENIC GLYCOSIDES.

lorchel   See TURBANTOP.

LSD *(lysergic acid diethylamide)*   [Other names: acid, blotter acid, haze, microdots, purple haze, sunshine, window panes.] LSD is a synthetic hallucinogenic drug usually found as a clear liquid and was the drug of choice during the 1960s. A synthetic derivative of ergot, it can be either injected or ingested (often in a soaked sugar cube). The drug has never been used medically, although it has been used to facilitate psychotherapeutic interviews. Its distribution and manufacture are governed by the Controlled Substance Act because of its potential for abuse.

Symptoms   Although its mechanism is not yet clear, LSD affects the brain and produces hallucinations, hyperexcitability, tremors, prolonged mental dissociation, psychopathic personality disorders, convulsions and coma, with a possible risk of suicide. There have been reports of numerous "flashbacks" many years after the final dose has been taken. Symptoms can appear within 20 minutes of ingestion, but there is no set toxic dose, since effects vary widely from one person to another depending on the situation and the person's current emotional state. However, hallucinations and visual illusions are dose related; the toxic dose may be only slightly greater than the therapeutic dose.

Treatment   There is no specific antidote, although Valium can control the hyperactivity or convulsions; coma is treated in the same way as barbiturate poisoning. Do not induce vomiting, since it is not effective and can worsen psychological distress; gastric lavage should be performed only if a massive dose has been ingested within 30–60 minutes. Administer activated charcoal.

lye   The common name for sodium hydroxide and one of a wide variety of caustic alkalies found in drain cleaners, oven cleaners and other household products, this is one of the most dangerous household poisons. Toddlers in particular are vulnerable to accidents, including burns to the eye, skin and esophagus. Because of the dangers of ingestion of lye in particular, federal legislation has required safety caps on containers of more than 2 percent concentrations of lye and banned use of more than 10 percent sodium hydroxide in household liquid drain cleaners.

Symptoms   In small doses, lye causes nausea, vomiting, coughing and the spitting of blood. Larger amounts can result in weakness, dizziness, slow, shallow breathing, and unconsciousness followed by convulsions and, sometimes, mild heart attack. Death is almost always a result of pulmonary problems. Inhalation causes lung damage.

Treatment   Gastric lavage only when preceded by endotracheal tube in comatose victims. *Do not induce vomiting.* Magnesium or sodium sulfate or citrate may be used as a cathartic. Oxygen and supportive therapy may also be needed.

See also ALKALINE CORROSIVES.

lysergic acid diethylamide   See LSD.

M

malathion This is an insecticide generally considered to be safe for use around people and animals to eliminate pests such as fruit flies, mosquitoes and boll weevils, in addition to household flies and lice on farm animals. Malathion is a colorless liquid with a definite smell, slightly soluble in water and sold as wettable powders, emulsifiable concentrates, dusts or aerosols. While it is possible to become sick after skin contamination or inhalation, fatal cases have been reported usually only after ingestion. If heated, malathion becomes extremely dangerous, emitting toxic phosphorous oxide fumes; the addition of water transforms this into phosphoric acid.

In addition, recent research has discovered that low doses of malathion *can* cause a response in mice similar to an allergic reaction. These studies were begun following reports of rashes and allergy symptoms in humans after aerial spraying of malathion, particularly following medfly spraying in the San Fernando Valley in southern California. Although scientists at the University of Southern California at Los Angeles say the effects of the pesticide are probably not life threatening, they are unsure how the chemical would affect those with impaired immune systems.

Symptoms Almost immediately to within several hours, symptoms begin: dermatitis, headache, nosebleeds, nausea, vomiting, diarrhea, blurred vision, excess salivation, bronchitis, shock, cardiac arrhythmias and pulmonary edema; death is caused by the muscle weakness that affects the lungs, interfering with breathing.

Treatment Respiratory support must be maintained to guard against respiratory failure.

See also INSECTICIDES; ORGANOPHOSPHATE INSECTICIDES.

mambas The black mamba *(Dendroaspis polylepis)* is one of the most dangerous of all snakes; a large black mamba can produce enough venom to kill 10 adults. Growing up to 14 feet, its color ranges from dull gray to greenish brown or black, depending on its age. This highly aggressive snake is found in savanna, rocky outcrops, thickets and remnant forest in Ethiopia, Somalia, and southwest Africa. Extremely agile and speedy, it is the most territorial of all the mambas; when cornered, it rears up to strike, biting a person's head or trunk. Its potent venom is neurotoxic and cardiotoxic; the fatality rate is nearly 100 percent without antivenin.

The green mamba *(D. angusticeps)* is smaller and less aggressive and prefers to live in trees. Highly agile, this snake is found in the forests and thickets and is highly dangerous when restrained.

The mambas have no upper jaw teeth behind their two fangs and are not aggressive unless provoked or restrained. Their color often conceals them until an unwary intruder gets too close.

Symptoms Local pain, swelling, paralysis of vocal cords, sweating, vomiting, restlessness, drowsiness, collapse, coma and death.

Treatment Antivenin is available.

See also ANTIVENIN; SNAKES, POISONOUS.

mandrake, American [Other names: devil's apple, hog apple, Indian apple, raccoon berry, umbrella leaf, wild jalap, wild lemon.] Also known as the mayapple *(Podophyllum pelatum)*, this plant produces fruit that, when ripe, can be eaten safely in moderation even by children. Eating the plant is fatal within 30 minutes.

The Middle Eastern variety was a famous love potion during the Middle Ages, when it was also considered to have magical properties. Some believed it would protect against evil spirits, and others believed that elves could not tolerate its smell. The ancient Greeks associated the mandrake with Circe, the witch. Because it was believed that touching the root would be fatal, dogs were trained to pull the dark brown root out of the ground, whereupon, according to legend, the root would shriek and the dog would die. Others believed that, pulled from the ground while muttering the correct incantation, the plant could bring forth the devil. In fact, the simple possession of mandrake could mark the owner as a witch, and three German women were executed in 1630 for just such a crime.

The American mandrake grows in moist woods and pastures. Found from Quebec to Florida, west to Ontario, Minnesota and Texas, it grows about one foot tall, with a jointed dark root about half the size of a finger, branching in a fork that resembles a pair of legs; in fact, it resembles a tiny human being. Leaves are deeply lobed with one white flower that appears in the spring, resembling a strawberry blossom; this is followed by a yellow fruit that is edible when ripe (and is sometimes used for preserves).

Poisonous part Rootstock, stem, flower, leaves and unripe fruit contain several hallucinogenic alkaloids, including hyoscyamine (atropine) and mandragorin; toxins also include podophylloresin and its glucoside, and alpha- and beta-peltatin. When green, the rhizome, foliage, seeds and green fruit are poisonous. Herbalists believe the best time for collecting the root is the latter part of October or early November, after the fruit is ripe.

Symptoms Within a few minutes to a half hour after ingestion of large amounts of the plant or topical application of the resin, mandrake poisoning causes severe diarrhea and vomiting, sedation, slowed heart rate, pupil dilation, coma and death. The mandrake's close relative, the mayapple, causes gastroenteritis, headache, and collapse and, when combined with alcohol, can be fatal within 14 hours.

Treatment   There is no specific antidote; give fluid replacement and blood transfusions if necessary.

manganese   Workers in mining, metalworking, foundry and welding occupations are generally the only people exposed to manganese toxicity from chronic rather than acute exposure.

Poisonous part   While the exact mechanism of manganese toxicity is not known, inhalation affects the central nervous system; manganese is not well absorbed from the gastrointestinal tract.

Symptoms   Although an acute intoxication is possible, causing pneumonitis, it is more likely that workers would be poisoned as a result of chronic exposure to low levels of manganese over a period of months or years. In the case of chronic exposure, manganese causes an affective psychiatric disorder (often misdiagnosed as schizophrenia or psychosis). This is followed by further signs of brain disease, such as parkinsonism or other similar movement disorders.

Treatment   For cases of acute inhalation toxicity, administer oxygen and treat symptoms. Long-term exposure should be treated with the typical drugs for psychiatric and movement disorders. Chelating agents have not been proven effective once chronic brain damage has occurred.

massasauga   *(Sistrurus catenatus)*   One of three rattlesnakes from the family Viperidae, this pygmy rattler ranges from the Great Lakes southwest to southeastern Arizona and Mexico. Its name, which is from the Chippewa language, means "great river mouth" and is thought to indicate the snake's habitat in the land of the Chippewa—swamps around rivers.

The massasauga has a stocky tail with a small rattle, and rounded dark blotches on its back and sides. A light-bordered dark bar runs from the eye to the rear of its jaw. The snake may grow to 40 inches. This "swamp rattler" is found in bogs, swamps, marshes, floodplains and dry woods in the East; grassy wetlands, rocky hillsides and the sagebrush and desert grasslands of the West. Unlike many snakes, massasaugas do not hibernate communally in an upland den but sleep alone in a mammal or crayfish burrow. They emerge in spring in response to the rains and rising water.

While fairly poisonous snakes, they are not aggressive and normally bite only when disturbed.

Symptoms   Symptoms appear within 15 minutes and include excessive thirst, nausea, vomiting, shock, paralysis, respiratory problems, anemia, necrosis, kidney problems and sometimes death. The bite of a rattlesnake is painful. Indications of a serious bite include swelling above the elbows or knees within two hours, hemorrhages, numbness at the puncture site, tingling around the mouth, yellow vision, vomiting and violent spasms.

Treatment   Antivenin is available.

See also PIT VIPER; RATTLESNAKE, CANEBRAKE; RATTLESNAKE, CASCA-

BEL; RATTLESNAKE, EASTERN DIAMONDBACK; RATTLESNAKE, MEXICAN WEST COAST; RATTLESNAKE, RED DIAMONDBACK; RATTLESNAKES; RATTLESNAKE, TIMBER; RATTLESNAKE, WESTERN DIAMONDBACK; SIDEWINDER; VIPER, GABOON; VIPER, JUMPING; VIPER, MALAYAN PIT; VIPER, RUSSELL'S; VIPERS; VIPER, SAWSCALE; VIPER WAGLER'S PIT; WATER MOCCASIN; WUTU.

matches   Serious cases of poisoning from ingesting matches are quite rare since the principal component of white or yellow phosphorus was replaced by red or by phosphorus sesquisulfide. The "strike anywhere" type of match is made of a nonpoisonous paste containing 6 percent phosphorus sesquisulfide and 24 percent potassium chlorate, plus zinc oxide, red ochre powdered glass, glue and water. "Safety" (or strike-on-box) matches are nonpoisonous; their chief ingredient is potassium chlorate. Book matches are similar to the safety type of match.

Accidental ingestion of matches by children often occurs, but it produces relatively insignificant side effects. Even if a child ate an entire book of 20 match heads, the total amount of potassium chlorate is still only 1/20 of the toxic dose.

meadow saffron   *(Colchicum autumnale, C. speciosum, C. vernum)*   [Other names: autumn crocus, fall crocus, naked ladies.] This crocus look-alike and ancient abortifacient is a member of the lily family and is often mistaken for an onion. It has long, tubular purple or white flowers that emerge from an underground bulb. Highly toxic, it is found in damp and woodsy areas in England, Wales and Scotland. Goats, which are immune to the poison, can eat the plant and pass on the poison in their milk, which will sicken anyone who drinks it.

Poisonous part   All parts (especially the bulbs) are toxic; tincture of colchicine is made from the seeds of *C. autumnale*, and the drug colchicine is used as a rheumatic.

Symptoms   Within two to six hours after ingestion, the victim begins to exhibit some symptoms similar to those of arsenic poisoning: burning throat, intense thirst, vomiting, difficulty in swallowing, bloody diarrhea, stomach pain, sensory disturbances, muscle weakness, delirium, cardiovascular collapse and respiratory failure. Meadow saffron poisoning is fatal in half of all cases, although it may not occur until three days after ingestion.

It is also possible to suffer chronic colchicine poisoning, with symptoms of hair loss and blood and protein in the urine and colchicine in the feces.

Treatment   Because colchicine is only slowly excreted, the victim is often ill for a long time. Painkillers and atropine may be given to alleviate stomach pain and diarrhea; fluids are required.

meclofenamate   See NONSTEROIDAL ANTI-INFLAMMATORY DRUGS.

medications as poisons   Even the most seemingly harmless over-the-counter medicine can be dangerous if used in the wrong amount or combined with the wrong products. Aspirin and acetaminophen, for example, take far too many lives each year from accidental overdose.

Poison control experts advise that all prescription and nonprescription drugs be stored out of the reach of children; never leave them casually on a kitchen table or counter, on a bedside table or in a pocketbook. Use only childproof packages. If medication must be refrigerated, keep it on the highest shelf out of the reach of children. If drugs are kept in drawers, lock them or install a childproof safety latch.

But children are not the only members of the family at risk for drug poisoning. Anyone who fails to read the instructions on the medicine label, or fails to follow a physician's instructions, is at risk for an overdose. Extra care must be taken particularly if a patient is taking multiple drugs. Some drugs that are completely safe on their own can become toxic if combined with another drug or drugs.

In addition, aging patients experience changes in the body that can also put them at greater risk for medication poisoning. The proportion of lean body tissue and water drops while the percentage of fat increases; drugs that dissolve readily in fat can be more easily stored there as well, building up as one grows older. Older patients sometimes have less efficient liver and kidneys and experience more problems breaking down and eliminating drugs.

Finally, some people experience drug allergies, so that even the normal recommended dosage becomes, for that person, toxic—even deadly. To a person sensitive to a particular medication, an allergy can produce hives, facial swelling, wheezing and problems in breathing, rashes, itching and shock and sometimes death.

meperidine   (Demerol) Introduced in 1939 as a means of reducing the pain associated with muscle spasms, this drug was later found to have many other painkilling abilities. It soon became almost as popular a drug as morphine, but it is only about one-tenth as potent. Still, meperidine is a fairly strong analgesic and is used for treatment of moderate to severe pain, to supplement anesthesia before an operation and to relieve the pain of labor during childbirth.

Symptoms   Large doses of meperidine can cause twitches, tremors and convulsions, and the drug is especially dangerous when mixed with monoamine oxidase (MAO) inhibitors (a class of antidepressants). In fact, if it is taken within two weeks of an MAO inhibitor, it can cause symptoms similar to those in acute narcotic overdose (including convulsions, high blood pressure, coma and death).

Treatment Medical help should be sought immediately. Stimulants such as strong tea and coffee will help to keep the victim awake. If the victim is discovered soon after ingestion and is conscious, induce vomiting.

See also MEDICATIONS AS POISONS.

mercury Every known form of this highly toxic, silvery liquid metal is poisonous, and since there are more than 115 known mercury compounds, there are many opportunities for mercuric poisoning to occur. It is widely used in skin and hair bleach, dusting or wettable powders and fumigants, cathartics, antiseptics and diuretics, and in explosives, tooth fillings, electrical lamps, batteries, paints and felt. In the past, many milliners used mercury to help shape hats; it has been suggested that Lewis Carroll's Mad Hatter may really have been suffering from mercury poisoning, as did many hatters of the 1800s.

Its toxicity depends on the chemical form in which it appears, and in its most common form, as a free metal in fever thermometers, mercury is not a serious threat if ingested, since it is not well absorbed by the body. However, breathing mercury vapor is more hazardous. Employees in dental offices may also be exposed to excess levels of mercury, via recirculation ventilation systems or sloppy conditions. Mercury chloride found in antiseptics is the most toxic of all mercury compounds. Organic mercurials that are used to treat seeds are highly toxic, and acute cases of poisoning have been reported from fish contamination or water pollution.

There is a large number of professions whose workers are exposed to mercury, including those who make barometers, batteries, boilers, calibration instruments, caustic soda, carbon brushes, ceramics, chlorine, dental amalgam, electrical apparatus, neon lights, pressure gauges, disinfectants, dyes, explosives, fireworks, inks, drugs, insecticides and pesticides and wood preservatives.

Symptoms Acute poisoning from inhaling mercury vapor occurs almost immediately, causing stomach problems, coughing, fever, nausea, vomiting and diarrhea. The vapor affects the brain and lungs, attacking the respiratory system and causing pneumonia, pulmonary edema and ventricular fibrillation followed by death. Chronic poisoning results in damage to the central nervous system and can cause psychosis. Ingestion of mercuric chloride and other soluble mercuric salts can cause thirst, abdominal pain, vomiting and diarrhea, followed by kidney damage and death. Skin contamination with mercury compounds causes a variety of symptoms, including depression, sleeplessness, weight loss and anorexia, headaches, anxiety, hallucinations, loose teeth and tremors.

Treatment Dimercaprol and treatment of symtoms.

See also FISH CONTAMINATION; MERCURY AND DENTAL FILLINGS.

mercury and dental fillings The field of toxicology is sharply divided over whether mercury contained in dental fillings poses a hazard to human health. Research does suggest that mercury can have subtle but damaging effects from kidney to brain. Humans are exposed to mercury by eating seafood and by the gases released from "silver" amalgam fillings.

However, toxicologists can't agree over whether the tiny amount of mercury vapor that escapes from a typical filling is dangerous. In 1991, experts at the Food and Drug Administration and the National Institutes of Health decided that amalgams are at least as safe as the available alternatives. But more recent research released in March 1992 at the Society of Toxicology meeting in Seattle suggested that mercury may have effects on reproductive health for workers exposed to the mercury in the fillings. Yet many dentists are unconvinced; the American Dental Association believes that amalgams are safe.

All sides of the controversy agree that more research will be needed to finally decide the question of how toxic silver fillings really are.

See also MERCURY; FISH CONTAMINATION.

metal cleaner   See ALKALINE CORROSIVES.

metaldehyde   This is type of inorganic chemical insecticide often used in combination with calcium arsenate and used to control slugs and snails. It is also sold as fuel for small heaters that can cause toxic vapors if not properly ventilated. Poison control centers report incidences of children being poisoned after mistakenly eating slug or snail bait or heater fuel tablets.

Ingestion of 100–150 mg/kg may cause convulsions, and ingestion of more than 400 mg/kg is potentially lethal.

Symptoms   Metaldehyde is a gastric irritant; between one and three hours after ingestion it causes symptoms including nausea, vomiting, abdominal pain, flushed face, fever, muscular rigidity and twitching. In severe poisonings, convulsions and coma are followed by death from respiratory failure. Liver and kidney damage have been reported.

Treatment   There is no specific antidote. Perform gastric lavage immediately after ingestion, followed by activated charcoal and cathartics, with supportive therapy including plenty of fluids. Do NOT induce vomiting. Demulcents (such as milk) may relieve gastric distress; sedation may also be required.

See also INORGANIC CHEMICAL INSECTICIDES.

methanol   See METHYL ALCOHOL.

methocarbamol   This centrally acting muscle relaxant is used in the control of painful muscle spasms following the bite of the black widow spider and strychnine poisoning. Onset of action almost immediately follows intravenous administration.

See also BLACK WIDOW SPIDER; STRYCHNINE.

methyl alcohol (wood alcohol) Also known as methanol, this common household solvent is related to ethyl alcohol and is found in solvents, perfumes, windshield washing liquids, duplicating fluid, antifreeze, shellac and paint removers.

It is far more poisonous than the ethyl alcohol found in cocktails, because it metabolizes into formaldehyde upon ingestion; it also takes far longer to eliminate methyl alcohol from the body. While it can produce intoxication, its metabolic products may cause metabolic acidosis, blindness and death.

Methyl alcohol is a liquid at room temperature, evaporates quickly and can be swallowed, inhaled as a vapor or absorbed through the skin. In the past, moonshine makers (who distill ethyl alcohol from fermented grain) sometimes mistakenly mixed wood shavings in with the brew, resulting in a toxic brand of moonshine. (Methyl alcohol is made from fermented wood.)

Symptoms   The fatal oral dose of methyl alcohol is estimated to be 30 to 240 m. Because methyl alcohol metabolizes slowly in the body, there is a latency period ranging from 12 to 48 hours between ingestion/inhalation and symptoms. In the first hours after ingestion, the primary symptom is intoxication because the body has not yet begun to break down the substance into more toxic products. Once methyl alcohol is transformed into formaldehyde in the body, it causes fatigue, headache, nausea and vomiting, vertigo, back pain, severe abdominal pain, vision problems, dizziness and blindness. (These symptoms will appear even later if ethanol has been drunk at the same time.) In large doses, symptoms progress to rapid, shallow breathing, cyanosis, coma, precipitous drop in blood pressure and death from respiratory arrest. An autopsy would show massive organ damage, especially in the eyes. Breathing fumes can cause headache, eye irritation, dizziness, visual disturbances and nausea. In extreme cases, inhaling these fumes can be fatal; it damages the liver, heart, kidneys and the lungs, predisposing them to pneumonia.

Treatment   Ethanol (100 proof) is administered to interfere with the metabolism of methyl alcohol; within two hours of ingestion, gastric lavage is preferred, but syrup of ipecac may be given at home to induce vomiting before medical help arrives. Ethanol is then administered orally or intravenously for the next four days until the methyl alcohol is excreted; kidney dialysis may also remove the alcohol from the blood. Folic acid may also be administered; and the experimental drug 4-methylpyrazole, while not yet available in the United States, can inhibit alcohol dehydrogenase and prevent methyl alcohol metabolism. Activated charcoal has not been shown to absorb methyl alcohol efficiently, and it may also delay the absorption of orally administered ethanol.

methyl bromide   This odorless, colorless gas is used in insecticidal fumigants and fire extinguishers and in the production of chemicals and dyes. It is considered to be a potential industrial carcinogen by the National Institute of Occupational Safety and Health (NIOSH). It can be inhaled or absorbed easily through the skin; methyl bromide also easily penetrates protective clothing and can be retained in boots and clothing for some time.

Symptoms Methyl bromide affects the central nervous system, the respiratory tract, the skin and the cardiovascular system. There is a wide variance in onset of symptoms, ranging from a few minutes to two days after ingestion. Methyl bromide irritates the eyes, skin and upper respiratory tract, which may lead to pulmonary edema; skin contamination can cause a rash or chemical burns. With acute exposure, there may be malaise, vision disturbances, headache, nausea, vomiting, vertigo, tremor, seizures and coma followed by death from pulmonary or circulatory failure. In addition, chronic exposure may lead to dementia or psychosis.

Treatment Some scientists recommend the use of dimercaprol or acetylcysteine, although their use has not been tested in controlled studies. Remove all contaminated clothing and wash the skin with soap and water; irrigate eyes with saline or tepid water.

methyl chloroform See TRICHLOROETHANE.

methyl mercury See FISH CONTAMINATION; MERCURY.

methylene chloride One of a group of chlorinated hydrocarbons, this chemical solvent is listed as a human carcinogen by the National Toxicology Program of the U.S. Department of Health and Human Services. It is encountered by millions of Americans every day in products ranging from paint strippers and thinners to paint, hair spray, antiperspirants, room deodorants and Christmas tree light sets. Upon combustion, it can produce phosgene, chlorine or hydrogen chloride; it was considered to be one of the least toxic of the chlorinated hydrocarbons, but now it is a suspected carcinogen.

Methylene chloride irritates mucous membranes and depresses the central nervous system. Carbon monoxide is generated within the body during metabolism of methylene chloride.

Symptoms Inhalation is the most common route of intoxication and causes skin irritation, nausea, vomiting and headache. Severe exposure may lead to pulmonary edema, heart problems and central nervous system depression with respiratory arrest. Ingestion can lead to corrosive injury and system intoxication. Chronic exposure is toxic to bone marrow, the kidneys and the liver.

Treatment Administer 100 percent oxygen by tight-fitting mask or endotracheal tube; if skin or eyes are contaminated, wash thoroughly. In case of ingestion, do NOT induce vomiting; perform gastric lavage if the victim has ingested within the past 30–60 minutes or has ingested a large amount. Administer activated charcoal and a cathartic, although the effectiveness of the former is not known.

metoclopramide   This antiemetic drug is used to control persistent nausea and vomiting often found in poisoning cases, especially when activated charcoal may not be given.

Mexican beaded lizard *(Heloderma horridum)*   One of only two poisonous lizards in the world out of more than 3,000 lizard species, the Mexican beaded lizard is found only in Mexico and is a relative of the Gila monster, also a member of the *Heloderma* genus. Slightly larger than the Gila monster, the Mexican beaded lizard is still not a very large animal—between 19 and 29 inches long; it is a mixture of black, yellow and pink and has knobby scales. Both lizards are sluggish but have a strong bite. Fatalities from the bite of a Mexican beaded lizard are rare.

Beaded lizards are nocturnal and mate during summer, laying between three and five eggs in autumn and winter. Although these lizards are relatively slow moving, they can bite quickly and hang on stubbornly. While biting, they chew so that the grooved teeth can allow the venom to flow from the glands at the base of the mouth. In general, the bite of the beaded lizard is not fatal, but it is quite painful. There have been only eight recorded deaths from bites of both these lizards.

Beaded lizards live underground, either in abandoned holes or ones they dig themselves; they locate their food by scent rather than sight, following a trail in much the same way as a bloodhound does.

See also GILA MONSTER.

Mexican hallucinogenic mushroom *(Psilocybe mexicana)*   Also known as "magic mushrooms," these are a species of mushrooms that contain the hallucinogenic substance psilocin-psilocybin, which American Indians have used for thousands of years in their religious ceremonies.

The *Psilocybe* genus includes more than 100 different species of the little brown mushrooms, which are found growing in grass and manure heaps—especially after spring rains. Though found primarily in the South, they grow almost everywhere in the United States. One of the easiest ways to identify the *Psilocybe* mushroom is by its blue-green discoloration in areas where it has been handled or damaged.

Symptoms   Within an hour of ingestion, its effects—which are usually considered pleasant—appear: euphoria, loss of sense of distance and size and hallucinations. Symptoms will last between four and six hours depending on the quantity of toxin ingested, the mood and personality of the person and, the setting of the experience. Effects lasting longer than 24 hours are not due to a natural toxin but to the consumption of a mushroom with another hallucinogen added (usually phencyclidine or PCP). The mushrooms can cause high fever, convulsions and death in children who have eaten them.

Treatment For those who seek medical assistance, treatment usually involves reassurance, although sedation (with diazepam) is sometimes necessary. In children, treatment includes external cooling and respiratory support; it may be necessary to administer diazepam to control convulsions.

See also HALLUCINOGENIC MUSHROOMS; MUSHROOM POISONING.

Mexican moccasin See CANTIL SNAKE.

midazolam This ultrashort-acting benzodiazepine is used to help manage anxiety, agitation and psychosis following overdose of hallucinogenic or stimulant drugs such as LSD or amphetamines. It is also used to induce sedation and amnesia during placement of an endotracheal tube.

See also BENZODIAZEPINES.

Minipress (prazosin hydrochloride) One of a group of antihypertensives, this toxic medicine is available as a white crystalline water-soluble capsule.

Symptoms Within 30 to 90 minutes after ingestion, Minipress overdose causes headache, drowsiness, weakness, nausea, vomiting, diarrhea, shortness of breath, nervousness, rapid heartbeat, depression, rash, itching, blurred vision, loss of consciousness and death.

Treatment Atropine is administered while monitoring the cardiorespiratory systems and the kidney function.

See also ANTIHYPERTENSIVE DRUGS; MEDICATIONS AS POISONS.

mirex This type of synthetic organic insecticide is a chlorinated hydrocarbon that is almost impossible to dissolve in water and is generally no longer used as an insecticides. Emergency exceptions for specific uses are allowed, however.

Mirex was used throughout the southeastern United States to control fire ants, other ant species and yellow jackets. It breaks down in the soil and forms kepone, a chlorinated organic insecticide banned from use in 1978.

Symptoms Inhalations, ingestion or skin contamination can cause chest pain, weight loss, rash and a range of neurological problems including tremors, mental alterations, weakness and slurred speech. Both mirex and its derivative, kepone, cause cancer in experimental animals.

Treatment Gastric lavage followed by saline cathartics. Avoid all fats and oils (including milk), since they increase the rate of absorption. Administer phenobarbital sodium for tremors and barbiturates for convulsions, and provide oxygen if necessary. If the skin has come in contact with these insecticides, wash with soap and water immediately to head off skin problems and systemic absorption. Remove contaminated clothing.

mistletoe (American: *Phoradendron rubrum, P. serotinum, P. tomentosum;* European: *Viscum album*) This popular winter holiday plant is a parasite of deciduous trees in the southeastern United States, and the whole mistletoe plant—especially the berries—is poisonous, although seldom fatal.

Mistletoe has thick, leathery leaves, with white translucent berries in the *P. serotinum* and *P. tomentosum* varieties and pink berries in the *P. rubrum* variety. *P. serotinum* is the variety typically sold as a decorative holiday plant at Christmas; it grows from New Jersey to Florida and west to southern Illinois and Texas. *P. tomentosum* is found from Kansas to Louisiana and west to Texas and Mexico.

V. album is a parasite found principally on apple trees and, although a European plant, has been introduced into Sonoma County, California. Its thick, leathery leaves are up to three inches long and yellow-green in color; the fruit is a sticky white berry.

Mistletoe is a plant steeped in legend and mystery. It is said that mistletoe was once a tree, the wood of which had been used to make Christ's cross, and was relegated to exist only as a parasite ever after. Similarly, it was an herb of the underworld in both Greek and Roman legends, while in Britain the Druid priests were said to use mistletoe in many important religious ceremonies. Tradition says that the mistletoe was the "golden bough" that the Trojan hero Aeneas, forefather of the Romans, carried with him on his descent into Hades. The bough opened the gates of hell for the hero and brought him safely back.

Its reputation as an herb of love, in which two people standing under it at Christmas must kiss, originated in Scandinavia, when Balder (the god of peace) was killed with an arrow dipped in mistletoe. When his fellow gods asked that his life be spared, mistletoe was given to the god of love, who announced that anyone who passed beneath it must be given a kiss as a symbol of love. It subsequently became a part of the Christmas celebrations when the Druids used the greens as a way of welcoming the New Year.

Poisonous part Stems, leaves and berries of this plant contain toxic amines and proteins called phoratoxins, toxic lectins that inhibit synthesization of proteins in the intestinal wall. They can cause hallucinations, slow heartbeat, high blood pressure, heart attacks and cardiovascular collapse. While poisoning is rarely fatal, there have been cases in which children have died after eating mistletoe berries. Tea brewed from the berries has also been fatal.

In the European variety *(V. album)* only the leaves and stems are toxic, containing a toxic lectin (toxalbumin) called viscumin, which interferes with protein synthesis. In addition, related lectins called viscotoxins are also found.

In addition to its own toxic properties, mistletoe may also take up poisonous substances from the tree on which it lives.

Symptoms Similar to those of poisoning by digitalis, symptoms appear after a delay of a few hours and include severe nausea, vomiting, diarrhea, stomach cramps, difficulty in breathing, slow pulse, delirium, hallucinations and coma.

In the European variety, poisoning symptoms are similar to, but less toxic than, those caused by the lectins in rosary pea *(Abrus prevatorius)* and castor bean *(Ricinus communis)*. Symptoms in this variety appear some time after ingestion and include abdominal pain and diarrhea together with lesions of the intestinal tract. Severe poisoning with this variety of mistletoe is rare.

Treatment Treat as for severe gastroenteritis, with replacement of fluids and electrolytes.

monkshood *(Aconitum)* [Other names: aconite, bear's foot, friar's cap, helmet flower, soldier's cap, western monkshood *(A. columbianum)*, wild monkshood *(A. uncinatum)*, wolfsbane, yellow monkshood *(A. lutescens)*.] Dubbed "queen mother of poisons" before the birth of Christ, this extremely poisonous plant may reach six feet in height with small blue, pink or white flowers and a unique hood-shaped upper petal appearing from June to September. According to legend, it is ruled by Hecate, goddess of the underworld, who supposedly poisoned her father with it.

Monkshood is a strikingly beautiful plant rich in myth and medicine, history and magic. Often grown as an ornamental perennial in shady borders around older homes, this plant has flowers that resemble delphiniums; the flowers are arranged on stems of equal height and distance from each other and blossom in an orderly fashion from stem base to tip. Although the plant is a perennial, the spongy root is an annual and sprouts tiny side roots, each capable of producing another monkshood plant. Together with larkspur and columbine, monkshood belongs to the buttercup family and includes about 100 species in the genus *Aconitum*.

The name may come from the Greek *akonitos*, "without struggle" or "without dust," or from the Greek city Acona, where a naturalist in the third century once identified the plant. Other sources suggest the name comes from the hill of Aconitus, where Hercules fought with Cerberus, the three-headed dog who guards the entrance to Hades. Saliva from this dreaded dog's mouth dripped onto monkshood, making it a deadly poison.

In mythology, monkshood formed the cup that Medea prepared for Theseus. In Rome, Nero ascended to the throne after poisoning Claudius by tickling his throat with a feather dipped in monkshood. While it is named for the shape of its flower, it was also associated with political intrigue among the ranks of the Roman Catholic clergy. Tradition holds that Romeo (of Shakespeare's *Romeo and Juliet*) committed suicide with monkshood.

Witches also make wide use of this plant in herbal preparations to induce supernatural experiences, combining it with belladonna in ointments the witches rubbed on their bodies to help them "fly." In fact, these two plants produce an irregular heart action and delirium, which is believed to have caused the sensation of flying. During the Middle Ages, the plant was widely feared because it was thought witches used it to summon the devil. In Shakespeare's *Macbeth*, the witches' brew calling for "tooth of wolf" refers to monkshood, which is also known as wolfsbane because arrows dipped in the poison kill wolves. (For this same reason, medieval folks believed monkshood would protect them against werewolves.)

Monkshood thrives naturally and is also cultivated as a decorative plant in Canada and the northern United States, including Alaska. Until the 1930s, monkshood was used as a painkiller, diuretic and diaphoretic. Ointments containing monkshood have been used externally to treat rheumatism, neuralgia and lumbago, and a tincture was used to lower pulse rate and fevers and treat cardiac failure. Because of its toxicity, monkshood is rarely used today in medicine, although it is still valued in homeopathy as an ointment for muscle and joint pain.

Poisonous part   The entire plant is poisonous. However, the roots and leaves contain the greatest concentration of the toxin aconitine and similar alkaloids, including picratonitine, aconine, benzoylamine and neopelline. The alkaloids first stimulate and then depress the central and peripheral nerves. One teaspoonful of the root is lethal to an adult, and even handling the plant is dangerous to highly sensitive people. Because of the root's similarity to Jerusalem artichoke or horseradish, monkshood should never be planted near a vegetable garden. Even touching the plant's juices to an open wound can cause pain, fainting sensations and suffocation.

But like many botanical toxins, the one in monkshood can be beneficial if administered in very small doses. In fact, 18th- and 19th-century physicians used monkshood as a cardiac sedative, although modern drugs have since replaced it.

Symptoms   If monkshood is eaten, symptoms start rapidly with a burning or tingling sensation of the lips, tongue, mouth and throat. Delayed-onset symptoms include excessive salivation, nausea, vomiting, tightness and numbness in the throat, impaired swallowing and possibly speech impairment. Intermittent visual disturbances can include blurred vision or color patches in the visual field and pronounced and prolonged pupil dilation. Dizziness, prickling skin sensation, muscle weakness and uncoordinated movements can also occur.

In critical cases there are heart rate and rhythm disturbances followed by convulsions and death. Death may occur as early as a few minutes after ingestion or as late as four days. Heart rate and rhythm disturbances can be serious.

Those who survive report odd hallucinations during the poisoning episode and sensory disturbances for a long time afterward. If the victim does not die, recovery occurs within 24 hours.

Treatment   There is no specific antidote, although gastric lavage and oxygen to help breathing, as well as drugs to stimulate the heart, may be used. Arrhythmias should be managed by electrocardiogram monitoring.

See also ACONITINE.

monoamine oxidase (MAO) inhibitors   A class of psychiatric drugs used to treat severe depression that also stimulate the central nervous system and affect the liver. MAO inhibitors may cause serious poisoning either by overdose or through interactions with other drugs or food.

For example, eating cheese or drinking alcohol (especially red wine) can cause hypertension, stroke and even death. Some MAO inhibitor drugs have been taken off the U.S. market because of extreme toxicity in combination with other drugs.

MAO inhibitors include furazolidone (Furoxone), isocarboxazid (Marplan), nialamide (Niamid), pargyline (Eutonyl), phenelzine (Nardil), procarbazine (Matulane) and tranylcypromine (Parnate).

Symptoms   In an acute overdose, symptoms may not appear for six to 24 hours, but they should be apparent quite soon after eating certain foods or taking certain other drugs. Symptoms include anxiety, flushing, headache, tremor, sweating, tachycardia and hypertension; severe poisoning causes severe high blood pressure, brain hemorrhage, delirium, high fever, cardiovascular collapse and multisystem failure.

Treatment   There is no specific antidote. Treat symptoms; monitor

DRUGS AND FOODS THAT DON'T MIX WITH MAO INHIBITORS

Drug	Food
Amphetamine	Beer
Buspirone	Beans
Dextromethorphan	Cheese
Ephedrine	Chicken livers
Fluoxetine	Pickled herring
Guanethidine	Snails
L-Dopa	Red wine
LSD (lysergic acid diethylamide)	Yeast
Meperidine (Demerol),	
Metaraminol,	
Methyldopa,	
Phenylephrine,	
Phenylpropanolamine,	
Reserpine,	
Trazodone,	
Tryptophan,	

temperature and vital signs, with an ECG for victims without symptoms. Do not induce vomiting because of the risk of seizures and worsening the high blood pressure; perform gastric lavage followed by activated charcoal and a cathartic.

See also ANTIDEPRESSANTS.

monomethylhydrazine   A propellant used in rocket fuel, this is also a decomposition product of the mushroom toxin gyromitrin and the primary toxic component of the gyromitra mushroom.

Symptoms   A strong convulsant, this substance can cause central nervous system depression, pulmonary edema and cardiovascular collapse, with some kidney damage and severe liver damage.

Treatment   The antidote is pyridoxine, which may help in the control of hyperexcitability and even coma but will not protect the liver from damage.

See also GYROMITRA; MUSHROOM POISONING; MUSHROOM TOXINS.

monosodium glutamate (MSG)   This natural salt is found in low amounts in seaweed, soybeans and sugar beets; refined, it is used to enhance the flavor of certain foods (especially red meat, poultry and fish). MSG is commonly used by the processed food industry and Asian restaurants as a flavor enhancer. The most common processed foods that use MSG include meat products, bouillons, precooked soups and gravies in packages, condiments, pickles, candy and baked goods.

Almost anyone who eats processed food, or dines at an Asian restaurant, will encounter MSG; most of the health complaints have come from people eating at Chinese restaurants. Soups and foods coated with a liquid sauce often contain the highest concentration of MSG, and rice used in Japanese sushi also contains high concentrations.

Labels must indicate which packaged foods contain MSG, but avoiding the additive is much more difficult in restaurants, since the menu most likely will not mention that the food contains this flavor enhancer. Unless it is explicitly stated otherwise, it should be assumed that Asian food contains MSG.

MSG contains the amino acid glutamate, which may be responsible for brain damage under certain conditions of oxygen deprivation in the brain (such as during a stroke), or when ingested in large quantities. While the glutamate in MSG is considered safe for adults, research at Washington University in St. Louis finding that large doses of glutamate may damage brain cells prompted the Food and Drug Administration to remove MSG from baby food in the mid-1970s.

Symptoms   Among certain individuals in a subgroup of the population, MSG causes "Chinese restaurant syndrome": tightness in the head and face, headache, chest pain, dizziness, sweating and numbness. According to the Food and Drug Administration, about 4 percent of the

population will have an occasional reaction to MSG; about 2 percent are highly sensitive to it.
Treatment Symptomatic.

moonseed *(Menispermum canadense)* [Other names: Canadian moonseed, Texas sarsaparilla, vine-maple, yellow sarsaparilla.] Sometimes mistaken for wild grapes, moonseed is a woody twining vine growing on stream banks and fences in eastern North America. Its Hawaiian relative, also called moonseed *(Cocculus ferrandianus)*, is used as a fish poison. A perennial, moonseed grows in the eastern part of the United States in moist woods, hedges and streams. Its woody root is very long and yellow, and its stem is a climbing vine with round, smooth leaves and yellow flowers appearing in July, followed by one seeded fruit.
Poisonous part Both leaves and fruit contain poisonous alkaloids.
Symptoms Within several hours after ingestion, moonseed grapes and leaves cause bloody diarrhea, convulsions, shock and death.
Treatment Gastric lavage.

moray eel *(Gymnothorax javanicus)* An eel of tropical oceans that is poisonous at certain times of the year. After eating, symptoms may develop quickly or slowly and include tingling sensations in the lips and mouth followed by numbness, nausea, vomiting, abdominal cramps, weakness, paralysis, convulsions, skin rash, coma and death in about 12 percent of cases.
See also CIGUATERA; DINOFLAGELLATE; FISH CONTAMINATION; FOOD POISONING.

morning glory *(Ipomoea)* [Other names: flying saucer, heavenly blue, pearly gates.] This is the common name for plants of the Convolvulaceae family, which are popular for their hallucinogenic properties. These viney plants have large, heart- shaped leaves and flaring, brightly colored flowers; the hallucinogenic part of the plant is the black or brown seeds. The seeds' hallucinogenic properties have been known since ancient times, when Aztecs and North American Indians used them as part of their religious ceremonies and in healing and divination. Not all species are toxic, however.
In recent times, the seeds of the morning glory have been advertised for sale in alternative publications as "hallucinogens" but also labeled "not for human consumption."
Poisonous part The seeds of this plant are poisonous and contain an active principle similar to that of LSD, but only one-tenth as toxic.
Symptoms Between 50 and 200 powdered seeds can produce symptoms similar to those caused by LSD, with feelings of depersonalization and visual hallucinations, in addition to psychoses and flashbacks later on.
Treatment Supportive and symptomatic. Do not induce vomiting;

gastric lavage should be performed within 30 minutes only in case of massive overdose.

morphine [Other names: lanthopine, laudanoisine, laudanum, meconidine, narcotine, protopine.] Considered to be supertoxic, this opiate is the principal alkaloid of opium and is the best-known narcotic painkiller. It is extracted from the unripe seed pods of the opium poppy. It has been used as a painkiller since 1886 and was often found in Chinese opium dens popular during the Victorian era.

A white crystalline alkaloid, it is available in liquid or tablet form and can be ingested or injected. Liquid morphine is a bluish syrup given to cancer patients to treat pain, sometimes mixed with a blue liqueur to strengthen the effects.

Morphine increases the effects of sedatives, analgesics, sleep-inducing drugs, tranquilizers, antidepressants and other narcotic drugs. It works faster if mixed with alcohol or other solvents. It works by blocking the transmission of pain signals at specific sites in the brain and spinal cord, preventing the perception of pain. Short-term use is not likely to cause dependence, but the euphoric effects of the drug have contributed to its long history as a street drug. Long-term abuse leads to a craving for the drug and a need to have ever-greater amounts. Sudden withdrawal of the drug can cause flu-like symptoms (sweating, shaking and cramping).

In addition, morphine cannot be used together with a wide range of drugs, including aminophylline, phenytoin, phenobarbital and sodium bicarbonate.

Symptoms Symptoms include sleepiness, physical ease, floating sensations, giddiness, unbalanced gait, dizziness, nausea, breathing problems, unconsciousness and coma. Depressant effects may last longer in those persons with liver or kidney problems. Death from morphine overdose occurs between six and 12 hours after ingestion and is almost always due to respiratory failure. If the victim survives for two days, the prognosis is good.

Treatment Naloxone is the antidote; recovery can be expected within one to four hours if administered soon after ingestion.

See also HEROIN; NARCOTICS; OPIUM.

mothballs See CAMPHOR; NAPHTHALENE.

mother-in-law plant *(Caladium)* This popular plant is cultivated both outdoors and as an indoor plant and can grow to about 16 inches. It is a deciduous plant with large, oval arrow-shaped leaves that can grow to be 14 inches long and come in a range of colors, including pink, red, white and green. The plants can be cultivated all year in subtropical gardens and during the summer in temperate zones.

Poisonous part All parts of the plant are toxic and contain raphides of calcium oxalate.

Symptoms   Ingestion causes pain, swelling and irritation of the mouth, lips, throat and the digestive tract, which leads to nausea, vomiting and diarrhea. Ingestion of a large amount can result in swelling of the tongue and throat, which can obstruct the airway.

Treatment   Pain and swelling subside on their own, but cool liquids and demulcents (such as milk) held in the mouth may help the pain. Painkillers are sometimes given, but the oxalates in this plant are insoluble and therefore do not cause systemic poisoning.

mountain laurel   See LAUREL, MOUNTAIN.

MSG   See MONOSODIUM GLUTAMATE.

multiple chemical sensitivity (MCS)   A physical illness clinical ecologists believe is caused by minute levels of toxic chemicals in the air, water and food. According to this theory, people with MCS suffer from fatigue, achy muscles, headaches, mental fogginess and other vague symptoms because of sensitivity to tiny amounts of toxic chemicals in the environment.

While many traditional physicians believe these ills are primarily psychosomatic, others believe there is evidence of a real chemical illness and that it may affect 15 percent of Americans. According to these clinical ecologists, the disease develops in one of two ways: through a slow buildup of chemicals over the years, or from one massive exposure such as an industrial chemical spill.

People are more vulnerable if they have nutritional deficiencies, a family history of allergies, a chronic disease or an infection that has weakened the immune system. Still, experts recommend that health problems must be ruled out before concluding that the environment is to be blamed for illness.

Even physicians who doubt the existence of MCS concede that it can't hurt to pay attention to chemicals and try to avoid overexposure. They recommend:

- Store insecticides, paint thinner and other toxic chemicals in an outside shed or garage; never keep them under the sink where the fumes can leak into the house.
- Choose electric appliances, 100 percent cotton or wool carpets, and furniture made of glass, chrome or solid wood instead of particleboard. Avoid "no chip" wood finishes that emit formaldehyde.
- Keep gas appliances repaired; replace filters regularly.
- Be cautious with chemicals used often: artists' oils, marking pens and typewriter correction fluid can be highly toxic.
- Air out the house often, especially when using appliances that burn gas, propane, wood or kerosene.
- Use your own nontoxic products: use fresh herbs and flowers as air

fresheners; dust with pure mineral oil sweetened with drops of lemon; soften fabrics by adding baking soda to rinse water.

- Air dry-cleaned clothes, bedspreads and drapes outside before bringing them into the house. If dry-cleaned goods have a chemical odor, refuse to accept them until they are properly dried; change cleaners if the problem persists.
- Read and follow labels; wear gloves and open windows when using mildew removers, rug shampoos or other household chemicals.
- Wash permanent-press clothes and sheets before using, or buy all-natural fibers (wool, cotton and silk).
- Avoid pesticides.
- Don't smoke. (Cigarette smoke contains 4,700 chemicals, according to the Environmental Protection Association).

muscarine   This alkaloid was isolated in 1869 as a minor toxic constituent in the mushroom *Amanita muscaria* (in fresh fungi, it is found in only a concentration of 0.0003 percent). It is found in much larger amounts in many species of *Inocybe* and some species of *Clitocybe* mushrooms. Eating mushrooms that contain muscarine is only rarely fatal; even without treatment, most symptoms fade within a few hours.

Symptoms   Muscarine, like pilocarpine, excites receptors of the parasympathetic nervous system and sympathetic nervous system. Within 15 to 24 hours after ingestion, muscarine poisoning produces profuse sweating and salivation, visual disturbances, nausea, vomiting, abdominal pain, diarrhea, headache and bronchospasm. Very high doses cause incontinence, slow heartbeat, low blood pressure and shock.

Treatment   Symptoms will disappear even without treatment in most cases. However, vomiting and gastric lavage may help together with the administration of atropine to suppress toxic symptoms.

See also AMANITA MUSHROOMS; FLY AGARIC; INOCYBE MUSHROOM; MUSHROOM POISONING; MUSHROOM TOXINS.

muscimol   This water-soluble toxin was first isolated in the early 1960s from the toxic mushrooms *Amanita muscaria* (or fly agaric) and *Amanita pantherina* (panther mushroom). Both muscimol and its metabolic precursor ibotenic acid are believed to be the primary cause for the toxicity of these two mushrooms and a few related species.

Symptoms   Within 20 to 90 minutes after ingestion, muscimol begins to affect the central nervous system, causing drowsiness, stupor, elation, hyperactivity, delirium, confusion, hallucinations, rapid heartbeat, gastroenteritis and urinary retention.

Treatment   Induce vomiting and perform gastric lavage; administration of physostigmine and diazepam (Valium) may help control symptoms and convulsions. Stimulants are not advised.

See also AMANITA MUSHROOMS; FLY AGARIC; MUSHROOM POISONING; MUSHROOM TOXINS; PANTHER MUSHROOM.

mushroom poisoning   There is a reason for the saying "There are old mushroom hunters, and bold mushroom hunters, but no old bold mushroom hunters." In the past 10 years, cases of mushroom poisoning have been on the increase, attributable to the rise of interest in "natural" foods and to better reporting of cases. At the same time, scientists have been learning more and more about the toxic properties of mushrooms, or "fungus fruit."

Out of the more than 5,000 varieties of mushrooms found in the United States, about 100 are toxic—but most of these cause only mild stomach problems. A few, however, can cause fatal reactions. Most of the toxic symptoms are caused by the gastrointestinal irritants that lead to the vomiting and diarrhea common in mushroom poisoning. In most cases, onset of stomach distress is rapid, but if the onset is delayed past six to 12 hours, the more serious amatoxin or monomethylhydrazine poisoning may be suspected. The stalk and cap of the mushroom that pops up after a spring rain are really the fruit of a vast underground network of microscopic filaments; therefore, picking a mushroom no more harms the plant than plucking an apple from a tree.

But despite the fact that scientists for the past hundred years have been trying to isolate the toxic principles in mushrooms, the exact chemistry behind the deadly poisons in these fungi is still unknown. While most of the species of mushroom are not poisonous, the few toxic ones that do exist are deadly and have been known since ancient times.

Since the first report of mushroom poisoning in 1871, much of the information about poisonous mushrooms is inaccurate—including the persistent belief that there are some ironclad "rules" that can be used to tell the difference between edible and toxic varieties. In fact, there is no rule that applies to all species of mushrooms.

For example, it's not true that a silver spoon or coin put in a pan with cooking mushrooms will turn black if the mushrooms are poisonous. *All* mushrooms will discolor silver in boiling water, if they are rotten, but *no* mushroom (toxic or edible) ever does as long as it is fresh. Toxic mushrooms won't get darker if soaked in water, nor will they get milky if soaked in vinegar.

A mycologist (mushroom expert) is the only one who can reliably detect poisonous mushrooms, and even mycologists make mistakes because the toxicity of mushrooms is complicated. Some are always deadly; others are poisonous sometimes but not others, depending on the stage of growth. And other poisonous mushrooms have never been regarded as toxic simply because no one has ever eaten them yet.

The most common poisonous mushrooms in the United States are those in the genus *Amanita* (including the world's deadliest mushroom, *A.*

phalloides); up to 90 percent of those who eat this mushroom will die if untreated.

Unlike most incidents of plant poisonings, which occur primarily in curious children, poisoning from mushrooms is generally found among adults who ingest them as a source of food or for their hallucinogenic effects. While it may be easier to obtain a history of the ingestion, it is usually almost impossible to identify the kind of mushroom eaten. It is possible, however, to identify the type of mushroom by evaluating the kinds of symptoms, since mushrooms produce only a small number of distinct toxic syndromes.

Identification   It's possible to identify the kind of mushroom ingested based on the following questions:

1. When was the mushroom eaten, and how long afterward did the symptoms appear? (When symptoms develop within two hours of ingestion, they are not often severe. Poisonings with a latency period of more than six hours may be severe or life threatening.)
2. What symptoms appeared first? If symptoms appeared quickly, are they primarily:

   • nausea and stomach pain with vomiting/diarrhea?
   • sweating?
   • intoxication or hallucinations but no drowsiness?
   • delirium and sleepiness or coma?

   If symptoms were delayed, did they produce:
   • a feeling of fullness and severe headache six hours later?
   • vomiting and watery diarrhea about 12 hours after eating?
   • extreme thirst and copious urination three days after eating?

If someone who did not eat mushrooms shows similar symptoms, it's possible the problem is bacterial food poisoning and not mushroom poisoning at all.

Symptoms   In general, symptoms that appear within two hours of eating poisonous mushrooms are rarely severe and require little intervention; symptoms that do not appear until six or more hours later are usually much more severe and can be life threatening. If more than one type of mushroom was eaten, several types of toxicity may occur. However, symptoms that appear after eating mushrooms may not be the result of systemic poisoning from a toxic mushroom. Some people are allergic to mushrooms, and others have a genetic deficiency of enzymes needed to metabolize the unusual sugars found in mushrooms; This deficiency causes gas and diarrhea. If alcoholic beverages were drunk within 72 hours of eating mushrooms, extreme nausea, vomiting and headache could occur as a result of the interference of edible mushrooms with the metabolism of alcohol.

Treatment   If someone becomes sickened and mushroom poisoning

MUSHROOMS GROUPED ACCORDING TO PRIMARY TOXIN

Amatoxins and Phallotoxins (Cyclopeptides)

Amanita phalloides
A. verna
A. virosa
A. bisporigera
A. ocreata
A. suballiacea

A. tenuifolia
Galerina autumnalus
G. marginata
G. venerata
Lepiota helveola,
Conocybe filaris

Muscimol and Ibotenic Acid

Amanita muscaria
A. pantherina
A. gemmata

A. cokeri
A. cothurnata
A. Strobiliformis

Monomethylhydrazine (gyromitrins)

Gyromitra esculenta
G. gigas
G. ambigua
G. infula
G. caroliniana

G. brunnea
G. fastigiata
Paxina
Sarcosphaera coronaria

Muscarine

Boletus calopus
B. luridus
B. pulcherrimus
B. satanas
Clitocybe cerrusata
C. dealbata
C. illudens
C. riuulosa
Inocybe fastigiata

Inocybe geophylla
I. lilacina
I. patouillardii
I. purica
I. rimosus
Amanita muscaria
A. pantherina

Coprine (and Cyclopropanone)

Coprinus atramentarius
Clitocybe clavipes

Indoles (psilocybin and psilocin)

Psilocybe cubensis
P. caerulescens
P. cyanescens
P. baeocystis
P. fimentaria
P. mexicana
P. pelluculosa

P. silvatica
Conocybe cyanopus
Gymnopilus aeruginosa
G. spectabilis
G. validipes,
Panaeolus foenisecii
P. subbalteatus

P. semilanceata
Stropharis coronilla

MUSHROOM TOXICITY

Mushroom	Toxin	Symptoms
Amanita muscaria, A. pantherina and others	Ibotenic acid, muscimol	Muscle jerks, hallucinations,
Amanita phalloides, A. ocreata, A. verna, A. virosa, Lepiota and *Galerina* species	Amatoxins	Vomiting, diarrhea, cramps, liver failure
Clitocybe dealbata, Inocybe species, *C. cerrusata, Omphalotus olearius*	Muscarine	Salivation, sweats, vomiting, diarrhea, miosis
Coprinus, Clitocybe clavipes	Coprine	Reaction with alcohol
Gyromitra (Helvella) esculenta and others	Monomethylhydrazine	Vomiting, diarrhea, weakness, seizures, hepatitis, hemolysis
Psilocybe cubensis and others	Psilocybin	Hallucinations

is suspected, first find out how many types of mushrooms were eaten, when they were eaten, the symptoms and if anyone else ate them. When determining symptoms, find out which ones appeared first. Gastrointestinal symptoms that appear more than six hours after ingestion are usually caused by a group of mushrooms including the deadly amanitas, or mushrooms containing monomethylhydrazine (including *Gyromitra* mushrooms, or false morels). If the victim has not already vomited, administer syrup of ipepac followed by activated charcoal and a cathartic. If possible, send vomited material, together with any remaining mushrooms, to a mycologist for identification. If ingested mushroom is of the *Amanita* species (except for *A. muscaria* or *A. pantherina*), the victim should be admitted to the hospital to monitor kidney and liver function.

See also AMATOXINS; COPRINE; GYROMITRA; MONOMETHYLHYDRAZINE; MUSCARINE; MUSCIMOL; MUSHROOM TOXINS.

mushroom toxins   Any illness due to the ingestion of a toxic mushroom (or toadstool) is known as mycetismus. Many species of wild mushrooms in many genera are poisonous; several of the toxins have been isolated and identified. It is important to remember that mushroom toxins differ among themselves and in the type of intoxication and symptoms they produce.

Poisoning by a mushroom toxin might range from mild symptoms of stomach upset to fatal disturbances of the body's major systems, including brain, heart, liver and kidneys.

It is estimated that between 50 and 300 people die from mushroom poisoning each year around the world; most of these are adults who have misidentified specimens.

See also AMANITA MUSHROOMS; AMATOXIN; COPRINE; FLY AGARIC; GALERINA MUSHROOMS; GYROMITRA; HALLUCINOGENIC MUSHROOMS; INKY CAP; INOCYBE MUSHROOM; LEPIOTA MUSHROOMS; MONO-METHYLHYDRAZINE; MUSCARINE; MUSCIMOL; MUSHROOM POISONING; TURBANTOP.

N

naloxone This opioid drug blocks the action of narcotic drugs and reverses breathing difficulty caused by a narcotics overdose. It is also given to newborn babies who are affected by narcotics during childbirth, and to patients who have received high doses of a narcotic drug during surgery. In addition, some reports suggest that naloxone may at least partially reverse the central nervous system and respiratory depression following clonidine and ethanol overdoses.

See also HEROIN; MORPHINE; NARCOTICS; OPIUM.

naphthalene More commonly known as mothballs or mothball flakes and toilet bowl cleaners, naphthalene is a white crystalline solid and a constituent of coal tar, which can be poisonous when eaten. The familiar mothball smell comes from naphthalene. In the past, naphthalene has also been used as an antiseptic. However, naphthalene is no longer commonly used because it has been replaced by the far less toxic paradichlorobenzene.

Too often, parents do not realize the toxicity of mothballs, and they are left where toddlers have access to them. In addition, it is not generally known that naphthalene does not easily dissolve in water and so may remain in clothes or blankets even after washing. It is even more dangerous to store baby clothes in mothballs, since naphthalene is very soluble in oil; the baby oil rubbed on an infant's skin acts as a solvent for the toxic substances in the clothes, which can then be absorbed in the baby's skin. Naphthalene products should never be used with children's clothes and diapers.

Symptoms Symptoms appear quickly, within five to 20 minutes depending on whether naphthalene was inhaled or eaten. First symptoms are nausea, vomiting, headache, diarrhea, fever, jaundice and pain while urinating. More serious poisoning causes excitement, coma and convulsions. Naphthalene causes kidney damage and destroys red blood cells, clumping them together and forcing the hemoglobins out. People with a hereditary deficiency of glucose-6-phosphate dehydrogenase (most often people of Mediterranean descent) are more susceptible to naphthalene poisoning. This same deficiency makes them sensitive to aspirin.

Treatment There is no specific antidote. If ingested, perform immediate gastric lavage followed by a saline cathartic; alcohol, milk, oil or fats should be avoided. Drink plenty of fluids to encourage the production of urine, and administer sodium bicarbonate orally and fluids with furosemide to stop kidney damage. With severe cases of poisoning with central nervous system problems, blood transfusions are given.

naproxen   (Naprosyn) See NONSTEROIDAL ANTI-INFLAMMATORY DRUGS.

narcissus *(Narcissus)*   This extremely toxic plant genus includes about 26 varieties of common flowering plants with hundreds of cultivars; they include popular plants such as the jonquil *(N. jonquilla)* and the daffodil *(N. pseudonarcissus)*—all of which are poisonous. While native to central Europe and North Africa, they are found throughout the United States.

Poisonous part   All parts of these plants—especially the bulbs—are poisonous and contain lycorine and other alkaloids.

Symptoms   Even small amounts of the bulbs can cause poisoning in adults within several hours to a few days, including symptoms of nausea, severe vomiting, diarrhea and colic. If eaten in large quantities, narcissus can cause convulsions, collapse, paralysis and death. Mortality is about 30 percent.

Treatment   Gastric lavage and fluid replacement.

narcotics   A group of depressants including codeine, opium, morphine, paregoric and heroin, which are used medicinally to relieve pain, coughing and vomiting. They require a doctor's prescription, since continued use can lead to dependence or addiction.

Depressants in addition to the above include fentanyl or Sublimaze; the eye drop DFP or diisopropylphosphate; Numorphan (oxymorphone); the painkiller Dilaudid (hydromorphone); the cough suppressant Hycodan or Dicodid; Lorfan (levallorphan); Levo-Dromoran (levorphanol); the painkiller Darvon (propoxyphene); the painkiller Talwin (pentazocine); the muscle relaxant Flexeril (cyclobenzaprine); Demerol (meperidine); and Dolantin (pethidine).

Symptoms   Soon after ingestion, the victim will become mentally stimulated and then quickly drowsy. As the body continues to absorb the narcotic, the victim will experience headache, slow, shallow breathing and finally unconsciousness and coma.

Treatment   Medical help should be sought immediately. Stimulants, such as strong tea and coffee, will help to keep the victim awake. If the victim is discovered soon after ingestion and is conscious, induce vomiting.

See also CODEINE; HEROIN; MORPHINE; OPIUM.

National Animal Poison Control Center   A 24-hour emergency center staffed by veterinary health professionals trained to handle pet poisonings. Pet owners who can't reach a vet or other local expert can call this center (at a cost of $2.95 per minute) by dialing 900-680-0000, or pay $30 per case by dialing 800-548-2423.

The nonprofit organization, affiliated with the school of veterinary medicine of the University of Illinois, was begun in 1978 and began charging for its services in 1990. All employees are veterinarians with clinical experience, with additional six months' training in toxicology; two are board certified with the American Board of Veterinary Toxicologists. In addition, the animal poison control center supports a backup laboratory to provide additional toxicological assistance.

The center fields calls equally from private pet owners and veterinarians and maintains an extensive log of poisoning cases from more than 4,000 different toxic agents. The kinds of animal poisoning cases vary according to the time of year: Pesticides and flea and tick poisonings in the summer; chocolate and poinsettia poisonings during the Easter and Christmas holidays. Most calls are due to insecticide poisonings used in and around the house or on the farm. The center handles livestock problems as well as household pets, from dogs and cats to canaries and pot belly pigs.

Poisonings with human medications make up as many as 20 percent of the calls to the animal poison center, especially heart pills and birth control pills left on nightstands. Toxic plants are a third major category.

See also PETS AND POISONING.

Nembutal   See BARBITURATES.

neostigmine   See PARASYMPATHOMIMETIC DRUGS.

neuromuscular blocking agents   A group of drugs that paralyze skeletal muscles, used to counteract excessive muscular activity, rigidity or seizures following overdoses involving stimulants (amphetamines, cocaine, phencyclidine) or strychnine. The drugs include succinylcholine, pancuronium and vecuronium. They are also used to help paralyze muscles prior to placement of an ototracheal tube.

neutralizers   Rarely used in modern hospitals, neutralizing agents at one time were sometimes employed instead of activated charcoal in certain poisoning cases: mercury and iron poisoning, iodine ingestion and strychnine, nicotine and quinine poisoning (see below).

Mercury   Sodium formaldehyde sulfoxylate neutralizes mercuric chloride and other mercury salts to metallic mercury, which cannot be absorbed by the body.

Iron   Gastric lavage with sodium bicarbonate converts the ferrous ion to ferrous carbonate, which is not well absorbed by the body.

Strychnine, nicotine and quinine   Administer potassium permanganate.

Iodine   Gastric lavage with a solution of starch and water, which is continued until the stomach contents are no longer blue.

See also IRON SUPPLEMENTS; MERCURY; NICOTINE; QUININE; STRYCHNINE.

nicotinamide   One of the B vitamins used to prevent toxic effects in the brain and endocrine system following the ingestion of the rat poison vacor. See also VACOR.

nicotine   A plant alkaloid found in several species of tobacco and an extremely fast-acting poison that, when eaten, can cause blood vessels to collapse and the muscles of respiration to fail in much the same way as does curare. While there is no medicinal use for nicotine, some of its derivatives are used as botanic insecticides; in fact, nicotine is the oldest insecticide known.

In those who ingest nicotine by smoking cigarettes or chewing the leaves, repeated small doses soon build up tolerance to the toxins. The primary danger of poisoning lies in the manufacture and use of insecticides containing nicotine.

Toxic doses vary and range from 4 mg to 2 g; generally 40 mg is considered fatal. Nicotine content in regular cigarettes averages about 15 to 20 mg per cigarette; cigars range from 15 to 40 mg. Eating tobacco is not generally a serious toxic risk, since the stomach does not absorb nicotine well from cigarettes.

Children may become poisoned with nicotine if they ingest tobacco or drink saliva spit out by a tobacco chewer (often collected in a spittoon or can). Adults may attempt suicide by ingesting nicotine-containing pesticides, or may be poisoned after coming in contact with tobacco while harvesting the plants.

Nicotine chewing gum (Nicorette) has been marketed as an aid for people to stop smoking, but its slow absorption makes nicotine intoxication from this product unlikely.

Symptoms   Nicotine's effects are extremely complex and vary from person to person, depending on the length of time following exposure, the amount of dosage and chronic use. Cigarette tobacco and moist snuff each contain about 1.5 percent nicotine; chewing tobacco contains 2.5 to 8 percent nicotine; nicotine gum contains 2 mg per piece in the United States (although bioavailability is only about 20 to 40 percent of that amount).

Rapid absorption of between 2 and 5 mg can cause nausea and vomiting, especially in a person unused to nicotine. Absorption of 40 to 60 mg in an adult may be lethal, although most smokers get this dose spread throughout the day. In a child, ingestion of one cigarette or three butts may be toxic, although serious poisoning from cigarette ingestion is rare.

Immediately after ingestion, nicotine causes a burning sensation in the mouth, throat, esophagus and stomach. Once in the bloodstream, whether after inhalation from tobacco smoke or though the mouth from chewing tobacco (or, more recently, in nicotine gum or the nicotine skin patch), the substance acts on the central nervous system until it is eventually broken down by the liver and excreted. It first stimulates, and then depresses, both the brain and spinal cord. It primarily affects the autonomic nervous system, which controls involuntary body activities (such as heart rate). While effects vary from person to person, it can slow the heart rate and cause nausea and vomiting.

In habitual users, however, nicotine increases the heart rate, narrows the blood vessels (thereby raising blood pressure) and stimulates the central nervous system, reducing tiredness and improving concentration. It is uncertain whether the nicotine contained in tobacco products is responsible for coronary heart disease, peripheral vascular disease and other heart problems.

Extremely large amounts of nicotine can affect breathing in ways similar to that of curare, paralyzing the breathing muscles and causing vomiting, seizures and death from respiratory arrest only minutes after ingestion.

Treatment In severe poisonings, artificial respiration and oxygen must be administered, since death occurs from respiratory paralysis. Nicotine is completely eliminated from the body within 16 hours, so victims who can be kept alive for that period may live. Mecamylamine (Inversine) is a specific antagonist of nicotine but is available only in tablets, which are not suitable for a victim who is vomiting, has low blood pressure or is having convulsions. Signs of parasympathetic stimulation (that is, slow heartbeat, salivation, wheezing, etc.) may respond to atropine.

For ingestion: gastric lavage followed by the administration of activated charcoal to absorb excess nicotine; pentobarbital, diazepam or inhalation anesthesia to control convulsions. For skin contamination: scrub skin with plenty of soap and water and remove contaminated clothing.

See also BOTANIC INSECTICIDES; NICOTINE GUM; NICOTINE PATCH; TOBACCO.

nicotine gum   (nicotine polacrilex) Popularly known by its trade name Nicorette, this is a nicotine resin that is used to help people stop smoking. It gradually releases nicotine when chewed. However, chewing too much of the gum will release too much nicotine and cause nausea. For this reason, heart patients, pregnant women and those with peptic ulcers should not chew the gum.

The gum was designed to be "parked" between cheek and gum, in order to maximize the nicotine's absorption. As the smoker begins to feel comfortable with the smoke-free behaviors, the amount of nicotine is decreased over a six-month period.

Symptoms The same as nicotine overdose: indigestion and upset stomach.

Treatment Symptomatic; decrease the amount of gum chewed.

See also NICOTINE; TOBACCO.

nicotine patch   The most recent innovation in the stop-smoking arsenal, the nicotine patch is one of the newest methods for timed-release medication. In this form, nicotine is gradually absorbed through the skin as a means to help a smoker stop using cigarettes.

However, recent research reports indicate that several patients wearing a patch have died from heart attacks because they have continued to smoke.

Symptoms Nicotine acts on the central nervous system until it is eventually broken down by the liver and excreted. It first stimulates, and then depresses, both the brain and spinal cord. It primarily affects the autonomic nervous system, which controls involuntary body activities (such as heart rate). In habitual users nicotine increases the heart rate and narrows the blood vessels (thereby raising blood pressure); it can also cause a heart attack.

Treatment The best treatment is preventive: *Never smoke cigarettes while wearing a nicotine patch.* In severe cases, artificial respiration and oxygen may need to be administered. Nicotine is completely eliminated from the body within 16 hours, so victims who can be kept alive for that period may live. Mecamylamine (Inversine) is a specific antagonist of nicotine but is available only in tablets, which are not suitable for a victim who is vomiting, has low blood pressure or is having convulsions. Signs of parasympathetic stimulation (that is, slow heartbeat, salivation, wheezing, etc.) may respond to atropine.

See also NICOTINE; NICOTINE GUM; TOBACCO.

nifedipine This calcium antagonist dilates the systemic and coronary arteries and is used to combat severe high blood pressure following overdose of vasoconstrictive substances such as phenylpropanolamine, cocaine, amphetamines, phencyclidine or other stimulants. It is also helpful to counteract peripheral or coronary artery spasms following poisoning by ergot or cocaine.

nightshade, bittersweet A member of the wide-ranging nightshade family (but a less deadly relative than deadly nightshade), bittersweet nightshade can also have poisonous effects.

Poisonous part The entire plant contains the toxin atropine and other belladonna alkaloids, including scopolamine, hyoscyamine, hyoscine and belladonna—but these are concentrated in the roots, leaves and berries. These alkaloids paralyze the parasympathetic nervous system (which controls the involuntary activities of the organs, glands, blood vessels and other body tissues). Atropine can directly stimulate the central nervous system and is eliminated almost entirely by the kidneys. Taken internally, as little as 0.1 g of atropine (one of the alkaloids extracted from nightshade) can cause poisoning.

Symptoms Symptoms appear between 15 minutes and a few hours after ingestion and include a scratchy or burning sensation in the throat with a loss of voice, rapid pulse, fever, nausea, vomiting, blurred vision, pupil dilation, inability to urinate, difficulty in swallowing, mental confusion, aggressive behavior, reduced secretion of saliva, convulsions, coma and death. The poison acts by paralyzing the nerve endings of the involuntary muscles. Mild poisoning acts as a euphoric, imparting a feeling of timelessness or giddiness to its victims. Severe poisoning causes blindness, rage and paralysis of the central nervous system. Coma is followed by death from respiratory failure.

Treatment Gastric lavage with 4 percent tannic acid solution and vomiting. Pilocarpine or physostigmine may be given for dry mouth and visual disturbances. There is no known antidote. There is risk of heart, kidney and urinary tract damage if symptoms are prolonged or severe. If treatment is initiated, prognosis is good.

See also ATROPINE; NIGHTSHADE; DEADLY.

nightshade, deadly (*Atropa belladonna* L.) [Other names: anuncena de Mejico, banewort, Barbados lily, belladonna lily, cape belladonna, dwale, English nightshade, lirio, naked lady lily, sleeping nightshade.] Also known as belladonna, deadly nightshade is a powerful drug plant (source of the drug atropine) with a history rich in magic, witchcraft and murder. It is a member of the Solanaceae family and is one of a group of nightshades.

However, the "true" nightshades contain the poison solanine, and they are closely related—the Jerusalem cherry, the woody nightshade or European bittersweet and the American, or black, nightshade. Deadly nightshade (the belladonna plant) belongs to another branch of the Solanaceae, and its chief poison is atropine.

Atropine and solanine have different effects on the body, so that reporting a poisoning with "nightshade" is not specific enough to determine correct treatment.

Native to Eurasia and North Africa, this three-foot, shrublike perennial herb is found in meadows, near old buildings and in shady, marshy places in North America and is cultivated commercially in Europe for medicinal purposes. While its fresh leaves have an unpleasant smell when crushed, the dried leaves are odorless; both have a bitter taste. Its alternate ovate leaves grow on multibranched stems, with glossy black, round berries and bell-shaped flowers that have an intensely sweet smell from July to September. A horizontal, underground, thickened plant stem produces shoots above and roots below and bears buds, nodes and scalelike leaves.

The name "belladonna" comes from the Italian, meaning "beautiful woman," a reference to its use during the Renaissance, when women used an extract to make their complexions luminous and to dilate their pupils for a wide-eyed, beautiful look. Rouge was also made from the berries. Its generic name *Atropa* comes from the Greeks, whose myth holds that when the thread of life was played out by the three Fates, Atropos cut it.

According to astrologists, deadly nightshade is ruled by Hecate and is popular in witchcraft as a shape changer, a flying ointment and a major hallucinogen. (Of 16 recipes for flying ointments, eight call for deadly nightshade.) It is also said that deadly nightshade can change into a beautiful enchantress on Walpurgis, the witches' sabbath.

There is also a place for nightshade in literature; it is believed Shakespeare intended it as the poison that Juliet takes in *Romeo and Juliet* so she will seem dead but is really just sleeping.

Poisonous part A single berry can be fatal, and the entire plant contains the toxin atropine and other belladonna alkaloids, including scopolamine, hyoscyamine, hyoscine and belladonna—but these are concentrated in the roots, leaves and berries. These alkaloids paralyze the parasympathetic nervous system (which controls the involuntary activities of the organs, glands, blood vessels and other body tissues). Atropine can directly stimulate the central nervous system and is eliminated almost entirely by the kidneys.

Taken internally, as little as 0.1 g of atropine (one of the alkaloids extracted from nightshade) can cause poisoning. The root is the most poisonous part, but the entire plant is deadly. A careful dose of deadly nightshade is antispasmodic, is a sedative and a diuretic and induces sweating; it also inhibits mucus and glandular secretions. At certain doses, the drug relieves pain and stimulates the central nervous system; it is classified as a narcotic. Its derivative atropine is considered an important drug today as an antidote for some types of nerve gas, and also as an antidote for depressant poisons such as muscarine, opium and chloral hydrate. Atropine is also an antispasmodic to treat gastritis, pancreatitis and chronic urethritis. Nightshade's leaves provide isolated compounds including hyoscyamine and scopolamine, and it was once used in ophthalmology for pupil dilation, although it has generally been replaced today by other chemicals.

The plant is often eaten by rabbits, which can then pass the poison on to anyone who eats the affected meat.

Symptoms Symptoms appear between 15 minutes and a few hours after ingestion and include a scratchy or burning sensation in the throat with a loss of voice, rapid pulse, fever, nausea, vomiting, blurred vision, pupil dilation, inability to urinate, difficulty in swallowing, mental confusion, aggressive behavior, reduced secretion of saliva, convulsions, coma and death. The poison acts by paralyzing the nerve endings of the involuntary muscles. Mild poisoning acts as a euphoric, imparting a feeling of timelessness or giddiness to its victims. Severe poisoning causes blindness, rage and paralysis of the central nervous system. Coma is followed by death from respiratory failure.

Treatment Gastric lavage with 4 percent tannic acid solution and vomiting. Pilocarpine or physostigmine may be given for dry mouth and visual disturbances. There is no known antidote for belladonna poisoning, and because the poison breaks down very slowly in the body, it is often impossible to save the victim. There is risk of heart, kidney and urinary tract damage if symptoms are prolonged or severe, and poisoning can be quickly fatal if treatment is not initiated. If treatment is initiated, prognosis is good.

See also ATROPINE; NIGHTSHADE, BITTERSWEET.

nightshade, yellow *(Urechites lutea)* This woody vine is found in Florida, the Bahamas and the Greater and Lesser Antilles south to St. Vincent. It has a milky sap and long, narrow leaves with yellow flower clusters. The fruit is contained in woody pods that can grow to eight inches, containing winged seeds.

Poisonous part The leaves of the yellow nightshade are poisonous, containing urechitoxin, a cardiac glycoside.

Symptoms Symptoms appear some time after ingestion, depending on the amount of material eaten. They include pain in the mouth; nausea and vomiting; abdominal pain; cramps and diarrhea; and heart problems (conduction defects and slow heartbeat).

Treatment Gastric lavage followed by activated charcoal and saline cathartics. For heart problems, atropine and phenytoin.

See also CARDIAC GLYCOSIDES; NIGHTSHADE, BITTERSWEET; NIGHTSHADE, DEADLY.

nitrogen oxides Nitric oxide and nitrogen dioxide are dangerous chemical gases released during a variety of chemical and industrial processes, including electric arc welding, electroplating and engraving. The oxides are found in engine exhaust, and they are produced when stored grain with a high nitrite content ferments in storage bins. Nitrogen dioxide is a colorless gas, arising from unvented gas stoves, that causes respiratory problems in children.

Slow accumulation and hydration to nitric acid in the alveoli cause delayed onset of chemical pneumonitis. Because nitrogen oxides do not dissolve well in water, there is very little upper respiratory irritation at low levels of exposure, and prolonged contact may occur with only a mild cough or nausea. However, with more concentrated exposures, upper respiratory symptoms such as burning eyes, sore throat and painful cough may be noted.

Symptoms After exposure, there may be a delay of up to 24 hours before chemical pneumonia may occur, with cough and pulmonary edema; following recovery there may be permanent restrictive and obstructive lung disease because of broncholar damage.

Treatment Administration of corticosteroids is the treatment of choice by many toxicologists, but there is no convincing evidence that this will improve the chances of avoiding chemical pneumonia or lung damage. Remove the victim from exposure and give oxygen; observe closely for signs of upper airway obstruction for at least 24 hours after exposure. Remove contaminated clothing and flush exposed skin with water; irrigate exposed eyes with saline.

nitroglycerin (glyceryl trinitrate) A vasodilating drug used to lower blood pressure and dilate coronary vessels; when taken with alcohol, it can cause a sharp drop in blood pressure. It is available in spray or tablet form and can be ingested, injected, inhaled or absorbed. Nitroglycerin is also given to treat coronary spasm in adults suffering from ergot poisoning.

Symptoms Immediately after ingestion the drug begins to dilate blood vessels throughout the body; overdose causes headache, flushing of skin, vomiting, dizziness, collapse, low blood pressure, coma and respiratory paralysis.

Treatment Induce vomiting with syrup of ipecac followed by activated charcoal.

nitroprusside Sodium nitroprusside is a vasodilator typically given to treat high blood pressure and heart failure and to induce hypotension for certain operations. Poisoning may occur with one single large overdose or with prolonged use. It is also used in the treatment of stimulant or mono-amine oxidase inhibitor overdose.

Poisonous part Nitroprusside releases free cyanide; acute cyanide poisoning may be produced with a high-dose infusion of nitroprusside. People with faulty kidneys may also have problems eliminating thiocyanate, which therefore accumulate and cause symptoms.

Symptoms The most common symptom is low blood pressure with reflex tachycardia. Cyanide poisoning includes symptoms of headache, hyperventilation, anxiety, agitation, seizures and metabolic acidosis.

Treatment In the case of cyanide poisoning, administer sodium thiosulfate; sodium nitrite may worsen low blood pressure and is not indicated. Hydroxocobalamin is available in Europe as a cyanide antidote. Continue to treat symptoms; hemodialysis may help eliminate thiocyanate and is helpful for victims with kidney problems.

See also CYANIDE.

nitrous oxide Also known as "laughing gas" widely used by dentists and available on college campuses, nitrous oxide is a general anesthetic and is used in a wide variety of commercial products, including whipped cream and cooking oil sprays.

Discovered in 1776, it was not used as an anesthetic until 23 years later; it was not widely used until 1860. It was, however, popular at parties; Sir Humphry Davy, the first person to synthesize the gas, enjoyed nitrous oxide parties as did the poets Samuel Coleridge and Robert Southey, and Peter Roget, author of *Roget's Thesaurus*. Reportedly, students in the early 19th century used nitrous oxide for recreational purposes, and one student actually quit medical school and began selling the stuff for 25 cents per dose.

However, this nonflammable, nearly odorless gas does not produce a complete anesthesia at safe levels and is therefore used as a painkiller or together with stronger anesthetic agents. It is often abused for the euphoria it produces and is easily available on the street.

Poisonous part Nitrous oxide depresses the central nervous system and, when used without enough oxygen, can be fatal.

Symptoms If used improperly (that is, without sufficient oxygen), nitrous oxide can cause irregular heart patterns, brain damage, death, headache, cerebral edema and permanent mental deficiency. Symptoms appear within a few seconds to several minutes.

Treatment There is no specific antidote. Administer oxygen; give symptomatic treatment. Chronic symptoms should disappear between two and three months after exposure has ended.

See also ANESTHETICS; GASEOUS/VOLATILE.

nonsteroidal anti-inflammatory drugs (NSAIDs)   This is a group of chemically diverse drugs widely used for the treatment of pain and inflammation. On their own, anti-inflammatory drugs are not very toxic, but victims with gastrointestinal tract disease, peptic ulcers or poor heart function and those on anticoagulant drugs should avoid them. Inflammation results in an increased blood flow, which in turn produces swelling, redness, pain and heat. Inflammation is one of the body's defense mechanisms in response to infection and certain chronic diseases such as rheumatoid arthritis.

NSAIDs include ibuprofen (Motrin, Rufen, Advil, Haltrin, Medipren, Nuprin), fenoprofen (Nalfon), meclofenamate (Meclomen), naproxen (Anaprox, Naprosyn), sulindac (Clinoril), indomethacin (Indocin), tolmetin (Tolectin), mefenamic acid, piroxicam (Feldene), oxyphenbutazone and phenylbutazone.

None of these should be taken with other nonsteroid analgesics or with warfarin or other oral anticoagulants, because bleeding time may be prolonged while on anti-inflammatory pain relievers. Antacids, however, may sometimes reduce the effects of an anti-inflammatory drug.

Symptoms While an overdose of most of the NSAIDs causes little toxicity beyond stomach pain, there are a few that do produce severe toxicity: oxyphenbutazone, phenylbutazone, mefenamic acid, piroxicam and diflunisal. In general, symptoms appear after ingesting more than five to 10 times the therapeutic dose.

If a person is allergic to aspirin or other nonsteroid analgesic drug, using another anti-inflammatory medicine could be fatal. Anti-inflammatory drugs become toxic when given to those with kidney problems, since the kidneys can't cleanse the blood. Overdose causes kidney failure and severe liver reactions, including fatal jaundice.

Normally NSAID overdose produces mild stomach upset, with nausea

NONSTEROIDAL ANTI-INFLAMMATORY DRUGS

Drug	Usual daily dose (adult)	Maximum recommended daily dose (adult)
fenoprofen	900-2,400 mg	3,200 mg
ibuprofen	900-2,400 mg	2,400 mg
indomethacin	50-150 mg	200 mg
meclofenamate	200-400 mg	400 mg
mefenamic	1,000 mg	1,000 mg
naproxen	500-1,000 mg	1,250 mg
piroxicam	20 mg	20 mg
sulindac	300-400 mg	400 mg
tolmetin	1,200-1,800 mg	2,000 mg

and vomiting plus abdominal pain. Occasionally, other symptoms might include sleepiness, lethargy, nystagmus, (an involuntary oscillation of the eyeball); tinnitus (ringing in the ears) and disorientation. However, with the more toxic drugs listed above and significant overdose of ibuprofen (in excess of 3,200 mg per day), symptoms may include seizures, coma, metabolic acidosis, kidney and liver failure and cardiorespiratory arrest. Diflunisal overdose resembles salicylate poisoning.

   Treatment   There is no antidote. Maintain symptomatic treatment together with antacids for mild stomach problems; perform gastric lavage, followed by the administration of activated charcoal and a cathartic. Research suggests charcoal hemoperfusion may help in the treatment of phenylbutazone overdose, although it has not been proven.

nontoxic plants   The following plants are considered nonpoisonous to humans, and toxic symptoms from eating them are rare. However, any plant can cause a reaction in certain sensitive or allergic people. Nonpoisonous plants include African violet, aluminum plant, aspidistra, aster, baby's tears, begonia, bird's nest fern, Boston fern, bougainvillaea, California poppy, camellia, Christmas cactus, coleus, creeping Charlie, dahlia, dandelion, Easter lily, gardenia, impatiens, jade plant, kalanchoe, lipstick plant, magnolia, marigold, nasturtium, Norfolk Island pine, pepperomia, petunia, poinsettia, prayer plant, purple passion, rose, sensitive plant, spider plant, swedish ivy, tiger lily, umbrella tree, violet wandering jew, wax plant, wild strawberry and zebra plant.

nontoxic substances The following substances are considered nontoxic and are harmful only in very large quantities: antacids, antibiotics, aquarium products, baby oil, birth-control pills, blackboard chalk, bubble bath, candles, caps for a cap pistol, castor oil, dehumidifying packets, denture adhesives, deodorants, diaper rash ointment, dry cell batteries, eye makeup, fabric softener, fishbowl products, glycerin, graphite (the "lead" in a pencil), hand creams and lotions, kaolin, lanolin, lauric acid, lipstick, makeup, modeling clay, multiple vitamins without iron, nail polish, petroleum jelly, putty, shaving cream, soaps, stearic acid, tallow, teething rings and watercolor paints. (Of course, any substance can sometimes cause an unexpected reaction in sensitive individuals.)

nutmeg *(Myristica fragrans)* In small quantities this common spice is edible, but in large doses it can be fatal. Produced from the dried seeds of the nutmeg tree, it is found in the South Pacific and the East Indies. Mace, another popular spice and the extract used as a spray to discourage attackers, is also obtained from this tree.

Nutmeg has been used since the seventh century A.D. to treat asthma and fever. It takes up to three whole nutmegs or up to 15 g of the grated spice to become intoxicated.

Symptoms Symptoms appear within two to six hours after ingestion and include sedation, euphoria and hallucinations, which can last up to two days. The stimulation of the central nervous system may be accompanied by tachycardia, skin flushing, decreased salivation and delirium, with nausea, vomiting and abdominal cramps. Other symptoms, much like those of intoxication with PCP, can include belligerent behavior and hyperactivity. Occasionally, complications can lead to coma, shock and death.

In very high doses, nutmeg is a hallucinogen that can cause liver damage and death. In fairly small amounts, it can cause severe headache, cramps and nausea.

Treatment Gastric lavage; supportive treatment including a cathartic. Administer barbiturates or diazepam to control convulsions.

nux-vomica *(Strychnos nux-vomica)* [Other names: strychnine.] Found in India and Hawaii, this "dog button plant" is actually a small tree, with oval leaves and yellow to white clusters of flowers. Its small, attractive fruit resembles a mandarin or Chinese orange and looks tempting to eat; the fruit contains seeds that look like gray velvet buttons.

Poisonous part The entire tree contains strychnine, but the seeds contain the greatest concentration of the poison. The blossoms, which smell of curry powder, can be mistaken by a child as edible and are therefore a potential cause of poisoning.

Symptoms Extreme irritability and restlessness followed by exhaustion, sweating, muscular rigidity, respiratory problems and death. In severe cases, there are often generalized spasms that last from a few seconds to several minutes and are caused by external sensory stimuli. Metabolic acidosis may also appear.

Treatment Establish an airway, provide oxygen if needed; convulsions may call for a general anesthetic and muscle relaxant; reduce fever and correct acidosis with intravenous sodium bicarbonate.

See also STRYCHNINE.

O

octopus, blue-ringed *(Hapalochlaena maculosa)* The only poisonous octopus, this small, harmless-looking marine animal looks playful and cute, but its bite can be fatal. The octopus is brown and speckled, with blue bands around its tentacles that glow just before the poison is released. Just four inches long, this unique octopod is usually found in shallow waters around the coast of Australia and can be deadly if provoked. It feeds on mollusks and crabs with its strong beak and can commonly be found under rocks at low tide.

Normally, both males and females are equally toxic, but when the female blue-ring begins brooding her eggs, her venom becomes even more potent. However, like most other female octopuses, she stops eating once she deposits her eggs and, soon after they hatch, she dies.

A relative, the Australian spotted octopus *(H. lunulata)*, lives near Queensland, New South Wales, Sydney and Victoria, in the Indian Ocean and Japan. Another relative, almost as deadly, is the North American west coast octopus *(Octopus apollyon)*, found from Alaska to Baja California.

Symptoms The bite of the blue-ringed octopus is often not even noticed and usually occurs when the creature is picked up or played with, as it is generally shy and stays away from humans. Immediately after the bite, the poison begins to affect the central nervous system, causing severe pain and paralyzing muscles of the entire body until breathing stops. Its poison can kill in minutes.

Treatment Immediately after the bite, it is important to maintain breathing through mouth-to-mouth resuscitation, since death usually occurs as a result of the neuromuscular poisons.

oleander *(Nerium oleander)* Also known as Jericho rose, this extremely deadly poisonous plant is a native of Asia and is widely cultivated in the United States as an ornamental shrub and houseplant. It is widely planted in the South and Southwest because of its beautiful flowers and is widely found in the South planted along driveways and property lines as a colorful hedging. This plant's toxic reputation has been known since ancient times, although the general population today may not be aware of its deadly properties.

Oleander is a fragrant evergreen shrub with narrow leaves and white, yellow, pink or red blossoms and leathery leaves that can reach 10 inches. Winged seeds are borne in long, narrow capsules.

Poisonous part   All parts of the oleander plant are poisonous; one leaf can kill an adult. Even the nectar from the flower, honey from the pollen, the smoke from the burning plant and the water in which flowers are placed are poisonous. The clear, gummy sap contains cardiac glycosides, oldendrin and nerioside, which stop the heart. Serious poisoning cases have been reported from using oleander twigs to roast meat; children can be poisoned by chewing on a single leaf or flower.

Symptoms   Onset of symptoms may be immediate: pain in the mouth and throat, nausea, severe vomiting, stomach pain, bloody diarrhea, dizziness, altered state of consciousness, slow or irregular heartbeat, dilated pupils, drowsiness, slow respirations, coma and death.

Treatment   Prompt gastric lavage is vital, together with cardiac depressants to control heart rhythm. The preferred antidote is dipotassium instead of calcium EDTA, since dipotassium chelates calcium in the body. Activated charcoal may be given later. Treatment is similar to that for digitalis poisoning.

See also CARDIAC GLYCOSIDES; FOXGLOVE.

oleander, yellow   *(Thevetia peruviana)*   While its action is the same as that of oleander and it is just as poisonous, its sap is milky. Growing to 20 feet tall, with leaves very similar to those of oleander, this plant has flowers that are yellow with a hint of peach. The small oval fruit contains up to four flat seeds. Yellow oleander is found in the southwestern United States, Florida, the West Indies, Hawaii and Guam.

Poisonous part   All parts of the oleander plant are poisonous—especially its seeds, which contain a glycoside similar to digitalis.

Symptoms   Onset of symptoms may be immediate or appear later, depending on the amount of toxin ingested: nausea, severe vomiting, stomach pain, bloody diarrhea, dizziness, altered state of consciousness, slow or irregular heartbeat, dilated pupils, drowsiness, and slow respirations.

Treatment   Prompt gastric lavage is vital, followed by activated charcoal, together with cardiac depressants to control heart rhythm. Treatment is similar to that for digitalis poisoning.

See also CARDIAC GLYCOSIDES; FOXGLOVE.

opium   *(Papaver somniferum)*   This sticky substance is found in the fruit and juices of the opium poppy, which grows throughout Europe, Asia and the tropics and can be combined with other drugs to form laudanum, paregoric and other medications.

It has been used in the Orient since 200 B.C., when it was mentioned in the writings of Theophrastus, a Greek philosopher who studied under Aristotle. At that time, opium was given through punctures in the skin or inhaled as a vapor into the nose and mouth, where it unpredictably produced either analgesia or death. In the second century A.D., the Greek physician Galen was treating his patients with opium, and in 700 years it had spread to Arabia.

In the 16th century, physicians figured out how to create laudanum from opium, but its use gradually evolved to include recreational abuse, and by the late 1600s opium smoking had spread everywhere. Opium was introduced as a medicine in Britain in 1680 by Thomas Syndenham, an English physician who proclaimed that opium was "universal and efficacious."

By 1729, however, its negative side was recognized in Asia, and opium smoking was outlawed in China and its import from India banned. Unfortunately, the British East India Company (which imported the drug) refused to stop and smuggled the drug into China—leading to the so-called opium wars between Great Britain and China in 1839 and again in 1856.

Opium's use reached a peak in popularity during Victorian times, when cities were honeycombed with opium dens and physicians prescribed laudanum for a variety of "female problems" (cramps, menstrual distress, etc.). Its use spread to the United States with the thousands of Chinese laborers imported to help build the western railroads in the middle of the 19th century.

Today, the extraction of morphine and the development of synthetic narcotics have rendered opium obsolete, and it is considered an old-fashioned remedy. It is used to treat infants who are born addicted because of their mothers' abuse of narcotics, usually in the form of paregoric, a mixture of opium, camphor, benzoic acid and alcohol. Opium is classified as a Schedule II or III drug depending on its form.

Symptoms Opium, which contains codeine, morphine, thebaine, papaverine and narcotine, is a central nervous system depressant that restricts pupil size, slows breathing, and causes nausea, vomiting, constipation, weak pulse, low blood pressure, dehydration and euphoria followed by cardiovascular depression, unresponsiveness, coma, respiratory failure and death within two to three hours of ingestion of a large dose.

Treatment Gastric lavage followed by activated charcoal and cathartics, with the administration of naloxone and other supportive and symptomatic treatment.

See also LAUDANUM.

oral contraceptives See BIRTH CONTROL PILLS.

organophosphate insecticides These extremely potent insecticides interfere with nerve signal transmission and, if ingested, can cause serious systemic poisoning and death. The most common organophosphate insecticide is parathion. An outgrowth of nerve gas research done in Germany during the 1930s, these insecticides are often used by commercial growers to control insect pests and are the most common sources of insecticide poisoning in humans. The Environmental Protection Agency has reported that more than 80 percent of all pesticide poisoning hospitalizations were caused by the organophosphates, mostly involving children, laborers and farmers.

Organophosphate insecticides like malathion and diazanon are also used by home gardeners to control spider mites, aphids, mealy bugs and other pests. They continue to be popular because they are effective and don't remain in body tissues or the environment, due to their unstable chemical structure that disintegrates into harmless radicals within days of application. The organophosphates have largely replaced banned DDT as an agricultural insecticide.

Still, the use of organophosphate pesticides can result in a buildup of residue on leaves and stems and—if used inside the home—can result in the release of noxious vapor into the air. Individual organophosphates vary widely in their toxicity; probably the most dangerous is TEPP (tetraethylpyrophosphate), the oldest known organophosphate; malathion lies at the other end of the spectrum as the least toxic of the group.

The organophosphates interfere with the enzyme cholinesterase, which helps to regulate the amount of acetylcholine in the body; this causes a buildup of acetylcholine, which interferes with the central nervous system and the parasympathetic nervous system.

Toxic levels of organophosphates occur in children who ingest pesticides or animal tick and flea killers; they also occur in agricultural exposure by farm workers and suicide attempts (the largest number of cases).

For those occupations involving exposure to organophosphates, such as factory workers producing lubricants, fire retardants and pesticides, it should be understood that these compounds are highly toxic and can penetrate the skin without producing sensations and can be fatal. These compounds are being investigated for delayed neurotoxicity.

Symptoms   Symptoms usually appear within 24 hours of exposure but vary according to the specific chemical, exposure and type of contamination. At first, symptoms include headache, cramps, vomiting, diarrhea, dizziness, weakness, sweating and salivation. In cases of severe poisoning, symptoms include coma, pulmonary edema, psychosis, convulsions, bradycardia, cyanosis, twitching and paralysis. Death usually occurs within 24 hours after complications occur in cases that have not been treated, or within 10 days in treated cases.

Treatment   Remove all contaminated clothes, wash thoroughly with soap followed by a second wash with alcohol. Administer syrup of ipecac (if victim is fully alert) and perform gastric lavage. Atropine is the antidote for organophosphate poisoning, with the possible administration of pralidoxime.

See also MALATHION; TEPP.

oven cleaner   See ALKALINE CORROSIVES.

oxalates   A class of compounds related to oxalic acid, named after the wood sorrel (Oxalidaceae) family, in which it was first identified. Oxalate salts and oxalic acid are found in philodendron, dieffenbachia and other plants and can be very irritating to the skin and mucous membranes. In severe cases, exposure to calcium oxalate can cause the throat to swell shut, resulting in suffocation. In addition, oxalic acid and many of the oxalate salts can become concentrated in the kidneys and cause systemic poisoning.

See also DIEFFENBACHIA; PHILODENDRON.

oxycodone   A semisynthetic derivative of codeine marketed in the United States as an ingredient of combination products only. (For example, Percodan contains oxycodone hydrochloride, oxycodone terrephthalate and aspirin.) Oxycodone is a Schedule II drug (drug with high potential for abuse) capable of inducing a morphine like dependence stronger than that associated with codeine. It has about the same painkilling ability as morphine when injected, and it retains half of its effectiveness when given by mouth.

Symptoms   Respiratory depression, stupor, cold and clammy skin, slow heartbeat, and low blood pressure. More severe overdoses can lead to apnea, circulatory collapse, coma, cardiac arrest and death.

Treatment   The antidote is naloxone. Do not induce vomiting. Gastric lavage may be effective even after several hours following ingestion; administer activated charcoal and a saline cathartic. Give supportive and symptomatic treatment; seizures may be controlled with intravenous diazepam.

See also CODEINE; MORPHINE; NALOXONE; NARCOTICS.

oxygen   This colorless, odorless gas is essential for all forms of life on earth, because it is necessary for the metabolic burning of foods to produce energy (aerobic metabolism). Oxygen is also used as a treatment following inhalation of toxic gases; 100 percent oxygen is indicated for carbon monoxide poisoning; hyperbaric oxygen (100 percent oxygen delivered to the victim in a pressurized chamber) is believed by some experts to more rapidly improve recovery from carbon monoxide poisoning.

oxymorphone   A semisynthetic derivative of oxycodone and a narcotic painkiller, oxymorphone has less of a depressing effect on the cough reflex; it is therefore used primarily as a painkiller for postsurgical patients. Reported to be more than 10 times stronger than morphine and almost twice as toxic, it is equally addictive.

Symptoms   Respiratory depression, stupor, cold and clammy skin, slow heartbeat, and low blood pressure. More severe overdoses can lead to apnea, circulatory collapse, coma, cardiac arrest and death.

Treatment   The antidote is naloxone. Do not induce vomiting. Gastric lavage may be effective even after several hours following ingestion; administer activated charcoal and a saline cathartic. Give supportive and symptomatic treatment; seizures may be controlled with intravenous diazepam.

See also NARCOTICS; OXYCODONE.

P

paint removers See HYDROCARBON.

paint thinner See PETROLEUM DISTILLATES.

panther mushroom *(Amanita pantherina)* Often confused with its close relative, fly agaric, the panther mushroom is a relatively small, squat plant with a cap surface colored from yellow to purple brown and covered with white warts. Raised in the United States, it is found in spring and fall in conifer woods west of the Cascade Mountains in Oregon and Washington.

    Poisonous part Muscimol is a water-soluble toxin first isolated in the early 1960s from both the fly agaric and the panther mushroom. Both muscimol and its metabolic precursor, ibotenic acid, are believed to be the primary cause for the toxicity of these two mushrooms and a few related species.

    Symptoms Deaths from eating the panther mushroom have occasionally been reported in the United States. Within 20 to 90 minutes after ingestion, muscimol begins to affect the central nervous system, causing drowsiness, stupor, elation, hyperactivity, delirium, confusion, hallucinations, heartbeat problems, gastroenteritis, urinary retention, blurred vision, watery diarrhea and convulsions.

    Treatment Induce vomiting and perform gastric lavage; administration of physostigmine and diazepam (Valium) may help control symptoms and convulsions. Stimulants are not advised.

    See also FLY AGARIC; MUSCIMOL; MUSHROOM POISONING; MUSHROOM TOXINS.

paradichlorobenzene One of two common ingredients in mothballs and toilet bowl cleaners (the other is naphthalene), this chemical has a pungent odor but is far less toxic than naphthalene. However, ingestion of large amounts can still cause stomach upset and central nervous system stimulation. Up to 20 g have been well tolerated by adults.

    Symptoms Nausea and vomiting very soon after ingestion.

    Treatment There is no specific antidote. Administer activated charcoal and a cathartic. Treat coma or seizures if they occur.

    See also NAPHTHALENE.

paralytic shellfish poisoning (PSP) PSP is the most serious of the three types of shellfish poisoning caused by toxic forms of dinoflagellates (one-celled plankton) found in a variety of shellfish. While shellfish by themselves are not poisonous, they can become contaminated by bacteria and other organisms from their environment and pass them on to humans when the shellfish is eaten. Oysters, clams and mussels are particularly prone to becoming contaminated because of their metabolic system, which pumps water across the gills to isolate plankton for their food. This system makes them vulnerable to bacteria, viruses or other contaminants in the water. Crustacean shellfish (such as lobsters) only very rarely transmit PSP.

Some types of toxic plankton multiply rapidly during the warm summer months; because their color is pink or red, this phenomenon has come to be called "red tide." These plankton (*Gonyaulax*) produce the deadly poison saxitoxin, which blocks nerve impulses and causes paralytic shellfish poisoning; it is so toxic that even one contaminated shellfish can be fatal if eaten. This is why clams, oysters and mussels are not sold during months without an "R" (the summer months).

In addition, most cases of shellfish poisoning have occurred when people ate raw shellfish; in any case, neither heat nor freezing will kill the toxins that cause PSP.

The first incidence of PSP was recorded as early as 1689, and further outbreaks have been recorded many times since then.

Poisonous part The toxin saxitoxin and its analogues stop the flow of sodium, preventing nerve conductance; it is not possible to build up immunity by becoming exposed to sublethal doses.

Symptoms Symptoms of shellfish poisoning resemble those of curare poisoning and develop within five to 30 minutes after eating contaminated oysters, clams or mussels. Oral ingestion of as little as 0.5 to 1.0 mg of contaminated shellfish can be fatal, and a victim's survival depends on how much he has consumed. Symptoms are characterized by gradual paralysis and trembling. Other symptoms include nausea, vomiting and diarrhea. If the victim survives the first 12 hours, prognosis for complete recovery (within a few days to two weeks) is good. Between 8.5 and 23.2 percent of PSP poisonings are fatal.

Treatment There is no known antidote to saxitoxin. As in any treatment of curarelike poisoning, administration of prostigmine may be effective, together with artificial respiration and oxygen as needed.

See also DINOFLAGELLATE; FISH CONTAMINATION; FOOD POISONING; SHELLFISH POISONING.

paraquat This powerful defoliant is not generally available on store shelves, as it can be toxic if inhaled, absorbed through the skin or ingested. Diquat, which is only half as toxic as paraquat, is used much more widely as a defoliant; the two are contained together in a 2.5 percent granular formulation known as Weedol.

Solutions available for home use are generally extremely dilute (0.2

percent), but the commercial varieties may contain up to 21 percent para-quat.

Symptoms Appearing two to five days after ingestion, symptoms include burning mouth and throat, vomiting, abdominal pain, swelling, diarrhea and fever. This is followed by liver and kidney damage and then respiratory problems, cyanosis and fatal lung deterioration. Ingestion of as little as 2 to 4 g (or 10 to 20 ml of concentrated 20 percent solution) has been fatal. Food in the stomach may bind paraquat, preventing its absorption and reducing its toxicity.

Poisoning with diquat may cause corrosive injury, with severe gastroenteritis, massive fluid loss and kidney failure.

Treatment For assistance with treatment, call ICI Americas, Inc., 24 hours a day at (800) 327-8633. There is no specific antidote. Induce vomiting with syrup of ipecac if gastric lavage is not possible or activated charcoal is not available (carefully, as paraquat can be corrosive). Immediately after vomiting, administer absorbent clay (or activated charcoal if clays are not available) plus a cathartic. Ingestion of any food or even plain dirt may give some protection if other absorbents are not immediately available. For skin contamination, remove clothes and wash thoroughly; in the event of eye contamination, wash eyes for 15 minutes and see an ophthalmologist. Avoid giving excessive oxygen and treat fluid and electroyte imbalances.

See also HERBICIDES.

parasympathomimetic drugs These drugs, including physostigmine, pilocarpine, neostigmine and methacholine, act on the parasympathetic nervous system and are administered by ingestion, injection or application to mucous membranes. They are used to treat glaucoma, myasthenia gravis, bladder problems and certain heart irregularities.

Symptoms Overdose produces breathing problems, tremor, involuntary defecation and urination, pinpoint pupils, vomiting, low blood pressure, bronchial constriction, wheezing, twitching, fainting, slow pulse, convulsions and death. Repeated small doses may mimic symptoms of acute poisoning.

Treatment Prompt administration of atropine results in immediate recovery.

See also MEDICATIONS AS POISONS.

parathion (0,0-diethyl 0-p-nitrophenyl phosphorothioate) This brown-yellow liquid is used as an insecticide and also as a deadly nerve gas that is fatal upon contact. Most fatalities have occurred while spraying into the wind, cleaning equipment (and airplanes) used for spraying or gathering produce that has been sprayed. Industrial poisonings have also occurred by workers who absorb the poison through the skin. It is also a common suicide choice in Europe.

Poisonous part The toxic compound includes muscarine and other poisonous principles that have not yet been fully identified.

Symptoms Parathion is highly toxic by skin contact, inhalation or ingestion. It destroys enzymes needed for proper functioning of nerves and muscles, causing contraction of pupils, headache, photophobia, spasms, abdominal pain, nosebleeds, nausea, muscle weakness, twitching, diarrhea, convulsions, heart block, paralysis, respiratory difficulty and pulmonary edema, ending in fatal respiratory failure. Death is usually quite painful, with tremors, muscle spasms and convulsions. Parathion used as a nerve gas is fatal upon skin contact, although it can also be absorbed by the lungs; it causes painful tremors, muscle spasms, convulsions and death.

Treatment The antidote is a huge dose of atropine for 48 hours plus treatment of symptoms.

See also MUSCARINE; ORGANOPHOSPHATE INSECTICIDES.

pavulon (pancuronium) See NEUROMUSCULAR BLOCKING AGENTS.

PCBs See POLYCHLORINATED BIPHENYLS.

PCP See PHENCYCLIDINE.

peach pit See PRUNUS.

penicillamine One of the derivatives of penicillin used, not for fighting microbes, but for chelating heavy metals such as lead, mercury, arsenic and copper. It is often used following an initial treatment with calcium EDTA or dimercaprol. Penicillamine is easily absorbed in the body, and the penicillamine and metal complex is then excreted from the body.

pennyroyal oil A volatile oil obtained from the pennyroyal plant (*Mentha pulegium*), one of a large number of plants belonging to the mint family. Pennyroyal has traditionally been used to bring on menstrual periods and as an abortifacient by the American Indians. A colorless liquid, pennyroyal oil readily evaporates at room temperature.

Symptoms In large doses, pennyroyal oil induces a fatal reaction due to kidney failure.

Treatment There is no known antidote for pennyroyal oil. Treatment is supportive and symptomatic.

See also VOLATILE OILS.

pep pills See AMPHETAMINES.

HOW TO USE CHEMICAL PESTICIDES

Like any tool, pesticides must be used with care. Follow these tips for safe use of such chemicals:

- Always read the label on each container before using, and follow directions.
- Store pesticides out of the reach of children, and keep in labeled, original containers.
- Avoid smoking while spraying or dusting; many of these chemicals are flammable.
- Wear protective clothing and masks. Keep your sleeves rolled down and your collar up. Wash immediately with soap and water if you spill pesticide material on your skin.
- Wash your hands thoroughly after spraying or dusting and before eating or smoking. Change your clothes, too.
- If you should feel sick while using a pesticide or shortly after, call your physician immediately.

Percodan (oxycodone) This narcotic painkiller derived from morphine is used in the treatment of severe pain; it is often combined with aspirin, phenacetin and caffeine. Percodan depresses the central nervous system and its sedative qualities are strengthened when taken together with tranquilizers, antihistamines, antidepressants, sedatives, sleeping pills, alcohol or narcotics. Combining this drug with phenytoin (Dilantin) can cause brain death.

Symptoms When Percodan is taken in overdose, symptoms include drowsiness, clumsiness, lightheadedness, dizziness, sedation, nausea and vomiting; severe overdose can produce weak muscles, stupor, coma, low blood pressure, respiratory depression and cardiac arrest within 30 minutes.

Treatment The antidote is naloxone.

See also MORPHINE; NARCOTICS; OXYMORPHONE.

pesticides Also known as "crop protectants," pesticides are chemicals used in protecting crops from predators, competitors and diseases that can cause major losses. Specific types of pesticides are used for different purposes: Insecticides control insects; fungicides control plant diseases; herbicides control weeds that compete with crops; and rodenticides control rodents that attack crops in storage.

American farmers use about five pounds of pesticides a year for every man, woman and child in the country. But according to the National Cancer

---

HOW TO REDUCE DANGER OF PESTICIDE CONTAMINATION

To reduce the danger from pesticide-contaminated food:

- Buy organic produce that has been grown without the use of pesticides. Look for the certification labels from organic farming associations (such as the California Certified Organic Farmers or the Organic Foods Production Association of North America).
- Rinse all produce under cold running water.
- Don't wash produce with soap; soap may contain chemicals that have not been approved for human consumption.
- Peel away outside layers of fruits and vegetables (plus outer leaves of leafy vegetables).

Institute, the health benefits from eating fresh fruits and vegetables outweigh possible dangers associated with pesticide residue.

In addition, the Food and Drug Administration monitors pesticide residues in domestic and imported produce by testing selected samples. In 1990, the FDA tested 6,602 samples and found no residues in 58 percent of the produce; 41 percent had residue within FDA safety guidelines, and 1 percent had unsafe levels of residue. When the FDA discovers such unsafe levels, it impounds the produce.

Acceptable levels of pesticides are set by the Environmental Protection Agency (EPA), based on current knowledge of the long-term effects of pesticide residues.

Since farmers in other countries do not have as strict residue requirements, all produce entering the United States must pass inspection by the FDA. In 1990, the FDA found that of 7,908 samples tested, 62 percent were residue free and another 34 percent had residue within accepted levels; about 4 percent had excess amounts of residue.

The alternative to buying produce that has been treated with pesticides is to buy organic food, although the term "organic" currently has no federal legal definition: It could mean that the farmer used naturally occurring pesticides, or no pesticides at all. To address this problem, the 1990 Farm Bill required the National Organic Standards Board to set guidelines for organic labeling and grower certification, a program that must be in place by October 1, 1993. At present, 26 states have enacted laws and standards for the term "organic."

See also ALAR; ALDICARB; ALDRIN; BACILLUS THURINGIENSIS; BENZENE HEXACHLORIDE; BOTANIC INSECTICIDES; CARBAMATE; CARBARYL;

CHLORDANE; CHLORINATED HYDROCARBON PESTICIDES; CHLOROBEN-
ZENE DERIVATIVES; CREOSOTE; DDT; DERRIS; DIELDRIN; ENDRIN; ETHYL-
ENE DIBROMIDE;   INDANE DERIVATIVES;   INORGANIC CHEMICAL
INSECTICIDES; INSECTICIDES; LINDANE; MALATHION; TEPP; TOXAPHENE.

petroleum distillates   A wide range of products can be distilled from
petroleum, but three of the most common liquids—and potentially toxic—
are paint thinner, kerosene and gasoline. Inhaling the fumes and ingesting
the liquids present toxic hazards. Each year, more than 28,000 children
under age five ingest these products, which accounts for up to one-fourth
of all poison deaths in this age group. Poison centers suspect the problem
may be even more widespread than this.
   Substances most commonly ingested (in order) are kerosene, mineral seal
oil, turpentine, gasoline, lighter fluid, and petroleum-based insecticides.
   Symptoms Petroleum distillates in small doses cause nausea and
vomiting, coughing and spitting blood. Larger amounts can result in
weakness, dizziness, slow, shallow breathing and unconsciousness followed
by convulsions and, sometimes, mild heart attack. Death from ingesting
petroleum distillates is almost always a result of pulmonary problems.
   Treatment Gastric lavage only when preceded by insertion of
endotracheal tube in comatose patients. *Do not induce vomiting* (unless an
insecticide or other poison also has been ingested with the petroleum
distillate). The victim's head should be kept lower than the hips to prevent
vomitus from being aspirated into the lungs. Magnesium or sodium sulfate
or citrate may be used as a cathartic. Oxygen and supportive therapy may
also be needed.

pets and poisoning   Pets are just as much at risk for common household
poisoning than any curious two-year-old; curious pets can leap up, paw open
cabinets and chew through child protective caps in a surprisingly short time.
Any products that would be considered poisonous to a tot should also be
locked away from pets, including medications, household and garden chemicals, insect and rat killers and automotive products.
   According to experts at the National Animal Poison Control Center, it
only takes a small amount of a potentially toxic substance to do serious harm
to a pet. For example, one extra-strength acetaminophen tablet or one
teaspoon of undiluted antifreeze can kill a seven-pound cat. In addition, an
animal's medicine should never be given to another species (cat medicine
for dogs or vice versa). Flea and tick products can be toxic if used incorrectly,
especially on cats (who are extremely sensitive to whole-house flea and tick
treatments).
   Among other common products, the caffeine in chocolate, if eaten in
sufficient quantities, is toxic to dogs. Unsweetened baking chocolate is the
most dangerous of all chocolate, as it contains 10 times the amount of

theobromine and caffeine as white or milk chocolate. About one ounce of baking chocolate can be fatal to a 10-pound dog (or about 1/4 ounce for every 2.2 pounds).

Symptoms   Although vomiting is the most common symptom, poisoning in animals may also cause diarrhea, anorexia or sudden behavior change (such as depression).

Treatment   According to veterinarians at the National Animal Poison Control Center, if the pet has not ingested a caustic or oily substance, the best emergency treatment is to induce vomiting. But because vomiting on an empty stomach will make the animal retch without bringing up the toxic substance, owners should feed the pet a soft diet (such as canned pet food or milk) before giving an emetic. Possible emetics for pets can include syrup of ipecac, saline or hydrogen peroxide.

When local expert help is unavailable, pet owners may call the National Animal Poison Control Center 24 hours a day for advice. Dial 900-680-0000 at a cost of $2.95 per minute or 800-548-2423 at $30 per call.

See also ANTIFREEZE; NATIONAL ANIMAL POISON CONTROL CENTER.

phencyclidine (PCP)   This former veterinary drug became popular as a cheap street drug during the late 1960s, when it was widely known as "angel dust." It may be snorted, smoked, ingested or injected and is often substituted for other illicit drugs such as THC (tetrahydrocannabinol, the active ingredient in marijuana), mescaline or LSD. It produces a dissociative state and inhibits pain perception in its street dosage of 1- to 6-mg tablets; ingestion of 6 to 10 mg causes toxic psychosis. Overdose (150 to 200 mg) is fatal. Although classified as a stimulant, PCP can both excite and depress the central nervous system.

PCP was developed in 1957 as an analgesic and short-acting intravenous anesthetic, but the side effects were so toxic that the drug was withdrawn for human use; it was later reintroduced in 1967 only to veterinarians as an anesthetic under the trade name Sernyl or Sernylan. It became popular in the late sixties and was mixed with THC, LSD, psilocybin or mescaline. PCP is sprinkled onto parsley or marijuana for recreational smoking. There have been reports that users have been able to snap out of handcuffs and have attacked large groups of people and the police unarmed. The loss of fear may cause individuals to try to stop a train by standing in front of it or mutilating themselves.

Symptoms   Mild use produces lethargy, euphoria, hallucinations and sometimes bizarre or violent behavior, with rapid swings between quietness and agitation. Severe overdose leads to high blood pressure, rigidity, high fever, rapid heartbeat, convulsions and coma; the pupils are often small, and death may occur as a result of self-destructive behavior or as a result of the high fever (kidney failure or brain damage).

Treatment   There is no specific antidote. Ammonium chloride is sometimes given to help remove the PCP from the central nervous system. Provide symptomatic treatment and sedation (benzodiazepines) to control agitated behavior; phenothiazines and other antipsychotics are ineffective and may induce low blood pressure or seizures. Do not induce vomiting because of the risk of rapid onset of seizures or coma. Perform gastric lavage only if ingestion has occurred during the past four hours, or when multiple agents have been ingested. Follow by activated charcoal and a cathartic. Mildly intoxicated persons should be managed with sensory isolation in a physically protected environment. Symptoms may last for several days as the drug empties into the stomach and is then reabsorbed through the intestines. Haloperidol or chlorpromazine are recommended for continued psychosis.

See also MEXICAN HALLUCINOGENIC MUSHROOM.

phenobarbital   This barbiturate is used primarily to control convulsions, although it has generally been replaced by newer anticonvulsant drugs. Because there is a delay in onset of the beneficial effects of this drug, other anticonvulsants (diazepam or phenytoin) are generally tried first.

phenol   Also known as carbolic acid, this is a white crystalline substance with a burning taste and a distinct acrid odor. It is used in the manufacture of fertilizers, paints, paint removers, textiles, drugs and perfumes and is widely used in the dye, agricultural and tanning industries. In addition, clove oil in clove cigarettes contains the phenol derivative eugenol and may cause severe tracheobronchitis.

Phenol is equally deadly whether inhaled, absorbed through the skin or eyes or ingested. It was once used in households to kill germs but has been replaced today by less toxic compounds. Hexachlorophene is a chlorinated biphenol that was used throughout the United States as a topical antiseptic and scrub until its adverse effects on the brain were recognized. Other compounds of phenol include creosote, creosol, hydroquinone, eugenol, dinitrophenol and pentachlorophenol.

Poisonous part   While the mechanism behind its toxicity on the central nervous system is not known, phenol can cause corrosive injury to the eyes, skin and respiratory tract. There are no minimum toxic levels, although there have been reports of infants dying after repeated skin applications of small doses. Adult deaths have occurred after ingestion of 1 to 32 g of phenol, although survival after ingesting 45 to 65 g has also been reported. There have been reports of infant deaths with as small as 50- to 500-mg doses.

Symptoms   Phenol is markedly corrosive on any tissue in which it comes in contact. Exposure to the eyes can cause blindness; contact with the skin (at even low vapor concentrations) can cause a delayed burning and gangrene, with paleness, weakness, sweating, high fever, shock, cyanosis, excitement, frothing, coma, kidney damage and death. Ingesting large amounts of phenol can severely burn the mouth and throat and can cause abdominal pain, nausea, corrosion of the lips, mouth, esophagus and stomach, cyanosis, muscle weakness, collapse, coma and death. Death from phenol poisoning is most likely during hot weather when loss of body heat is inhibited.

Treatment Do NOT induce vomiting, because phenol is corrosive and may induce seizures. Ingested poison can be treated with milk, olive oil or vegetable oil followed by repeated gastric lavage. (Neither mineral oil nor alcohol should be used, since they speed up the absorption of phenol, although some medical texts still recommend them.) Castor oil dissolves phenols and interferes with absorption. Follow with activated charcoal and a cathartic.

For skin contact, wash the area for 15 minutes followed by the application on the skin of castor oil, olive oil or petroleum jelly. For eye contact, immediately flush with tepid water or saline.

See also CREOSOTE.

phentolamine This vasodilator acts on both venous and arterial vessels with a rapid onset of action (within two minutes) and is used to treat high blood pressure following overdose of phenylpropanolamine or stimulant drugs such as amphetamine, cocaine, ephedrine, etc.

phenurone See SLEEPING PILLS.

phenylpropanolamine See DECONGESTANTS.

phenytoin (Dilantin) This epileptic drug is used to prevent seizures and may easily cause an accidental overdose in persons in chronic therapy because of drug interactions or slight dosage adjustments. Poisoning may occur either by an acute overdose by mouth or by chronic overmedication. Poisoning may also occur following rapid intravenous administration. Persons with kidney problems may experience toxicity at lower levels.

Symptoms Mild symptoms include nystagmus, (involuntary movement of the eyeball), nausea, vomiting, agitation, irritability and hallucinations. At high levels of overdose, symptoms include stupor, coma and respiratory arrest. The toxicity to the heart that occurs with rapid intravenous injection does not result from oral overdose.

Treatment There is no specific antidote. Treat symptoms, induce vomiting or perform gastric lavage followed by the administration of activated charcoal and a cathartic orally or by gastric tube.

philodendron (*Philodendron*) This is the most popular houseplant in the United States, but eating the leaves can cause painful swelling and blisters in the mouth. This climbing vine has aerial roots and large, heart-shaped or notched leaves, sometimes with variegated patterns.

Poisonous part   The leaves contain raphides of calcium oxalate and other, unidentified proteins. The oxalates are insoluble and therefore do not cause systemic poisoning.

Symptoms   Pain and swelling of the lips, mouth, tongue and throat; contact dermatitis is also possible.

Treatment   Pain and swelling fade by themselves, but keeping cold liquid in the mouth (such as milk) can help.

See also OXALATES.

philodendron, split leaf *(Monstera deliciosa)* [Other names: breadfruit vine, cut leaf philodendron, fruit salad plant, hurricane plant, Mexican breadfruit, shingle plant, swiss cheese plant, window plant, windowleaf.] This woody climber has thick leaves with irregular holes. Grown as an indoor plant in the United States and native to Mexico, it is also cultivated in the West Indies, Hawaii and Guam.

Poisonous part   The leaves are toxic and contain raphides of calcium oxalates.

Symptoms   After eating, the lips, mouth and tongue begin to burn and swell followed by an acute inflammatory reaction. Because eating the leaves of this plant is quickly painful, there is little danger that large amounts will be ingested.

Treatment   The pain and swelling will fade by themselves, but cool liquids (such as milk) held in the mouth, together with painkillers, may help ease the pain. The insoluble oxalates in these plants don't cause systemic poisoning.

See also OXALATES.

phosgene   Once manufactured as a weapon for chemical warfare, phosgene is now used as an industrial gas to manufacture dyes, resins and pesticides. In addition, it is often produced during fires or while welding metal that has been cleaned with chlorinated solvents.

An irritant, it does not immediately cause symptoms at low doses; for this reason, a person may unknowingly inhale the gas over a period of time, injuring the lungs.

Symptoms   Exposure to mild amounts causes cough and some irritation. After 30 minutes to eight hours (depending on how long the person was exposed) further symptoms develop: labored breathing and swelling in the lungs; and permanent lung damage may result because phosgene is changed in the alveoli into hydrochloric acid, causing damage and inflammation of the small airways and tissue.

Treatment   There is no specific antidote. Treat symptoms and give supplementary oxygen if needed.

phosphate esters   A group of highly toxic compounds that are used as insecticides and are extremely poisonous to humans and animals; they are quickly absorbed from the skin, lungs and gastrointestinal tract. The greatest hazard to humans from these insecticides is through breathing the compounds, which is three times more toxic than oral exposure and 10 times more toxic than skin absorption. These esters were discovered accidentally by the Germans during World War II in their search for poison gas.

Symptoms   Weakness, unsteadiness, blurred vision, vomiting, abdominal cramps, diarrhea, salivation, sweating, tremors and problems in breathing.

Treatment   Administration of atropine, supportive therapy as required.

See also INSECTICIDES.

phosphine   This colorless gas is heavier than air, and, while rarely causing poisoning in the general public, it does present a hazard to metal refiners, acetylene workers, fire fighters and pest-control operators. Phosphine is a highly toxic gas of particular danger to the lungs, brain, kidneys, heart and liver. Chronic exposure to less-than-lethal dosages can also produce toxic symptoms.

Symptoms   Inhalation causes severe lung irritation, cough, labored breathing, headache, dizziness, lethargy and stupor followed by seizures, gastroenteritis and kidney and liver problems. Symptoms usually appear fairly soon after inhalation, except in the case of chronic low-level exposure.

Treatment   There is no specific antidote. Treat symptoms, and provide supplemental oxygen if needed.

phosphorus   A chemical used as an inorganic insecticide and also in the manufacture of fertilizers and fireworks. As a red, granular insoluble substance, phosphorus is nontoxic, but its yellow or white form is highly poisonous and ignites on contact with moist air and water, trailing white fumes and burning with an eerie green light. At one time, phosphorus was used on the tips of matches, but it has since been replaced because of its toxicity.

Phosphorus is highly corrosive and a general cellular poison; the fatal dose of white-yellow phosphorus is about 1 mg/kg, although deaths have been reported from ingesting as little as 15 mg.

Symptoms   Immediately after ingestion, yellow phosphorus begins to affect the digestive tract, causing abdominal pain, nausea, vomiting luminescent material and diarrhea. Cardiac collapse may occur because of fluid loss from vomiting and diarrhea and because of direct toxicity on the heart. It is possible that death may occur within 12 hours after ingestion. If not, there may follow one to three days with no symptoms, during which time phosphorus begins to damage the liver and muscle, heart, kidney and nervous system; after about three days the symptoms will return, much more serious this time with liver enlargement, jaundice, delirium, convulsions and coma.

Death may not occur until three weeks following ingestion. Phosphide (rat poison) ingestion causes jaundice, pulmonary edema and cyanosis and can be fatal within one week.

There is also a problem with skin contamination: If yellow phosphorus dries on the skin, it can cause a second- or third-degree burn.

If the phosphorus vapor is inhaled, symptoms appear within two days and include conjunctivitis, nausea, vomiting, fatigue, coughing, jaundice, tremors, numbness, low blood pressure, pulmonary edema, collapse, heart problems, convulsions and coma. Inhalation may be fatal within four days to two weeks. The classic sign of chronic poisoning is called "phossy jaw," an aching and swelling of the jaw followed by deterioration of the jawbone, in addition to weakness, weight loss, anemia and spontaneous fractures.

Treatment There is no specific antidote. Eliminate exposure and give oxygen. With ingestion, perform gastric lavage followed by the administration of activated charcoal and a cathartic, although there is no evidence that charcoal absorbs phosphorus. Provide symptomatic and supportive treatment. Do not induce vomiting. For skin contamination, wash with plenty of water. For chronic poisoning causing jaw necrosis, surgical excision of affected jawbone may be required.

See also INSECTICIDES.

physostigmine A treatment used in poisoning cases with symptoms of severe anticholinergic syndrome (agitated delirium, sinus tachycardia, high fever with no sweating). It is NOT used as an antidote for cyclic antidepressant overdose, nor at the same time as certain neuromuscular blockers such as succinylcholine.

See also PARASYMPATHOMIMETIC DRUGS.

phytonadione See VITAMIN K_1.

phytotoxins Also called toxalbumins, these are extremely deadly protein molecules (similar to bacterial toxins) that are produced by a few plants, including the castor bean, rosary pea and black locust. In a manner similar to that of bacterial toxins, the phytotoxins elicit an antibody response after ingestion. Eating just one seed from a plant containing these toxins can be fatal. Most phytotoxins are destroyed by heat.

Interestingly, however, different people will react differently to the presence of phytotoxins. Symptoms include gastrointestinal irritation, with lesions and swelling of organs.

See also CASTOR BEAN; ROSARY PEA; BLACK LOCUST.

pilocarpine See PARASYMPATHOMIMETIC DRUGS.

pit vipers   Seventeen of the 19 venomous snakes in North America belong to this family of dangerous poison snakes, which includes about 290 species. There are three genera in the family: *Agkistrodon* (copperheads and cotton-mouths), *Crotalus* and *Sistrurus* (both rattlesnakes).

Pit vipers seem to be extremely highly evolved snakes very well designed for capturing, killing and eating fairly large, warm-blooded prey. Most have stout bodies with wide heads, patterned with crossbands and blotches and with retractable hollow fangs in the front of the upper jaw. The fangs can be folded back and then positioned forward as the mouth opens to strike. The pit viper's name comes from the heat-sensitive pits located on each side of the head between the nostril and the eye, which is used to locate its prey.

Seriousness of the bite depends on a wide variety of variables, including the snake's size (usually the larger, the more venomous) and whether the snake is hungry or alert. The angle of the bite and its depth and length also affect the seriousness of the bite. In addition, the size of the victim can be important (children and infants are at greater risk), and the health of the victim at the time of the bite will also affect the outcome. Persons with diabetes, hypertension or blood coagulation problems and the elderly are particularly sensitive to snake venom, and menstruating women may bleed excessively following the bite of a pit viper. Several cases of miscarriage have been reported when pregnant women have been bitten. Finally, the location of the bite itself is crucial to its seriousness; venomous snake bites on the head and trunk are twice as serious as those on the extremities, and bites on the arms are more serious than those on the legs.

Poisonous part   The venom of the pit vipers is a mixture of proteins that acts on a victim's blood. Even snakes that appear to have been killed by the side of the road have been reported to bite. The size of the snake can give an idea of its potential dangerousness and can be judged by the distance between the fang marks. Fang marks less than 8 mm apart would be a small snake; between 8 to 12 indicates a medium-size snake, and more than 12 mm suggests a large venomous snake. Even snakes that have been "de-fanged" can be dangerous, since all snakes grow new fangs from time to time.

Symptoms   Swelling, internal bleeding, changes in red blood cells, central nervous system symptoms including convulsions and sometimes psychotic behavior, muscle weakness and paralysis. In addition, there are general systemic symptoms of fever, nausea, vomiting, diarrhea, pain and restlessness. Tachycardia and bradycardia can develop, and kidney failure has been reported.

Treatment   Within the first 30 to 45 minutes after the bite of a pit viper, apply a venous tourniquet a few inches above the bite, loosening it every 15 to 30 minutes and reapplying it above the level of progressive swelling. Keep the victim quiet, lying down to decrease metabolic activity (which affects the spread of the venom). The wound area (especially if it is an arm or leg) should be kept lower than the heart. Within 30 minutes, trained individuals can incise the wound area and apply suction. Antivenin is available but should be administered within four hours; antivenin is rarely helpful if given more than 12 hours after the bite. Tetanus prophylaxis is advisable; other treatment might include blood transfusions, intravenous fluids, treatment for convulsions and antihistamines to control itching. In addition, broad-spectrum antibiotics may be administered, since snakebites are notorious for becoming infected. If antivenin has not been administered (or was given hours after the bite), sloughing of the skin around the bite is common.

While certain anecdotal reports in the popular press have reported that some individuals become immunized after many bites of the pit viper, scientifically controlled attempts to develop immunity in human beings have failed.

See also COPPERHEAD SNAKE; RATTLESNAKE, CANEBRAKE; RATTLESNAKE, CASCABEL; RATTLESNAKE, EASTERN DIAMONDBACK; RATTLESNAKE, MEXICAN WEST COAST; RATTLESNAKE, RED DIAMONDBACK; RATTLESNAKE, SOUTH AMERICAN; RATTLESNAKE, TIMBER; RATTLESNAKE, WESTERN DIAMONDBACK; SNAKES, POISONOUS; WATER MOCCASIN.

plum cherry pit   See PRUNUS.

poinsettia *(Euphorbia pulcherrima)*   This popular Christmas plant has a long-standing poisonous reputation, but there are only two cases of fatal poisoning by poinsettia in toxicological literature. All references to poinsettia as potentially lethal have been traced to one case in 1919 when a Hawaiian child was reported to have died after eating poinsettia. However, researchers in the 1970s found that poinsettia was not lethal; several rat studies showed that large amounts of poinsettia could be eaten without harm. While some authorities and many popular magazines still report poinsettia as poisonous, most experts now agree that it is virtually certain poinsettia is not.

In the 1988 annual report of the American Association of Poison Control Centers National Data Collection System, there were no serious poisonings reported out of 3,001 exposures during the rating period.

However, it may be possible that the plant's milky sap may cause mild abdominal pain with vomiting and diarrhea if ingested. Locally, this sap can cause skin and mucous membrane irritation.

poison ivy *(Toxicodendron radicans)*   Poison ivy is one of the most common plants in the United States that are poisonous to touch; it causes a contact dermatitis in most people—as many as 87 million Americans.

The leaves of the poison ivy plant are glossy green, may be notched or smooth and almost always grow in groups of three—two leaves opposite each other and one at the end of the stalk. However, according to some experts there are exceptions, and leaves may sometimes appear in fives, sevens or even nines. In early fall, the leaves may turn bright red. Although it usually grows as a long, hairy vine—often wrapping itself around trees—it can also be found as a low shrub growing along fences or stone walls. Poison ivy has waxy yellow-green flowers and greenish berries that look rather like a peeled orange. These berries can help in identification of the plants in late fall, winter and early spring before the leaves appear.

Poison ivy is found throughout the United States, but it is most common in the eastern and central states.

Poisonous part   Poison ivy, poison oak and poison sumac are closely related species, all three containing a colorless or slightly yellow resin called urushiol, which comes from a Japanese word meaning "lacquer." Skin contact with urushiol causes an allergic reaction known as contact dermatitis in many individuals. While each of these three plants contains a slightly different type of urushiol, they are so similar that individuals sensitive to one will react to all three. The entire plant contains urushiol and is therefore poisonous: leaves, berries, stalk and roots.

Urushiol is easily transferred from an object to a person, so anything that touches poison ivy—clothing, gardening tools, a pet's fur, athletic equipment, sleeping bags—can be contaminated with urushiol and cause poison ivy in anyone who then touches the object. Urushiol remains active for up to one year, so any equipment that touches poison ivy must be washed. Even the smoke from burning poison ivy is toxic and can irritate the skin of the face, eyes and lungs, since urushiol can be carried in smoke. Individuals should never burn poison ivy plants as a way to get rid of them, since the smoke given off by these burning plants is particularly dangerous and can enter the nasal passages, throat and lungs of anyone who breathes it.

As the leaves die in the fall, the plant draws certain nutrients and substances (including the oil) into the stem. But the oil remains active, so that even in winter it may cause rash if the broken stems are used as firewood kindling or vines on a Christmas wreath.

Symptoms   While not every person is allergic to poison ivy, about seven out of 10 Americans are sensitive to urushiol and will develop contact dermatitis if exposed to a large enough dose.

Symptoms vary from one person to the next; some people exhibit only mild itching, while others experience severe reactions, including severe burning and itching with watery blisters. The skin irritation, swelling, blisters and itching may appear within hours or days, usually developing within 24 to 48 hours in a sensitized person. The skin becomes reddened followed by watery blisters, peaking about five days after contamination and gradually improving over a week or two, even without treatment. Eventually, the blisters break, and the oozing sores crust over and then disappear.

Despite common misconception, poison ivy is *not* spread by scratching open blisters or skin-to-skin contact but by the oil (urushiol) found in the plant. Anything that brushes against this oil is contaminated and can pass on poison ivy if it brushes the skin. Poison ivy is not spread from person to person, by touching blisters, since only the oil spreads the rash. For this reason, doctors recommend not scratching blisters because any remaining urushiol that hasn't been washed off can be transmitted to another part of the body. In addition, scratching blisters may cause infection from germs on the fingernails. Animals can also transmit poison ivy from their fur to their owners' skin. Any animal suspected of coming in contact with poison ivy should be given a bath; wear protective gloves when bathing affected animal.

In addition, allergy to poison ivy, oak and sumac may also mean a person is allergic to related plants, including cashews, pistachios, mangos and Chinese or Japanese lacquer trees.

Treatment The best treatment is to wash the affected area immediately after contact (within 10 minutes, if possible) with yellow laundry soap and *cold* water, or water from a shower. Do not bathe in a tub, as this could spread the oil. Do not scrub with a brush. If contaminated while in isolated areas, wash in a cold running stream. Any clothing that might have come in contact with urushiol must be washed several times. If the urushiol is washed off, there is little further treatment needed of mild cases of the rash. Remove rings, watches, bracelets, etc., before washing hands. Wash contaminated jewelry.

Early application of topical steroids minimizes the severity of dermatitis; systemic steroids given during the first six hours after exposure are the most effective.

Itching can be treated with compresses soaked in cold water. A calamine lotion spread over the rash will help relieve the itching and burning and dry the area. Products containing local anesthetics (such as benzocaine) or irritants (camphor or phenol) should be avoided. Systemic antihistamines do not work against the rash, although their sedative action may help the person sleep. In the case of a severe reaction, a physician may prescribe corticosteroid drugs by mouth or injection.

Extremely sensitive individuals can be desensitized to the effects of poison ivy with allergen extracts, although results have been sometimes disappointing and desensitization does not last longer than one season. The procedure requires a great deal of time (three to six months) and effort. Adverse reactions to the desensitization include swelling, dermatitis, gastroenteric disturbances, fever and inflammation at the injection site. Because of these problems, immunization is only recommended for those sensitive people who live or work near poison ivy. Convulsions have occurred in children following oral administration of the plant's extract. No cream, lotion or spray has yet proved effective to protect against the allergen, although studies are continuing.

Alternatively, recent research suggests that a vaccine may be available for millions of Americans tormented with the itchy rash each summer. Researchers at the University of Mississippi have developed an experimental vaccine that seems to prevent an allergic reaction and may shorten the painful symptoms after the rash appears. Researchers explain that the vaccine works best as an injection and probably would be most helpful for those who are highly sensitive to the plants. The agent has been tested on animals but has not yet been tested on humans. Researchers at the university have been studying the oily compounds of the plants that make the skin blister and itch. From these, they created less toxic forms, which allow the body to tolerate the plants in the laboratory.

See also POISON OAK; POISON SUMAC; URUSHIOL.

poison oak *(Toxicodendron diversilobum)* A plant poisonous by touch, this is one of three closely related species containing similar forms of the resin urushiol. Urushiol causes a contact dermatitis in seven out of 10 Americans who come in contact with it. The leaves of poison oak occur in groups of three and are very similar to oak leaves, from which the plant gets its name. The underside of the leaves are much lighter green than the tops because of the thousands of tiny fine hairs that cover them. Berries may be greenish or creamy white, although not all plants bear fruit. Poison oak usually grows as a low shrub on the west coast from Mexico to British Columbia.

Symptoms Symptoms vary from one person to the next, ranging from mild itching to severe burning and itching with watery blisters, and usually develop within 24 to 48 hours in a sensitive person. Symptoms usually peak about five days after contamination and gradually improve over a week or two even without treatment. Eventually, the blisters break, and the oozing sores crust over and then disappear. Poison oak is *not* spread by scratching open blisters but by the urushiol found in the plant. Anything that brushes against this oil is contaminated and can pass on poison oak if it brushes the skin. For this reason, doctors recommend not scratching blisters, since any remaining urushiol that hasn't been washed off can be transmitted to another part of the body. Animals can also transmit poison oak from their fur to their owners' skin. Any animal suspected of coming in contact with poison oak should be given a bath (gloves should be worn).

Treatment The best treatment is to wash the affected area immediately after contact with yellow laundry soap and *cold* water, lathering several times and rinsing the area in running water after each sudsing. Do not scrub with a brush. If contaminated while in isolated areas, wash in a cold running stream. Any clothing that might have come in contact with urushiol must be washed several times. If the urushiol is washed off the skin, there is little further treatment needed in mild cases. Itching can be treated with compresses soaked in cold water, and calamine lotion spread over the rash will help relieve the itching and burning. In the case of a severe reaction, a physician may prescribe corticosteroid drugs by mouth or injection.

See also POISON IVY; URUSHIOL.

poison sumac   *(T. vernix* [L.] Kuntzel (= *Rhus vernix* L) This poisonous tree, a relative of poison ivy and poison oak, has seven to 13 long, narrow leaves growing in pairs with a single leaf at the end of the stem. In the spring, the leaves are bright orange and look something like velvet; as the season progresses, they become dark green and glossy on the upper surface of the leaf and light green on the underside. In the fall, the leaves turn red or orange. Poison sumac can be differentiated from nonpoisonous sumacs by its drooping clusters of green berries—nonpoisonous sumacs have red, upright clusters of berries. Poison sumac can grow to be 25 feet tall, although it is more often found between five and six feet. It is found in swampy areas throughout eastern United States.

Symptoms   Symptoms vary from one person to the next, ranging from mild itching to severe burning and itching with watery blisters, and usually develop within 24 to 48 hours in a sensitive person. Symptoms usually peak about five days after contamination and gradually improve over a week or two even without treatment. Eventually, the blisters break, and the oozing sores rust over and then disappear. The poison sumac rash is *not* spread by scratching open blisters but by the urushiol found in the plant. Anything that brushes against this oil is contaminated and can pass on the rash if it brushes the skin. For this reason, doctors recommend not scratching blisters, since any remaining urushiol that hasn't been washed off can be transmitted to another part of the body. Animals can also transmit poison sumac from their fur to their owners' skin. Any animal suspected of coming in contact with poison sumac should be given a bath; gloves should be worn while bathing.

Treatment   The best treatment is to wash the affected area immediately after contact with yellow laundry soap and *cold* water, lathering several times and rinsing the area in running water after each sudsing. Do not scrub with a brush. If contaminated while in isolated areas, wash in a cold running stream. Any clothing that might have come in contact with urushiol must be washed several times. If the urushiol is washed off the skin, there is little further treatment needed in mild cases. Itching can be treated with compresses soaked in cold water, and calamine lotion spread over the rash will help relieve the itching and burning. In the case of a severe reaction, a physician may prescribe corticosteroid drugs by mouth or injection.

See also POISON IVY; URUSHIOL.

poisoning   Poison can be inhaled, absorbed through the skin, or—most often—swallowed (either intentionally or accidentally). Most accidental poisonings can be prevented simply by keeping harmful substances out of the reach of children. The most important thing to remember in a poisoning case is not to make the problem any worse. Minutes can spell the difference between life and death, so prompt treatment is important. First aid is most effective, however, if you can identify the drug or chemical that caused the poisoning and contact your poison control center. If you can't, bring the container to the emergency room. Life support measures take precedence in the case of an unconscious person, but the poison must be identified if proper therapy can take place.

All cases of poisoning should be reported to a physician and treatment advice followed. With most poisons, emptying the stomach will remove any poison that has not been absorbed. The exceptions: acids, alkalies and petroleum-based products. Vomiting is considered to be more effective—and safer—than "pumping the stomach" (gastric lavage).

POISONING DON'TS

- Don't induce vomiting without medical advice.
- Don't give saltwater solution, especially to a child. While sometimes recommended in the past, salt walter is potentially dangerous, and if given repeatedly, it can cause salt intoxication, seizures and death.
- Don't neutralize by giving fruit juice or vinegar after an alkali has been swallowed. Studies show that giving an acid to neutralize a base produces heat, increasing the possibility of a burn injury.
- Don't give sodium bicarbonate, chalk or soap after an acid poisoning. Studies suggest that giving a base to neutralize an acid can release carbon dioxide gas, stretch the stomach and even cause it to rupture.
- Don't give milk to coat the digestive tract. Milk may bind syrup of ipecac and interfere with vomiting. And if a petroleum substance has been swallowed, milk may cause vomiting, which could introduce the substance into the lungs. Giving milk to coat the digestive tract is not a good idea unless a corrosive or highly irritating substance has been swallowed.
- Dilution with water or milk should not be a standard first aid practice unless a corrosive poison has been swallowed. For other types of poison, however, milk or water will actually increase the rate of absorption of the poison by causing the substances to dissolve more rapidly. A stomach that is filled with water or milk will force the contents through the sphincter between the stomach and the small intestines, where it will be absorbed faster. However, water can be given when using syrup of ipecac.
- Don't rely on first aid instructions on warning labels. They are often outdated and inaccurate. Follow only the advice of a poison control center or your physician.

HOW TO PREVENT POISONING

There are a wide range of toxic products found in any home. Those with small children must be particularly aware of potential hazards, since small children are at special risk for a fatal accident: their curiosity is relentless, and their bodies are small enough so that a relatively small amount of toxin can be fatal.

Make a rule that all hazardous items must be kept in high cupboards, on tall shelves in closets or in locked drawers or cabinets. Place all hazardous materials in one such area in your kitchen or utility room for cleaners, one in the garage for garden and auto poisons and another in your bathroom. Make sure all toxic products are always returned to the secure cabinet in which they belong.

Here is a sampling of common potentially dangerous products found in almost every home:

Cleaning products

- products containing chlorine bleach, ammonia and detergents
- toilet bowl cleaners
- drain cleaners
- furniture polish
- floor polish and waxes

Household goods

- nail polish and nail polish remover
- shoe polish
- rubbing alcohol
- hair dye
- hair spray

Medications

- aspirin
- acetaminophen
- prescription medications
- cough medicines
- cold pills

Garden products

- roach powders/baits
- rat pellets
- rose dust
- weed killers
- flower, garden and shrub sprays
- lime
- treated seeds

Garage products

- Antifreeze
- kerosene or gasoline
- paint thinners and strippers

AGE AND SEX DISTRIBUTION OF HUMAN POISON EXPOSURE CASES

Age	Male #	Male %	Female #	Female %	Total #	Total %
<1	75,339	4.1	69,201	3.8	146,178	8.0
1	181,667	9.9	158,699	8.6	342,396	18.6
2	185,337	10.1	161,542	8.8	348,923	19.0
3	86,411	4.7	72,109	3.9	159,525	8.7
4	37,242	2.0	30,065	1.6	67,786	3.7
5	20,175	1.1	16,102	0.9	36,525	2.0
6–12	57,870	3.1	43,892	2.4	102,700	5.6
13–19	43,069	2.3	61,388	3.3	104,906	5.7
20–29	57,796	3.1	67,487	3.7	125,702	6.8
30–39	46,970	2.6	59,746	3.3	106,990	5.8
40–49	23,531	1.3	33,171	1.8	56,834	3.1
50–59	10,566	0.6	15,917	0.9	26,536	1.4
60–69	7,341	0.4	12,177	0.7	19,563	1.1
70–79	4,647	0.3	8,565	0.5	13,243	0.7
80–89	2,132	0.1	5,014	0.3	7,162	0.4
90–99	399	0.0	1,029	0.1	1,433	0.1
unknown	69,055	3.8	93,879	5.1	171,537	9.3
TOTAL	909,547	49.5	909,983	49.5	1,837,939	100.0

Source: American Journal of Emergency Medicine 10 no. 5 (September 1992).

poisonwood *(Metopium toxiferum)* One of a group of plants that are poisonous on contact, poisonwood is found in the West Indies and in Florida.

Poisonous part Any part of this tree is poisonous on contact, especially the sap.

Symptoms Upon contact, the individual's skin turns black, causing a rash and blisters. Smoke from a burning tree can cause temporary blindness.

Treatment Symptomatic.

pokeweed *(Phytolacca americana)* [Other names: American nightshade, cancer jalap, crow berry, Indian polk, inkberry, pigeon-berry, pocan bush, poke, pokeberry, red ink plant, red weed, scoke.] This unpleasant-smelling plant is found in damp, woodsy areas from Maine to Minnesota, south to the Gulf of Mexico, Florida and Texas and also in California and Hawaii; it can also be found in parts of Canada, Europe and southern Africa. It is commonly found along fields and fences, growing 12 feet tall with white to

DISTRIBUTION OF REASON FOR POISONING AND AGE FOR 764 FATALITIES

Reason	<6 years	6–12	13–17	>17 years	TOTAL
Accidental					
General	30	0	0	8	38
Environmental	6	3	1	20	30
Misuse	3	1	2	29	35
Occupational	0	0	0	12	12
Unknown	0	0	0	2	2
TOTAL	39	4	3	71	117
Intentional					
Suicide	0	0	23	385	408
Misuse	1	0	0	24	25
Abuse	0	0	16	66	82
Unknown	0	0	5	56	61
TOTAL	1	0	44	531	576
Adverse reaction	2	0	0	15	17
Unknown	2	0	1	51	54
TOTAL	44	4	48	668	764

Source: American Journal of Emergency Medicine 10 no. 5 (September 1992).

purple drooping flowers, black berries and a large perennial rootstock. Young leaves and stems are sometimes eaten as cooked greens, and these can be eaten safely if cooked twice in two different pans of water.

Poisonous part   All parts of the pokeweed plant contain the poison laccine, saponins and glycoproteins, especially the roots and leaves—and the seeds are almost as toxic as the roots. Only two or three unriped berries can be fatal if eaten by a child, although mature berries are relatively nontoxic. Poisonings usually occur from eating uncooked leaves in salads or by mistaking the roots for parsnips or horseradish.

Symptoms   Symptoms begin about two hours after ingestion and include burning and bitterness in the mouth, nausea, vomiting and diarrhea; occasionally, spasms, convulsions and death occur.

Treatment   Gastric lavage; replacement of fluids and electrolytes.

polychlorinated biphenyls (PCBs)   This group of chlorinated hydrocarbon compounds consists of nonflammable liquids widely used as insulators for electric equipment and in the manufacture of some carbonless copy papers and some inks and paints; they were also used in heat exchangers, electrical condensers, adhesives, paints and hydraulic and lubricating fluids.

They may be clear, amber colored or dark and oily, and some (containing chlorobenzenes) smell like mothballs; others smell like motor oil. Until recently, microscope immersion oils contained 40 to 50 percent PCBs. They were widely used since the 1930s because of their excellent electrical and insulating abilities, but the Environmental Protection Agency banned further manufacture of PCBs in 1978 because of their suspected role in cancer. Many uses have been halted because of their chronic toxicity and danger to the environment.

PCBs cause problems in the environment because they have a long half-life, are very stable and are readily taken up by living organisms, accumulating in higher levels of the food chain. While equipment manufactured since 1979 doesn't usually contain PCBs, most pre-1979 capacitors do, and it is considered safe to assume that anything leaking from a pre-1979 transformer, capacitor or light ballast contains PCBs unless there is a "no PCB" label on the equipment.

PCB contamination is almost universal, and they are found in human milk, in human adipose tissue and in the brain and liver of small children. While little is known of the toxic effects of PCBs in humans, rhesus monkeys given 25 parts per million (ppm) showed signs of PCB intoxication. Infants exposed to PCBs before birth frequently were born dead or with birth defects.

In 1968, 15,000 people in Japan ate rice bran oil contaminated with PCBs from a leaking heat exchanger; 1,000 of them were poisoned in the largest episode of PCB food contamination. As little as 500 mg ingested over a 50-day period prompted symptoms (even liver damage) in some victims. Infants exposed in the uterus were born with swollen eyelids, facial swelling, growth and mental retardation, neonatal jaundice and a peculiar type of skin discoloration known as "cola babies." Follow-up studies in the Japanese poisonings showed that victims still had high levels of PCBs in their body fat four years after the poisoning incident.

Currently, the Food and Drug Administration recommends that food products not contain more than 5 ppm of PCBs; since the 1977 Environmental Protection Agency's ban on the manufacture of PCBs, occupational exposure and environmental damage have been drastically reduced.

Symptoms   PCBs are readily absorbed when inhaled, ingested or absorbed through the skin. They are also well absorbed from the gastrointestinal tract and are stored in fat. Both skin contact and ingestion cause the skin disease chloracne and damage to the liver, skin hyperpigmentation, blindness, swelling, nausea, vomiting and abdominal pain. PCBs are far more likely to cause poisoning as a result of long-term exposure rather than with a single acute overdose. Chronic exposure may cause symptoms as much as six weeks or longer after the onset of exposure.

Treatment   There is no way to remove PCBs once they have entered the body. Treatment is supportive and symptomatic, aimed at preventing liver damage. If inhaled, give supplemental oxygen. Wash contaminated skin or eyes; if ingested, induce vomiting or perform gastric lavage followed by the administration of activated charcoal and a cathartic.

See also SAPONIN.

Portuguese man-of-war *(Physalia palagica)* The best-known member of the jellyfish family (also known as a bluebottle), the Portuguese man-of-war gets its name from the floating portion of its body that appears above the surface of the sea, resembling the rigging of a caravel. While its bite is rarely fatal, it can be quite painful. Technically, the Portuguese man-of-war is not a jellyfish but a hydroid—a polyp that lives cooperatively in colonies. Each of the small, separate animals has an assigned task—some direct the movement of the whole complex, others catch food, some paralyze prey and others digest it and distribute it throughout the entire group.

Poisonous part The tentacles of the Portuguese man-of-war trail several feet below its body, floating on the surface of the water; some tentacles will be markedly longer than the others and are called "fishing tentacles." These poisonous tentacles may extend from the central float bag for 50 feet or more. All the tentacles are covered with many thousands of stinging cells that emit a coiled hollow thread that can penetrate skin. Venom in these coils is injected through the thread. The man-of-war is found throughout the world in warm waters, and its sting is far more severe than those from the more common jellyfish.

Symptoms Toxicity depends on the sensitivity of the victim and the number of stings. Symptoms include immediate and intense stinging or throbbing, a radiating sensation similar to being stung by hornets, causing wheals and blisters, severe chest and abdominal pain, shock and collapse. The pain has been compared to an electric shock, with the sensation extending up the extremity. More generalized symptoms include headache, shock, cramps, nausea and vomiting, and recent reports have noted the possibility of acute kidney failure.

Treatment There is no known specific antidote. Alcohol, ammonia or vinegar and salt water (DO NOT USE FRESH WATER) poured over the site of the sting will deactivate the tentacles, which should then be scraped off with a towel, *not the hand.* Pull off (do not rub) the tentacles. The tentacles will continue to discharge their nematocysts as long as they remain on the skin. Watch carefully for signs of shock or breathing problems.

Baking soda in a paste with water should be applied to the sting to relieve pain; after an hour, moisten again and scrape off the baking soda with an object to remove any remaining nematocysts. Calamine lotion also will help ease the burning sensation, and painkillers may help with the stinging pain; other treatment includes administration of a local anesthetic and muscle relaxants to relieve cramps. Alcohol and compresses of aromatic spirits of ammonia help relieve pain, as does meat tenderizer. If given early, the calcium blocker verapamil may be effective. Morphine may be necessary to relieve pain.

See also JELLYFISH.

potassium hydroxide See ALKALINE CORROSIVES.

potassium or sodium thiocyanate This drug, traditionally given for high blood pressure, has been replaced by safer drugs, although sodium thiocyanate is still prescribed by a few physicians.

Symptoms Almost immediately upon ingestion of large amounts, the drug begins to depress metabolic cellular activity of the heart and brain, causing disorientation, weakness, low blood pressure, confusion, psychotic behavior, convulsions and death. Even when the victim begins to recover from thiocyanate poisoning, death can still occur after a sudden relapse as much as two weeks after poisoning.

Treatment Perform peritoneal dialysis.

potassium permanganate A disinfectant and astringent that can be used to treat skin inflammation, potassium permanganate is sometimes applied to a dressing or may be applied directly to the skin. It is sometimes used in the treatment of strychnine, nicotine and quinine poisoning, although it is always hazardous to use. Mistakes in mixing the crystals in water make this a hazardous drug, since, if prepared in too concentrated a dose, it can destroy cells of the mucous membranes by its alkaline caustic action. In solutions of greater than 1 to 5,000 parts strength, the solution will cause corrosive burns.

Although it has a reputation as an abortifacient when introduced in the vagina (as a douche to induce abortion), it can cause serious injury to the vaginal walls and massive hemorrhaging.

Symptoms While symptoms vary depending on the dose, low concentrations cause a burning feeling in the throat, nausea, vomiting, difficulty in swallowing and some gastroenteritis. In stronger concentrations (2 or 3 percent solutions), symptoms will also include swollen throat and dry mouth, making swallowing difficult. At even greater concentrations (4 to 5 percent), kidney damage will occur and there may be possible disorientation, low blood pressure and rapid, shallow pulse; death may follow from circulatory failure or pulmonary complications.

Treatment In cases of skin contamination, wash affected area repeatedly with warm tap water, and treat perforations surgically. For ingestion, do NOT induce vomiting; perform gastric lavage cautiously. Activated charcoal and cathartics are not useful. Give large amounts of fluid and supportive therapy. Cold milk is also suggested as a way to oxidize organic material.

See also MEDICATIONS AS POISON.

potato   This cousin of deadly nightshade is a popular vegetable the world over, but it can also be poisonous if eaten raw and unripe. Although the skin of a potato has more fiber, iron, potassium and B vitamins than the flesh, diners must avoid potato skins with a greenish tinge—which indicates the presence of chlorophyll, a sign that the potato has been exposed to too much light after harvest. The presence of this greenish tinge means that there may be larger amounts of the naturally occurring toxin solanine in the skin, which may cause cramps, diarrhea and fatigue.

Poisonous part   The leaves, stems, skin and sprouts contain solanine, a naturally occurring glycoalkaloid, and other toxins. Although undamaged potatoes contain some solanine, the concentration is very low and a person would have to eat about 12 pounds of them to be poisoned. If a potato has greenish skin, pare away the green areas and gouge out all sprouts. Solanine has a stronger effect on children.

Symptoms   A fast-acting toxin, solanine causes symptoms including burning and rawness in the throat, headache, vomiting, abdominal pain, diarrhea, swelling of the brain, stupor, coma, convulsions and death (usually in children).

Treatment   Gastric lavage, emetics, cathartics and fluid and electrolyte monitoring.

See also NIGHTSHADE, DEADLY.

pothos   (*Epipremnum aureum*)   [Other names: devil's ivy, golden Ceylon creeper, golden hunter's robe, golden pothos, ivy arum, Solomon Island ivy, taro vine, variegated philodendron.] This popular indoor plant often found in hanging baskets grows outdoors throughout subtropical climates of southern Florida, Hawaii, Guam and the West Indies, where it twines on trees up to 40 feet high.

Poisonous part   The entire plant is toxic and contains calcium oxalate raphides and other, unidentified irritants.

Symptoms   Skin contact causes dermatitis, and ingestion by children results in diarrhea.

Treatment   There is no specific treatment, but guard against dehydration in children with diarrhea.

See also OXALATES.

pralidoxime   This drug is used as an antidote to organophosphate insecticide poisoning and is most effective if treatment is begun within 24 hours after exposure. Its use in the treatment of carbamate poisoning is still controversial; it may not be harmful, but it is not often used because of its short duration.

Preludin   (phenmetrazine hydrochloride) One of the appetite-suppressant drugs of high toxicity, Preludin is a white water-soluble powder and is available in tablets or injectables. Similar to amphetamines, Preludin activates the central nervous system and raises blood pressure; rapid heartbeat and addiction are quite common. Within a few weeks of using this drug, tolerance begins to develop.

Symptoms Appetite suppression, impaired judgment, incoordination, palpitations, high blood pressure, restlessness, dizziness, dry mouth, euphoria, insomnia, tremors, confusion, headache, hallucinations, panic, fatigue and depression. Psychotic episodes are possible even at recommended doses, together with an unpleasant taste in the mouth, diarrhea or constipation and other stomach problems. Overdose may cause circulatory collapse, coma, high or low blood pressure followed by death. Abruptly stopping the drug causes depression, fatigue, irritability, hyperactivity and psychosis (sometimes confused with schizophrenia).

Treatment Sedation with barbiturates.

See also AMPHETAMINES.

privet *(Ligustrum vulgare)* This common hedge plant is a deciduous shrub with small, white clustering flowers and blue or black waxy berries that appear throughout the winter. Native to the Mediterranean, privet hedges are grown throughout the United States and Canada.

Poisonous part The entire plant, including the berries, contain the irritant glycoside syringin (ligustrin), nuzhenids and secoiridoid glucosides.

Symptoms A large number of berries can cause diarrhea, colic and gastroenteritis; poisoning can be fatal in young children.

Treatment Fluid replacement to prevent dehydration.

procaine A local anesthetic and related to cocaine, this drug is a synthetic version of the coca bush alkaloids. It is used to control possible irregular heartbeat following poisoning by a variety of cardioactive drugs and toxins (such as digoxin, cyclic antidepressants, stimulants and theophylline). It is also used to relieve pain and irritation caused by sunburn or hemorrhoids, to numb tissues before minor surgery and as a nerve block. It is used topically to relieve pain when inserting needles, and it is given intravenously as an antiarrhythmic agent following a heart attack to reduce the danger of ventricular arrhythmias (irregular heartbeat).

Although procaine is used to treat poisoning by other drugs, it is also toxic itself if used excessively.

Symptoms Immediately upon ingestion, procaine causes giddiness followed by dizziness, blue color, low blood pressure, tremors, irregular and weak breathing, collapse, coma, convulsions and respiratory arrest. Procaine is considered to be the most dangerous of all the cocaine derivatives; even a small amount can cause fatal shock.

Treatment Efforts to remove the drug after 30 minutes are useless. The ingested drug must be removed immediately and absorption from the injection site limited by tourniquet and wet cloths. Give oxygen and artificial respiration until the nervous system depression lifts. If the victim survives for one hour, recovery outlook is good.

See also ANESTHETICS, LOCAL; LIDOCAINE.

propane   The principal ingredient in bottled gas in northern states, which (in low concentrations) is physiologically inert. However, high concentrations of the gas may cause narcosis (a state of sleep or drowsiness). A concentration of 10 percent propane causes slight dizziness in a few minutes; displacement of air by this gas can cause shortness of breath, unconsciousness and death. The principal toxic effects from gases are from carbon monoxide.

See also CARBON MONOXIDE.

propranolol   This beta adrenergic blocker is used to control heart irregularities caused by overdose of theophylline, caffeine, amphetamines, ephedrine or cocaine.

Prunus   A genus of trees and shrubs that includes apricot, cherry, choke cherry, peach, plum and sloe, whose chewed pits are poisonous and posses cyanogenic glycosides. The *Prunus* species have white or pink flowers and a fleshy fruit over a stone or pit. They are widely cultivated throughout the northern temperate zone, and a large number of these fruit trees are available commercially.

Poisonous part   The kernel of the pit is poisonous, containing the cyanogenic glycosides (amygdalin) that liberates hydrocyanic acid on hydrolysis. Of all the poisonings with the entire genus, the most fatal cases involve ingestion of apricot pits.

Symptoms   Hours may pass between ingestion of the pit and toxic symptoms, because the glycosides must be hydrolyzed in the gastrointestinal/tract before cyanide is released. Once this occurs, symptoms include abdominal pain, vomiting, lethargy and sweating. Cyanosis (blueness of the skin) may or may not occur. In severe cases, the victim may lapse into a coma and experience convulsions, flaccid muscles and incontinence.

Treatment   If conscious, perform gastric lavage. Although activated charcoal absorbs cyanide, it releases it slowly during its passage through the intestine; instead, give a 25 percent solution of sodium thiosulfate after lavage. If unconscious, correct acidosis, treat for shock and administer oxygen; administer cyanide antidote.

See also CYANOGENIC GLYCOSIDES.

Psilocybe mexicana   See MEXICAN HALLUCINOGENIC MUSHROOM.

ptomaine poisoning   Ptomaines are substances produced by decaying animal or vegetable proteins; ptomaine poisoning is not the same as food poisoning. Foods that contain ptomaines are far from appetizing; they look, smell and taste completely unpleasant and therefore are not usually a danger to humans. Most ptomaines aren't harmful; most ptomaine poisoning is actually staphylococcal poisoning. Ptomaine poisoning is also an obsolete term for food poisoning caused by bacterial poisons.

See also FOOD POISONING.

pufferfish   This exotic food fish, considered a delicacy in Japan, where it is known as "fugu," can cause poisoning if improperly prepared and cooked. It can also inflict a painful sting. There are more than 90 species of puffer, all belonging to the family Tetraodontidae; they are considered to be one of the most poisonous fish in the world, with a 60 percent fatality rate even with treatment. In Japan, there have been hundreds of deaths; at least three have been reported in Florida. Usually eaten only during the winter months (which is not its reproductive season), pufferfish is still the primary cause of death from food poisoning in Japan. From 1955 to 1975, 3,000 Japanese were poisoned by eating fugu and 1,500 died.

In Japan, cooks and restaurants that serve fugu must have a special license and training to prepare this sometimes deadly dish. Still, about 10 Japanese diners die each year from eating the wrong parts of the fish. Fugu lovers say that the fish tastes like chicken and that it produces a mild intoxication, feelings of warmth and euphoria. In the United States, one species of puffer (called the blowfish) is served in restaurants under the name of "sea squab."

Pufferfish get their name from their ability to inflate themselves when threatened, puffing themselves up to several times their normal girth until they are almost spherical. Puffers are most toxic just before and during their reproductive season, because of the interaction between gonad activity and toxicity, although the same species found in different locations at the same time could vary widely in its toxicity. They are commonly found in warm or temperate regions around the world, including the west coast of Central America, throughout the Indo-Pacific, Japan and from Australia to South America.

Puffers are very territorial and seek rocky crevices to hide in. A close relative is the deadly porcupine fish, which not only inflates when threatened but also erects sharp quills all over its body.

Poisonous part   The poison found in the pufferfish is tetrodotoxin, a basic compound that does not deactivate when heated and carries a high fatality rate when eaten. This nerve poison is 150,000 times more deadly than curare; it is contained in the entrails and is not destroyed by cooking. There is evidence that the toxin is used as part of the Haitian voodoo potion used in the zombie ritual.

Symptoms   While death from a puffer *sting* is rare, it causes an immediate severe throbbing pain that may stay at the site of the wound or spread throughout the body and last for several hours or days. There may be redness and swelling at the site of the sting, and the area may become numb.

Improperly preparing or cooking this fish causes a far more serious type of poisoning. Within minutes to hours, symptoms include numbness and tingling beginning in the extremities and spreading over the body together with a floating feeling. There is nausea and vomiting, and other gastrointestinal symptoms appear. Paralysis in an ascending pattern appears, and the victim finds it difficult to breath, which progresses to coma, convulsions, respiratory arrest and death. The first 24 hours after ingestion are critical; there is a high fatality rate.

Treatment   For a puffer sting, contact medical help immediately; flush the wound with fresh or salt water and then soak the affected area in hot water or put hot compresses on it. The water should be very hot (122°F), so that the heat will deactivate the poison. Continue applying hot water for 30 minutes to an hour.

There is no antidote to tetrodotoxin ingestion, and there is great controversy over the relative benefits of the administration of atropine, edrophonium or pyridostigmine. Otherwise, treatment is supportive and symptomatic. Induce vomiting or perform gastric lavage if ingestion occurred within the preceding hour, followed by the administration of activated charcoal.

See also FOOD POISONING; TETRODO TOXIN.

pyrethrin   The active chemical derived from pyrethrum (extracted from chrysanthemums grown in Zaire and Kenya), pyrethrin is one of the oldest known botanic insecticides. It was used hundreds of years ago in China, and the plants were cultivated in Europe more than a century ago. Pyrethrin and pyrethrum come from two strains of chrysanthemum (roseum and carneum). To make the insecticide, pyrethrum flowers are ground and then used either undiluted or mixed with inert ingredients or other insecticides to kill a variety of garden and household insect pests.

While pyrethrin has largely been replaced by more toxic insecticides, it is still often found in pesticide preparations for fighting fleas in dogs. Both pyrethrum and pyrethrin are the most widely used natural insecticides because they are deadly to a wide range of insects—possibly as effective in controlling pests as Sevin (carbaryl), a popular synthetic pesticide.

Pyrethrin is stronger than its dried flower source, since it has been strengthened to prevent insects from recovering from the effects of the poison. These synergists (derived from sesame) are somewhat controversial today because in large quantities they can affect the human nervous system. They can kill or incapacitate beetles, caterpillars, flies, wasps, bees, moths, fruit flies, butterflies, borers, whiteflies, chafers, leaf rollers and many other insects.

Symptoms   Breathing pyrethrin causes the most toxic reaction because of its highly allergic properties; skin contact can cause dermatitis in about half of those sensitive to ragweed. Severe poisoning with pyrethrin is unusual, although it can cause nausea, vomiting, gastroenteritis, excitability, incoordination, muscular paralysis and death from respiratory failure. Symptoms may last between two days and two weeks. Less serious poisoning results in reddened skin, burning and itching, swelling cheeks, headache, stomach problems and numb lips and tongue.

Treatment Atropine therapy may control gastroenteritis. Wash pyrethrin from eyes and skin, as it can cause a severe local dermatitis. Treat symptoms.

See also BOTANIC INSECTICIDES; PYRETHRUM.

pyrethrum A wide-spectrum botanic insecticide used for hundreds of years in China, pyrethrum is a powder made from one of two forms of chrysanthemums (roseum and carneum). Pyrethrin is the active chemical derived from pyrethrum and is also used as an insecticide.

Pyrethrum is a widely used natural insecticide because it can kill a wide variety of insects while posing little harm to humans and animals. Pyrethrum is more benign than its chemical ester pyrethrin and breaks down much faster (usually within 24 hours). It does not kill some insect pests but only stuns them for a period of time.

See also BOTANIC INSECTICIDES; PYRETHRIN.

pyridoxine (Vitamin B$_6$)   See VITAMINS.

Q

quaalude (methaqualone) Used to relieve anxiety and tension and as a sleeping pill, quaaludes have been taken off the American market but are still available on the street as a drug of abuse.

Symptoms Within five to 30 minutes, depending on whether the drug was injected or taken in the more common pill form, symptoms of overdose appear and include nausea, vomiting, stomach irritation, pulmonary edema, convulsions and death.

Treatment Gastric lavage and symptomatic treatment.

See also NARCOTICS.

quicklime (calcium oxide) Also called unslaked lime, this very powerful caustic is a component of portland cement and liberates heat in contact with water. It can cause serious damage if ingested, inhaled or allowed to contact the eyes. Note: Slaked lime (calcium hydroxide) is a simple alkali, and because of its low solubility in water, it is not greatly corrosive.

Symptoms Contact with the skin may produce first-, second- or third-degree chemical burns; eye contact may produce severe conjunctivitis as well as damaged corneas. Ingestion produces burning pain from mouth to stomach, with marked difficulty in swallowing. Mucous membranes are soapy and white and then turn brown and become ulcerated. Vomit is bloody and may contain shreds of mucous membrane. Pulse is feeble and rapid, breathing is rapid and collapse may follow. Death may result from shock, asphyxiation from swelling and intercurrent infections; pneumonia may occur in 48 to 72 hours. Esophageal stricture may develop within weeks, months or even years after ingestion.

Treatment Cold milk, water or tea should be given immediately. Irrigate the mouth with water; the damage to the esophagus from caustic alkalies occurs within the first minute, and therefore first aid measures after that are of doubtful value. DO NOT give carbonated beverages, and DO NOT induce vomiting or attempt gastric lavage (the small amount of alkali that usually reaches the stomach is quickly neutralized by the acid gastric juice). Olive oil may temporarily ease pain but should not be given in large amounts.

See also ALKALINE CORROSIVES.

quinidine This is one of a group of antiarrhythmic drugs commonly used to control arrhythmias and malaria and other infections. Acute ingestion of one gram of quinidine should be considered potentially lethal.

Symptoms   This drug primarily affects the cardiovascular and central nervous systems. Symptoms include heart problems, dry mouth, dilated pupils, delirium, seizures, coma and respiratory arrest. In addition, there may be nausea, vomiting and diarrhea after acute ingestion, and with chronic doses there may be tinnitus (ringing in the ears), vertigo, deafness and visual disturbances.

Treatment   Most therapies have proven ineffectual, and there is no known antidote. The primary goal is to keep the heart functioning until the drug is eliminated, which usually occurs within a few hours. Treat heart problems with hypertonic sodium bicarbonate. Do not induce vomiting; perform gastric lavage followed by the administration of activated charcoal and a cathartic. Quinidine is not effectively removed by dialysis. Treat low blood pressure, arrhythmias, coma and seizures as they occur; treat recurrent ventricular tachycardia with lidocaine or phenytoin.

See also ANTIARRHYTHMIC DRUGS.

quinine   A former drug treatment for malaria, quinine has largely been replaced by chloroquine but is still used for cases resistant to the newer drug. It is still prescribed for the treatment of nocturnal muscle cramps and has also been used as an abortifacient. The chief alkaloid of cinchona bark, quinine also contains related drugs (including quinidine).

The quinine content of "tonic" water is usually no larger than 30 mg/100 ml, although this small amount can produce symptoms in very sensitive people. Dubonnet contains 7 mg/100 ml.

The mechanism behind quinine's toxicity is believed to be similar to that of quinidine, although quinine is much less toxic to the heart. It is available in capsules and tablets of 130 to 325 mg; the minimum toxic dose for an adult is 3 to 4 g (one gram has been fatal to a child), although some people have taken much larger doses and survived.

Symptoms   Quinine depresses the cell function throughout the body, affecting the heart, kidney, liver and central nervous system. Quinine toxicity causes a syndrome called cinchonism, which causes tinnitus (ringing in the ears), blurred vision, weakness, nausea, vomiting, low blood pressure and heart problems. Evidence of the drug's effect on the brain can be seen in the resulting apprehension, confusion and excitement. Convulsions and respiratory arrest have also been reported, and death occurs from respiratory or circulatory collapse in a few hours to a few days.

If the victim recovers, there may be residual damage to the eyes and ears—even causing deafness.

Treatment   There is no antidote to quinine. Perform gastric lavage, followed by the administration of magnesium sulfate or activated charcoal. Do not induce vomiting. Give hypertonic sodium bicarbonate for cardiotoxicity.

See also QUINIDINE.

R

radiation poisoning Although excessive exposure to radiation is rare, it is a potentially catastrophic possibility in the nuclear age. Radiation poisoning may occur from internal or external contamination and from particle-emitting solids, liquids or gases (including beta and alpha particles, neutrons, protons and positrons) and electromagnetic sources (such as X rays or gamma rays).

Radiation interferes with the function of the body and damages RNA and DNA. Cells that turn over quickly, such as those found in the skin or gastrointestinal tract, are affected first. While contact with electromagnetic sources of radiation does not make the victim radioactive or dangerous to others, exposure to particle-emitting sources can be very contaminating to anyone who comes in contact with the victim.

Radiation dose is expressed in various terms, but rad (radiation absorbed dose) is the most common.

Symptoms Symptoms are dose related: Exposure to 100–200 rads causes nausea, vomiting, abdominal cramps and diarrhea; 200 rads is potentially fatal, and 600 rads is nearly always fatal within a few days, causing severe gastroenteritis and marked dehydration. Brief exposure to excessive amounts (5,000 rads or more) causes confusion and lethargy followed within minutes to hours by convulsions, coma, cardiovascular collapse and death.

In addition, exposure from anywhere between 200 and 1,000 rads often depresses the bone marrow function, opening the way to infections. Other symptoms include skin burns and hair loss.

Treatment For expert assistance in evaluation and treatment, contact the federal Oak Ridge Radiation Emergency Assistance Center and Training Site (available 24 hours a day) at (615) 576-3131 or (615) 481-1000, ext. 1502. Chelating agents may be useful for ingestion or inhalation of certain particles. Treat symptoms, maintain airway and replace fluid losses.

For particulate exposure, move the victim from the area, remove all clothing and wash the skin with soap and water; all water and clothing must be properly destroyed. Rescuers and hospital personnel should wear protective gear. Induce vomiting or perform gastric lavage in cases of ingestion. The effectiveness of activated charcoal and cathartics is unknown.

radon This invisible, odorless radioactive gas is created by the natural decay of radium and uranium found in rocks and soil. It is relatively harmless out of doors; it is most dangerous once it has seeped inside a house, where it breaks down into harmful elements that attach to dust particles that can enter the lungs. Once in the lungs, the elements decay in minutes, releasing alpha radiation. This radiation can cause cell damage possibly leading to lung cancer, and is among the most dangerous of toxic substances because of the number of cases of cancer it is estimated to cause each year.

According to the Environmental Protection Agency, it is estimated that one in 15 American homes has levels of radon high enough to pose a health risk. And another study of 552 homes suggested that there are about one million homes in the United States where the chances of developing lung cancer from radon are at least as great as one in 40 over a lifetime.

But in a 1991 survey by the American Lung Association, only 11 percent of Americans had tested their homes for radon. Further, animal studies suggest that in an average home in the United States, an individual has about a 1 in 300 chance of developing lung cancer in his or her lifetime from indoor radon—or that about 10 percent of all cases of lung cancer in this country are caused by this gas. (It must be remembered, however, that smokers are more susceptible to cancer from radon than nonsmokers.)

Radon is able to enter a building because of the small difference between inside and outside air pressure, which draws in the radon in much the same way as a fire draws heated air up a chimney: A heated house draws cool air from the basement or ground floor, where the pressure is low, and sends it to the upper floors, where the pressure is higher.

There are two types of kits available: carbon kits, use carbon to trap the radon gas and take a week or two to work; alpha-track monitors measure the alpha particles emitted by rado decay and must be left in place one to three months. Both kinds can be installed by a consumer but must be sent to a lab for analysis. They cost between $15 and $25. The EPA recommends that the lowest lived-in area of the house be tested, including the basement, if it is frequently used. Kits that have been evaluated and approved by the EPA are marked "EPA approved" on the package.

If radon is found in the home, there are several options to deal with it. The basement or crawl spaces of most houses have a slightly lower air presssure than the soil beneath, and this speeds the rate at which the gas can enter the house through the foundation. One way to cut down on the problem is to install pipes to the outdoors that ventilate the soil beneath the house. Or, consumers could pressurize the basement or crawl space with an air blower, flushing out the radon. Sealing cracks in the foundation and basement floor has not been shown to be an effective way to reduce the inflow of radon.

See also APPENDIX A.

ragwort *(Senecio)* [Other names: butterweed, squaw weed, stinking willie, tansy ragwort. In the United States, groundsel, ragwort and butterweed are commonly applied to many different varieties of *Senecio*.] There are about 3,000 species of *Senecio*, including threadleaf groundsel *(S. longilobus)* and common groundsel *(S. vulgaris);* many of the varieties contain poisonous alkaloids.

Ragwort is a four-foot-tall biennial or perennial herb with yellow flower clusters that has become naturalized in parts of Canada south to Massachusetts and in Washington and Oregon west of the Cascades.

Threadleaf groundsel is a shrubby perennial with white flowers found in Colorado and Utah south to western Texas and northern Mexico.

Common groundsel is a smaller annual with soft, fleshy leaves and yellow flowers that has become naturalized in Alaska and throughout Canada south to North Carolina and west to Wisconsin; it is also found in California, New Mexico and Texas.

Poisonous part   The entire plant is poisonous; honey made from the nectar and milk from animals who have grazed on these plants also contain the poisonous pyrrolizidine alkaloids. In general, poisonings have occurred from excessive drinking of herbal teas made from this plant, which causes Budd-Chiari syndrome, a liver disease leading to cirrhosis.

Symptoms   Abdominal pain; anorexia with nausea, vomiting and diarrhea. Chronic use of tea made from these plants can result in fatal cases of cirrhosis.

Treatment   There is no treatment for this type of liver disease caused by the pyrrolizidine alkaloids.

See also ALKALOIDS.

rat poison   Most rat poisons (or rodenticides) that are the most toxic to humans and pets are restricted for use only by commercial exterminators and government agencies. Inorganic rat poison compounds include arsenic, thallium, phosphorus, barium carbonate, zinc phosphide and vacor. Organic compounds include sodium fluoroacetate, alphanaphthylthiourea, warfarin, red squill, strychnine sulfate and dicarboximide.

There are two types of rodenticides: single dose (or acute) compounds and chronic varieties, such as the anticoagulant rat poisons. Acute poisons kill rats after a single feeding and usually include red squill, zinc phosphide, strychnine, arsenic, phosphorus and thallium sulfate. Chronic rat poisons, on the other hand, are preferred, since they do not produce symptoms in the rat that make it stop eating before acquiring a fatal dose, and anticoagulants are less toxic to humans and animals.

Poisoning with anticoagulant rodenticides is extremely rare, since huge doses would be needed in order to be toxic. When it occurs, the treatment is the administration of vitamin K_1 or blood transfusions.

See also ARSENIC; PHOSPHORUS; RED SQUILL; THALLIUM; VACOR; WARFARIN.

rattlesnake, canebrake   *(Crotalus horridus atricaudatus)*   This snake is one of a number of species of rattlesnakes known as pit vipers because of their heat-sensing pits behind the eyes and nose, with tail rattles that hiss before striking. The canebrake is the southern United States' version of the timber rattler.

Symptoms Symptoms appear within 15 minutes and include excessive thirst, nausea, vomiting, shock, paralysis, respiratory problems, anemia, necrosis, kidney problems and sometimes death. The bite of a rattlesnake is painful. Indications of a serious bite include swelling above the elbows or knees within two hours, hemorrhages, numbness at the puncture site, tingling around the mouth, yellow vision, vomiting and violent spasms.

Treatment Antivenin is available. Local care of the bite is essential. Antibiotics and tetanus vaccine should be given.

See also MASSASAUGA; PIT VIPERS; RATTLESNAKE, CASCABEL; RATTLE-SNAKE, EASTERN DIAMONDBACK; RATTLESNAKE, MEXICAN WEST COAST; RATTLESNAKE, RED DIAMONDBACK; RATTLESNAKE, TIMBER; RATTLE-SNAKE, WESTERN DIAMONDBACK; RATTLESNAKES; SIDEWINDER; SNAKES, POISONOUS; VIPER, GABOON; VIPER, JUMPING; VIPER, MALAYAN PIT; VIPER, RUSSELL'S; VIPER, SAWSCALED; VIPER, WAGLER'S PIT; VIPERS; WATER MOC-CASIN; WUTU.

rattlesnake, cascabel *(Crotalus durissus)* Also known as the tropical or South American rattler, the cascabel is one of the two most deadly rattle-snakes in the world and is found in tropical South America.

Poisonous part Crotamine, a toxin that causes convulsions, is found in the venom of this snake, which also relaxes the victim's neck muscles, causing the head to flop and adding to this snake's reputation as a neck breaker.

Symptoms Symptoms appear within 15 minutes and include excessive thirst, nausea, vomiting, shock, paralysis, respiratory problems, anemia, necrosis, kidney problems and sometimes death. The bite of a rattlesnake is painful. Indications of a serious bite include swelling above the elbows or knees within two hours, hemorrhages, numbness at the puncture site, tingling around the mouth, yellow vision, vomiting and violent spasms.

Treatment Antivenin is available.

See also MASSASAUGA; PIT VIPERS; RATTLESNAKE, CANEBRAKE; RATTLE-SNAKE, EASTERN DIAMONDBACK; RATTLESNAKE, MEXICAN WEST COAST; RATTLESNAKE, RED DIAMONDBACK; RATTLESNAKE, TIMBER; RATTLE-SNAKE, WESTERN DIAMONDBACK; RATTLESNAKES; SIDEWINDER; SNAKES, POISONOUS; VIPER, GABOON; VIPER, JUMPING; VIPER, MALAYAN PIT; VIPER, RUSSELL'S; VIPER, SAWSCALED; VIPER, WAGLER'S PIT; VIPERS; WATER MOC-CASIN; WUTU.

rattlesnake, eastern diamondback *(Crotalus adamanteus)* Also called the Florida diamondback, this snake is considered to be the most dangerous in North America, with a venom highly destructive to blood tissue. The largest of all the rattlesnakes and heavier than its western relative, the eastern diamondback has large dark brown or black diamonds with light centers on a body color of olive, brown or black and grows to be eight feet long. There are also prominent light diagonal lines on the side of its head. It has a heavy body with a large, sharply distinct head.

It is found in sparse woodland, dry pine flatwoods, abandoned farms and lowland coastal regions of the southeastern Gulf states of the United States and is found throughout Florida. However, the population has been reduced by hunters and land development.

Symptoms Symptoms appear within 15 minutes and include excessive thirst, nausea, vomiting, shock, paralysis, respiratory problems, anemia, necrosis, kidney problems and sometimes death. The bite of a rattlesnake is painful. Indications of a serious bite include swelling above the elbows or knees within two hours, hemorrhages, numbness at the puncture site, tingling around the mouth, yellow vision, vomiting and violent spasms.

Treatment Antivenin is available.

See also MASSASAUGA; PIT VIPERS; RATTLESNAKE, CANEBRAKE; RATTLE-SNAKE, CASCABEL; RATTLESNAKE, MEXICAN WEST COAST; RATTLESNAKE, RED DIAMONDBACK; RATTLESNAKE, TIMBER; RATTLESNAKE, WESTERN DI-AMONDBACK; RATTLESNAKES; SIDEWINDER; SNAKES, POISONOUS; VIPER, GABOON; VIPER, JUMPING; VIPER, MALAYAN PIT; VIPER, RUSSELL'S; VIPER, SAWSCALED; VIPER, WAGLER'S PIT; VIPERS; WATER MOCCASIN; WUTU.

rattlesnake, horned See SIDEWINDER.

rattlesnake, Mexican west coast *(Crotalus basiliscus)* The world's second most deadly rattlesnake, the Mexican west coast rattlesnake is found in western Mexico.

Symptoms Symptoms appear within 15 minutes and include excessive thirst, nausea, vomiting, shock, paralysis, respiratory problems, anemia, necrosis, kidney problems and sometimes death. The bite of a rattlesnake is painful. Indications of a serious bite include swelling above the elbows or knees within two hours, hemorrhages, numbness at the puncture site, tingling around the mouth, yellow vision, vomiting and violent spasms.

Treatment Antivenin is available.

See also MASSASAUGA; PIT VIPERS; RATTLESNAKE, CANEBRAKE; RATTLE-SNAKE, CASCABEL; RATTLESNAKE, EASTERN DIAMONDBACK; RATTLE-SNAKE, RED DIAMONDBACK; RATTLESNAKE, TIMBER; RATTLESNAKE, WESTERN DIAMONDBACK; RATTLESNAKES; SIDEWINDER; SNAKES, POI-SONOUS; VIPER, GABOON; VIPER, JUMPING; VIPER, MALAYAN PIT; VIPER, RUSSELL'S; VIPER, SAWSCALED; VIPER, WAGLER'S PIT; VIPERS; WATER MOC-CASIN; WUTU.

rattlesnake, red diamondback *(Crotalus ruber)* This rattler looks very much like the western diamondback rattlesnake, but its body color is more reddish or pinkish and its markings less distinct. It has diamond shapes down its midline, usually edged in lighter colors. Black and white rings circle the tail.

This snake prefers arid and semidesert, cold coastal regions in the foothills and mountains in southern California, Baja California and northern Mexico. It is most often seen during the spring sheltering in the sun or crossing the road at night.

Symptoms Symptoms appear within 15 minutes and include excessive thirst, nausea, vomiting, shock, paralysis, respiratory problems, anemia, necrosis, kidney problems and sometimes death. The bite of a rattlesnake is painful. Indications of a serious bite include swelling above the elbows or knees within two hours, hemorrhages, numbness at the puncture site, tingling around the mouth, yellow vision, vomiting and violent spasms.

Treatment Antivenin is available.

See also MASSASAUGA; PIT VIPERS; RATTLESNAKE, CANEBRAKE; RATTLE-SNAKE, CASCABEL; RATTLESNAKE, EASTERN DIAMONDBACK; RATTLE-SNAKE, MEXICAN WEST COAST; RATTLESNAKE, TIMBER; RATTLESNAKE, WESTERN DIAMONDBACK; RATTLESNAKES; SIDEWINDER; SNAKES, POI-SONOUS; VIPER, GABOON; VIPER, JUMPING; VIPER, MALAYAN PIT; VIPER, RUSSELL'S; VIPER, SAWSCALED; VIPER, WAGLER'S PIT; VIPERS; WATER MOC-CASIN; WUTU.

rattlesnake, South American See RATTLESNAKE, CASCABEL.

rattlesnake, timber *(Crotalus horridus)* The only rattler found in the pop-ulated northeastern United States, the timber rattlesnake has a range extending into much of the central and southern states except for Florida. As a result of urban pressure, this species has been exterminated in many parts of its range.

There are two distinct races of the timber rattler: *C. h. horridus,* found in the northern part of the species' range in pine forests and wooded slopes; and the canebrake rattlesnake, *C. h. atricaudatus,* found in southern lowlands in cane thickets and swamps. The timber rattler is large, with a robust body and a large, flat unmarked head. Its color is yellow brown or dark brown, with darker crossbands; completely black snakes are not uncommon. The canebrake rattler is more brightly marked, with a pink buff or brown color with bold black crossbands and an orange or red dorsal stripe. Both types have a black tail.

The timber rattler is often seen coiled up and motionless waiting for prey in the daytime during spring and fall, and on summer nights. In the north, large groups of timber rattlers can be seen in rocky dens, sometimes with copperheads.

Symptoms Symptoms appear within 15 minutes and include excessive thirst, nausea, vomiting, shock, paralysis, respiratory problems, anemia, necrosis, kidney problems and sometimes death. The bite of a rattlesnake is painful. Indications of a serious bite include swelling above the elbows or knees within two hours, hemorrhages, numbness at the puncture site, tingling around the mouth, yellow vision, vomiting and violent spasms.

Treatment Antivenin is available.

See also MASSASAUGA; RATTLESNAKE, CANEBRAKE; RATTLESNAKE, CAS-CABEL; RATTLESNAKE, EASTERN DIAMONDBACK; RATTLESNAKE, MEXICAN WEST COAST; RATTLESNAKE, RED DIAMONDBACK; RATTLESNAKE, TIMBER; RATTLESNAKES.

rattlesnake, tropical See RATTLESNAKE, CASCABEL.

rattlesnake, western diamondback *(Crotalus atrox)* Also called a coon tail rattler, this is the largest rattlesnake of the North American West. The western diamondback has a heavy body, with a large, spade-shaped head that is distinct from the neck. The body color is gray-brown or pink, with light-bordered, dark diamond blotches on the back. The diamonds are often covered with small dark spots, which are often faded and dusty looking. The tail is distinctive, ringed boldly with black and white. There are two light diagonal lines on the side of its face, and the stripe behind the eye meets the upper lip in front of the jaw angle.

The western diamondback is found in the semidesert and dry arid areas, rocky canyons, river bluffs and some cultivated areas in much of the southwestern parts of the United States from southeastern California east to central Arkansas, and as far south as central Mexico. Toxicologists consider this snake to be the most dangerous snake in the United States.

When threatened, the western diamondback stands its ground, lifts up its head and sounds a "rattling" warning. It is most active late in the day during the hot summer months.

Symptoms Symptoms appear within 15 minutes and include excessive thirst, nausea, vomiting, shock, paralysis, respiratory problems, anemia, necrosis, kidney problems and sometimes death. The bite of a rattlesnake is painful. Indications of a serious bite include swelling above the elbows or knees within two hours, hemorrhages, numbness at the puncture site, tingling around the mouth, yellow vision, vomiting and violent spasms.

Treatment Antivenin is available.

See also MASSASAUGA; PIT VIPERS; RATTLESNAKE, CANEBRAKE; RATTLE-SNAKE, CASCABEL; RATTLESNAKE, EASTERN DIAMONDBACK; RATTLE-SNAKE, MEXICAN WEST COAST; RATTLESNAKE, RED DIAMONDBACK; RATTLESNAKE, TIMBER; RATTLESNAKES; SIDEWINDER; VIPER, GABOON; VIPER, JUMPING; VIPER MALAYAN PIT; VIPER, RUSSELL'S; VIPER, WAGLER'S PIT; VIPERS; WATER MOCCASIN; WUTU.

rattlesnakes Rattlesnakes resemble any other viper except that they almost all have a rattle at the end of the tail formed by a series of dry, horny segments that vibrate with a rattling sound when shaken by the snake as a warning of its presence. Each time the snake loses its skin, a new segment is added. More than 98 percent of the snakebites in the United States are from rattlesnakes, which are found in two separate snake families: the Crotalidae (the eastern and western diamondbacks, the timber rattler, the canebrake rattler, the pacific rattler, and the mojave rattler), and the Viperidae (the sidewinder, or horned, rattler, and two types of pygmy rattlers—the massasauga and the pygmy. They are all considered pit vipers because of the heat-sensing pits between each nostril and eye.

Outside the United States, the cascabel rattler (also known as the tropical or South American rattler) is found in tropical South America and is one of the two most dangerous rattlers. The Mexican west coast rattler is the second most dangerous rattler and is found in western Mexico. The Brazilian rattler is found in southeastern Brazil, Argentina and Paraguay.

Although rattlesnakes are poisonous, fatalities in the United States are rare because antivenin is usually available immediately.

Poisonous part Rattlesnake venom includes the toxin acetylcholinesterase, and in some tropical varieties the convulsion-inducing toxin crotamine also appears.

Symptoms Within 15 minutes to an hour after being bitten, the victim will begin to experience thirst, nausea, vomiting, paralysis, shock, respiratory distress and drooping eyelids. Death follows malfunction of the kidneys. Tingling around the mouth, yellow vision and a numbed wound site all are indicative of a serious bite with a large amount of venom. In cases of severe poisoning, there will be swelling caused by hemorrhages above the elbows or knees within two hours.

Treatment Antivenin is available.

See also MASSASAUGA; PIT VIPERS; RATTLESNAKE, CANEBRAKE; RATTLESNAKE, CASCABEL; RATTLESNAKE, EASTERN DIAMONDBACK; RATTLESNAKE, MEXICAN WEST COAST; RATTLESNAKE, RED DIAMONDBACK; RATTLESNAKE, TIMBER; RATTLESNAKE, WESTERN DIAMONDBACK; SIDEWINDER; SNAKES, POISONOUS; VIPER, GABOON; VIPER, JUMPING; VIPER, MALAYAN PIT; VIPER, RUSSELL'S; VIPER, SAWSCALED; VIPER, WAGLER'S PIT; VIPERS; WATER MOCCASIN; WUTU.

red squill This botanic rat poison is one of the least toxic of all the organic rodenticides available. When ingested in large doses, it can interfere with the function of the heart; it is also an irritant and central-acting emetic.

Symptoms Acute poisoning causes nausea, vomiting, diarrhea, abdominal pain, cardiac irregularities, convulsion and death from ventricular fibrillation.

Treatment Induce vomiting with syrup of ipecac followed by gastric lavage. Administer lidocaine or phenytoin; monitor electrolytes.

See also RAT POISON.

resins   Also called resinoids, these compounds are made up of a wide variety of substances that are both resinous and semisolid at room temperature, and include potent toxins such as those found in rhododendron and laurel. Symptoms of resin poisoning include stomach irritation, vomiting, diarrhea, headache, weakness, irregular heartbeat, convulsions, coma and, sometimes, death.

See also LAUREL, MOUNTAIN; RHODODENDRON.

rhododendron *(Rhododendron)*   Once considered as belonging to two separate genera, rhododendron and azalea are now both considered to be in the *Rhododendron* genus. There are about 800 *Rhododendron* species, which are subdivided into eight subgenera.

This extremely common evergreen, semievergreen and deciduous shrub is found everywhere throughout Canada, Britain and the United States (except for the north central states and subtropical Florida). Rhododendrons are odorless, with bell-shaped flowers that come in a variety of colors; azaleas are sweet smelling with funnel-shaped flowers. Both are deadly narcotics said to have poisoned Xenophon's army from honey made from the flowers' nectar.

Poisonous part All parts of the plant are poisonous and contain carbohydrate andromedotoxin—the same poison as in mountain laurel. Honey made from the plant's nectar has also caused poisoning. Children who have chewed on the leaves have become seriously poisoned.

Symptoms Burning in the mouth, followed within six hours of ingestion by increased salivation, vomiting, tearing eyes, nasal discharge, prickling skin, difficulty in breathing, slow heartbeat, muscle weakness progressing to paralysis, convulsions, coma and death.

Treatment Fluids and electrolyte replacement; atropine for bradycardia; ephedrine for hypotension.

See also LAUREL, MOUNTAIN.

rhubarb *(Rheum rhabarbarum;* sometimes incorrectly referred to as *R. rhaponticum)* [Other names: pie plant, wine plant.] This common perennial, grown for its tasty stalk, has poisonous leaves that can be fatal if mistakenly cooked along with the rhubarb stalks or eaten raw.

Several feet tall at maturity, the plant has large, wavy oval leaves and is cultivated across the United States for its edible stalk.

Poisonous part The leaves are the only poisonous part of the rhubarb plant and contain oxalic acid, potassium and calcium oxalates and anthraquinone glycosides. They must be removed before eating or cooking.

Symptoms Several hours after ingestion, the digestive irritant in the leaves can cause stomach pain, nausea, vomiting, hemorrhage, respiratory problems, burning mouth and possibly cardiac or respiratory arrest following a drop in the calcium content of the blood. Without treatment, death or permanent kidney damage may occur. It is believed that symptoms are almost completely caused by the anthraquinone cathartics in the leaves.

Treatment Gastric lavage and emesis, together with calcium salts, calcium gluconate and other forms, to help precipitate the oxalate. Fluids must be replaced to prevent kidney malfunction.

ringhals *(Hemachatus hemachatus)* One of the spitting cobras, this brick-red snake is found in South Africa and prefers to spray venom toward the eyes rather than bite. The openings of the venom ducts are on the front of its fangs, so that when faced with an enemy the ringhal can apply muscular pressure on the gland to force the liquid in a stream straight at the enemy's eyes. The aim of the ringhals is absolutely deadly, and they are a real threat because they have a range of up to 10 feet. Spitting cobras can also bite, but they seem reluctant to do so.

Symptoms When contact is made with the eyes, there is excruciating pain and sometimes permanent blindness; there is also weakness, respiratory distress, collapse and death.

Treatment Antivenin is available, but only the specific antiserum for the type of cobra involved should be used, and victims are often tested for sensitivity before being treated. If the eyes are contaminated, they should be immediately flushed out and treated or blindness may result.

See also COBRA; COBRA, SPITTING; SNAKES, POISONOUS.

Ritalin Known chemically as methylphenidate, this drug is a stimulant but is ironically given to hyperactive children to calm down. In adults, it acts as a central nervous system stimulant and, if taken with monoamine oxidase (MAO) inhibitors, can drastically increase blood pressure. It is well absorbed when taken by mouth and is metabolized extensively by the liver. It has a low therapeutic index (that is, toxicity occurs at levels only slightly above the usual doses). A high degree of tolerance can occur after continued use.

Symptoms Overdose can cause agitation, nausea, vomiting, hyperthermia, tremors, seizures, hypertension, coma and convulsions; if taken with anticonvulsants, it may change seizure pattern.

Treatment Treat symptoms if they occur. There is no specific antidote for Ritalin; hypertension may be treated with a vasodilator such as phentolamine. Do not induce vomiting; perform gastric lavage and administer activated charcoal.

rosary pea *(Abrus precatorius)* [Other names: bead vine, black-eyed Susan, coral bead plant, crab's eyes, Indian licorice, jequirity bean, licorice vine, love bean, lucky bean, mienie-mienie Indian bean, paternoster pea, prayer bead, precatory bean, red bead vine, rosary bean, Seminole bead, weather plant, wild licorice.] This climbing, woody vine is found in tropical regions in Africa and Asia, and in Florida, Hawaii, Guam, Central America, southern Europe and India. Its leaves have short leaflets that droop at night and in cloudy weather, and its pea-shaped fruit pod holds five scarlet, pea-sized seeds with hard seed coats and a small black spot. Its seeds are used in rosaries, bracelets, leis, good luck charms and children's toys, but the seeds are harmless unless chewed.

Poisonous part   Seeds, or beans, if chewed. If swallowed whole, the hard seed coat prevents absorption and poisoning. The toxalbumin called abrin, one of nature's most poisonous substances, is the poison in rosary pea; the tetanic glycoside abric acid is found in the seeds. Abrin interferes with the protein synthesis in cells of the intestinal wall.

Symptoms   The severity of symptoms, which appear from several hours to several days after eating, depends on the number of beans eaten and how much they were chewed. Symptoms include mouth irritations, nausea, vomiting, severe diarrhea, acute gastroenteritis, chills, weakness, clammy skin with perspiration, weak, rapid pulse, and convulsions ending in death from heart failure. One seed chewed by a child can be fatal despite intensive care.

Treatment   The long time between ingestion and symptoms allows for the removal of the poisonous substance; convulsions are treated as they occur, together with a high carbohydrate diet to head off liver damage.

See also GLYCOSIDE.

roseum   A variety of chrysanthemum used in the production of the botanic insecticide pyrethrum.

See also PYRETHRUM.

rotenone   Also known as derrin or derris, rotenone is a broad-spectrum botanic insecticide derived from the derris root and used in lotions and ointments to treat chiggers, scabies and head lice; in dusts, washes and dips against animal parasites; and in insecticide sprays for home and agricultural use. Once believed to be harmless, it is now known to be more toxic than pyrethrin. While it has been used for many years, it has regained popularity in the last decade because it kills a wide variety of insects and is easy to make. This white, odorless crystal is sold in a 1 percent and 5 percent powder or spray.

Symptoms   Rotenone affects the nervous system and is most toxic when inhaled; skin contamination can cause a local irritation, and ingestion will cause stomach irritations but is rarely fatal. If inhaled, it can cause vomiting, abdominal pain, tremors and incoordination and can lead to convulsions and death from respiratory failure. Skin contact causes local irritation and dermatitis; ingestion produces nausea and vomiting. Chronic poisoning can cause kidney and liver damage.

Treatment Symptomatic.

See also BOTANIC INSECTICIDES.

rubbing alcohol See ISOPROPYL ALCOHOL.

rust remover See ALKALINE CORROSIVES.

S

saccharin Known by the trade name Sweet-N-Low, saccharin is an artificial sweetener discovered by accident in 1878 that is 400 times as sweet as sugar; American consumers ate or drank more than five million pounds of it a year before it was banned. Although the Food and Drug Administration announced a ban in March 1977, because it is mutagenic and causes cancer in laboratory animals, it is still an ingredient in many packaged foods and probably all toothpastes in the United States. Its name is derived from the Latin word *saccharun*, meaning "sugar"; pure saccharin is an odorless white power that easily dissolves in warm water but is destroyed by high heat. It has been criticized almost from the beginning of its use, first because it offered no food value and later because of its animal carcinogenicity.

Symptoms Ingestion of large amounts can produce toxic symptoms such as vomiting diarrhea, abdominal pain, frothing, muscle spasms, convulsions and stupor. In hypersensitive persons, even small doses may cause gastrointestinal symptoms such as vomiting and diarrhea, and allergic skin reactions.

Treatment Gastric lavage or induced vomiting for large overdoses, followed by a saline cathartic; symptomatic treatment.

See also SWEETENERS, ARTIFICIAL.

salicylates Widely valued for their painkilling and anti-inflammatory properties, the salicylates are found in a wide variety of over-the-counter preparations and cold products. The substance is an ingredient in aspirin and in most other analgesic preparations, and before the introduction of child-resistant caps, salicylate poisoning was one of the leading causes of accidental death in children. Oil of wintergreen, found in many skin ointments, is also high in salicylate content and can be fatal if ingested.

Aspirin should never be taken with acetaminophen (Tylenol), since it increases the liver toxicity of the Tylenol. Aspirin also increases the activity of anticoagulants. Vitamin C in large doses taken with aspirin can cause poisoning, but this is not usually fatal. Aspirin also interferes with the utilization of vitamin K in the liver.

Symptoms Salicylate poisoning causes a wide range of symptoms depending on the person's age and the amount swallowed. Two distinct syndromes may occur depending on whether the exposure is chronic or acute: acute ingestion of 150–200 mg/kg will produce a mild reaction; ingestion of 300–500 mg/kg will produce a more serious response. Chronic intoxication may occur with ingestion of 100 mg/kg for two or more days.

Onset of symptoms may be delayed for 12 to 24 hours. In cases of acute poisoning, vomiting is followed by ringing in the ears and lethargy; severe poisoning, causes coma, seizures, low blood sugar, high fever and pulmonary edema followed by death due to central nervous system failure and cardio-vascular collapse.

Chronic poisoning may result with older persons who have become confused over their dosage, or with young children. Symptoms include confusion, dehydration and metabolic acidosis, which may often be misdi-agnosed. With chronic poisoning, death rates are much higher and cerebral and pulmonary edema are more common.

Treatment There is no specific antidote for salicylate poisoning, but sodium bicarbonate is often given to help the kidneys eliminate the drug. Treat symptoms, replace fluid and maintain electrolyte balance; induce vomiting or perform gastric lavage followed by the administration of activated charcoal and a cathartic. With very large ingestions of salicylate, very large doses of activated charcoal are also needed to absorb the salicylate. Hemodialysis can be effective in removing salicylate. The victim should be treated for shock until medical care is available.

See also ASPIRIN; MEDICATIONS AS POISONS.

Salmonella Bacteria (including *S. enteritidis, S. cubana, S. aertrycke, S. choleraesius*) that multiply rapidly at room temperature and cause salmonellosis, an illness characterized by nausea, vomiting and diarrhea. Salmonella is found in raw meats, poultry, eggs, fish, raw milk and foods made from them, as well as in pet turtles and marijuana.

See also FOOD POISONING; SALMONELLOSIS.

salmonellosis One of the major types of food poisoning, salmonellosis is caused by *Salmonella* strains of bacteria *(S. enteritidis, S. cubana, S. aertrycke, S. choleraesius)*, which multiply rapidly at room temperatures. They are found in raw meats, poultry, eggs, fish, raw milk and foods made from them, as well as in pet turtles and marijuana. While salmonellosis is fatal in only 1 percent of cases, it is very dangerous in the elderly, pregnant women, young children and persons with cancer or AIDS.

Salmonellosis is common in this country; in 1963 there were 2,300 cases reported, with substantial increases each year. Bone meal, fertilizer and pet foods may all be implicated in the spread of salmonellosis. In particular, recent outbreaks have been linked to chickens and eggs; it is estimated that 60 percent of chicken carcasses in processing plants harbor the bacteria.

In the fall of 1992 the U.S. Department of Agriculture's Food Safety and Inspection Service approved two new methods to combat the rising level of salmonella on chicken: the use of trisodium phosphate in a rinse to destroy bacteria, and the use of irradiation to control potential contamination on poultry.

Food-grade trisodium phosphate is a federally approved ingredient that, according to tests, has no discernible effect on the taste, texture or color of chicken. The compound destroys salmonella by stripping a thin, exterior fat coating on the chickens. No residue is absorbed in the skin or meat of the birds. In one study, when carcasses were submerged in a water solution containing 8 percent trisodium phosphate at the end of the slaughter line, only 1 percent of the birds still contained salmonella organisms. By comparison, untreated carcasses in the same study had an 18 percent positive rate for salmonella.

No special labeling will be required for trisodium phosphate–treated chickens, but irradiated chicken must prominently carry the international symbol for the process with the words "treated with irradiation" on labels.

There are additional things consumers can do to help stop the spread of the disease at home. Proper refrigeration and cooking methods for meat and eggs must be observed at all times. Eggs should be refrigerated and not used raw (such as in Caesar salad or eggnog). Raw chicken should never touch any other food or utensils during preparation, and cooks should wash their hands after touching raw chicken.

Symptoms   While small amounts of salmonella can be ingested in otherwise healthy people without problem, elevated levels cause symptoms that appear from 12 to 48 hours after eating, smoking marijuana or handling turtles. They include severe headache, nausea, vomiting, fever, stomach cramps and diarrhea. Symptoms usually last two to seven days and can be fatal in infants and the elderly.

Treatment   Symptomatic, including bland diet (liquids and soft solids) and plenty of fluids to offset dehydration. Antibiotic treatment (chloramphenicol, ampicillin or a tetracycline) should be administered only in cases of severe infection.

See also FOOD POISONING.

saponin   One of the toxic glycoside compounds that vary in strength in any particular plant depending on the plant part and time of the year. While saponins are not easily absorbed by a healthy digestive tract, in the presence of other substances irritating to the digestive tract they can be absorbed, causing pain, vomiting and diarrhea similar to gastroenteritis. There is still much to be learned about the saponins, and many of the plants whose toxicity is a result of this compound have not been extensively studied. The saponin content of any one plant changes according to the part of the plant, its stage of growth and the season.

Plants that contain saponins include the corn cockle, tung tree, beech, English ivy and pokeweed.

See also GLYCOSIDE.

savin   (*Juniperus sabina*)   This extremely common shrub is found throughout the world and is an ancient abortifacient; oil made from the shrub is used to counteract overdose of cardiac medications like digitalis.

Poisonous part The entire savin plant is toxic.

Symptoms In small doses, ingestion causes water loss and starts menstruation; in large doses, it causes gastroenteritis with hemorrhages, vomiting, polyuria (excessive urine), oliguria (reduced urine) and anuria (absence of urine) and convulsions. Topically, savin oil causes blisters. Death from respiratory arrest occurs from 10 hours to several days later.

Treatment Castor oil followed by gastric lavage or emesis; follow immediately with a saline cathartic. Treat symptoms; give milk and plenty of fluids.

saxitoxin A deadly neurotoxin that is produced by plankton and causes paralytic shellfish poisoning (PSP). This poison gets its name from the Alaskan butter clam *(Saxidomus giganteus)*, from which it is extracted; it blocks nerve impulses, causes paralysis of the respiratory muscles and can be fatal if even one contaminated shellfish is eaten. It has minimal effects on the cardiovascular system. Although there is no antidote to saxitoxin, it is readily absorbed by activated charcoal.

See also DINOFLAGELLATE; FOOD POISONING; PARALYTIC SHELLFISH POISONING.

scombroid poisoning A type of poisoning caused by eating one of a group of scombroid fishes (including mackerel, swordfish, moray eel, mahimahi, tuna, bluefish, etc.), which contain a chemical called histidine. When these fish are allowed to stand at room temperature for several hours, histidine interacts with bacteria to form a histaminelike substance called saurine, which is the toxin involved in scombroid poisoning.

Scombroid fish are more susceptible to the development of saurine poison than most other kinds of fish because there is a great percentage of histidine in their musculature. All of the species that are potentially toxic live in temperate or tropical waters, especially around California and Hawaii; even commercially canned tuna can become toxic, although the most common fish responsible is mahimahi. Scombroid poisoning can be prevented simply by adequately refrigerating fish.

Symptoms Symptoms of saurine poisoning resemble those of a severe allergy: soon after eating the affected fish (which is said to have a sharp, pungent taste), the victim begins to experience headache, throbbing blood vessels in the neck, nausea, vomiting, burning throat, massive welts and itching; recovery occurs after 8–12 hours.

Treatment Gastric lavage; administration of antihistamines or the histamine blocker cimetidine (Tagamet).

See also FISH CONTAMINATION; FOOD POISONING; SHELLFISH POISONING.

scorpion   Looking like a little crab with eight legs (in fact, scorpions are cousins to the sea-dwelling crustaceans), the scorpion has a segmented tail that curls over the body and ends in a poison reservoir and stinger. This tail is so flexible that it is almost impossible to pick up a scorpion with the bare hands and avoid a sting. The scorpion of the Southwest inflicts severe pain with its neurotoxic venom and is especially dangerous to children.

Because of its eight legs, it belongs to the Arachnida family (as do tarantulas and spiders). Most of the more than 700 species are about three inches long, are either black or yellow and are found in most warm regions of the world.

Some of the most poisonous species are found in Mexico, North Africa, South America, parts of the Caribbean and India. About 40 species live in the United States, and though the stings of most scorpions are more or less harmless, the venom of one found in the southern states—the sculpturatus scorpion *(Centruroides exilicauda)*—contains a neurotoxin and can be lethal. Other poisonous scorpions in the United States include the brown scorpion *(C. gertschii)* and the common striped scorpion *(C. vittatus).*

Poisonous scorpions in Mexico and Brazil are the *Tityus bahiensis* and *T. serrulatus;* the most deadly scorpions in North Africa, India and Pakistan are *Androctonus asutralis* and *Buthus occitanus.*

While scorpions don't attack humans, they like dark, moist places and hide in clothing or shoes, where they will sting if stepped on. Because of their fondness for the dark and the wet, they often crawl into shoes at night, where they present a dangerous hazard. In areas with heavy infestations of scorpions, residents spread out a wet burlap sack at night; scorpions crawl in and can then be easily located and destroyed in the morning.

Poisonous part   In equal amounts, scorpion venom is proportionately more poisonous than snake venom; however, scorpions inject a smaller amount of venom when they sting. The pale yellow desert scorpion is about two inches long and is more lethal than the big black scorpion, and the red scorpions are not deadly. The poison of the scorpion carries a neurotoxin that destroys nerve tissue and disturbs the heart.

Symptoms   The first symptom is a severe, sharp and burning pain, similar to a bee sting. If the sting was of a nonlethal scorpion, the area of the sting will become swollen and discolored and may form a blister; symptoms will last for eight to 12 hours. If the sting was of the lethal species, the sharp pain produced by the sting is quickly followed by a pins-and-needles sensation at the sting site. The area of the sting will not become swollen or discolored; within one to three hours the following symptoms will appear: itchy eyes, nose and throat; tightness of jaw muscles and difficulty in speaking; extreme restlessness and muscle twitching; muscle spasms with pain; nausea, vomiting, and incontinence (caused by stimulation of the autonomic nervous system); drowsiness, difficulty in breathing and irregular heartbeat.

Because scorpion toxicity is dose related, fatalities are uncommon in adults; the smaller the victim, the greater the danger of death. Therefore, children and the elderly are at higher risk. Symptoms appearing within two to four hours after a lethal scorpion sting indicate a serious medical problem. Fatalities have occurred as much as four days after a scorpion sting. However, it is not true that any scorpion sting brings death, since very few species are toxic enough to be fatal. Only one out of a thousand stings is fatal. Interference with the absorption of venom will head off serious symptoms.

Treatment   Contact medical help immediately whether or not it is a lethal scorpion sting. Have the person lie still, with the bitten part immobile and lower than the heart. Apply ice packs to the wound, and apply a constricting band two to four inches above the bite, snug but loose enough to allow a pulse farther out on the limb. If swelling reaches the band, tie another band two to four inches higher up, and then remove the first one. After 30 minutes, remove the band. If pain is the only symptom, a cold compress and painkillers may be enough. More severe cases call for local anesthetics and powerful painkillers, plus an antivenin to deactivate the venom. Antivenins against the venoms of local, deadly species of scorpion are available in most parts of the world where the creatures are found. *Not recommended:* hot packs, alcohol, morphine or incisions.

See also SCORPION, BROWN; SCORPION, COMMON STRIPED; SCORPION, SCULPTURATUS.

scorpion, brown   *(Centruroides gertschii)*   One of three species of poisonous scorpions in the United States, the brown scorpion lives primarily in the Southwest—especially in Arizona.

Poisonous part   The sting of the brown scorpion carries a deadly neurotoxin far more lethal than snake venom, which can destroy nerve tissue and cause heart problems.

Symptoms   Intense pain, numbness and hemorrhage of the intestines and stomach; lung and seizure activities. There is generally only a mild tingling at the wound site, followed by throat spasms, restlessness, muscular spasms, stomach cramps, convulsions, blood pressure abnormalities, pulmonary edema and respiratory failure. Symptoms usually begin in one to two days, but death can come as much as four days after a sting. Still, only one of a thousand stings is fatal.

Treatment   Antivenin is available.

See also SCORPION.

scorpion, common striped   *(Centruroides vittatus)*   One of three poisonous scorpions living in the United States, the common striped scorpion lives primarily in Arizona and other areas of the American Southwest. Scorpions live near homes and like the dark warmth of shoes and closets; they are not aggressive toward humans unless suddenly disturbed. When attacking, the scorpion's front pincers grab on and its tail flings forward to sting (once or repeatedly).

Poisonous part   The sting of the common striped scorpion carries a deadly neurotoxin far more lethal than snake venom, which can destroy nerve tissue and cause heart problems.

Symptoms   Intense pain, numbness and hemorrhage of the intestines and stomach; lung and seizure activities. There is generally only a mild tingling at the wound site, followed by throat spasms, restlessness, muscular spasms, stomach cramps, convulsions, blood pressure abnormalities, pulmonary edema and respiratory failure. Symptoms usually begin in one to two days, but death can come as much as four days after a sting. Still, only one of a thousand stings is fatal.

Treatment   Antivenin is available.

See also SCORPION.

scorpion, sculpturatus *(Centruroides exilicauda)*   One of three poisonous scorpions is found in Arizona, New Mexico and parts of California. The bite from the sculpturatus scorpion contains a powerful neurotoxin that can be lethal. Scorpions live near homes and like the dark warmth of shoes and closets; they are not aggressive toward humans unless suddenly disturbed. When attacking, the scorpion's front pincers grab on and its tail flings forward to sting (once or repeatedly).

Poisonous part   The sting of the sculpturatus scorpion carries a deadly neurotoxin far more lethal than snake venom, which can destroy nerve tissue and cause heart problems.

Symptoms   Intense pain, numbness and hemorrhage of the intestines and stomach; lung and seizure activities. There is generally only a mild tingling at the wound site, followed by throat spasms, restlessness, muscular spasms, stomach cramps, convulsions, blood pressure abnormalities, pulmonary edema and respiratory failure. Symptoms usually begin in one to two days, but death can come as much as four days after a sting. Still, only one of a thousand stings is fatal.

Treatment   Antivenin is available.

See also SCORPION.

scorpionfish   The family of scorpionfish includes about 350 species, some of them as venomous as a cobra, that are found in oceans throughout the world. The scorpionfish proper is closely related to other poisonous members of the Scorpaenidae family, including the zebrafish, waspfish, butterfly fish, rockfish, stonefish, and lionfish.

The scorpionfish is found in the reefs and coral caves of the Pacific ocean and is about four to eight inches long with a large head and big mouth, colored in red-brown and white bands. Scorpionfish look so much like stones that they can be almost unnoticeable and can be easily stepped on when a person walks in shallow water. Most scorpionfish stings, however, are reported after handling of the fish when taking them off the hook or out of a net; there are about 300 cases of scorpionfish poisoning reported yearly in the United States. Depending on the species, scorpionfish have 17 or 18 venomous spines that are covered by a layer of skin called the integumentary sheath. As each spine enters a person's skin, its sheath is pushed down, releasing the venom from a gland that lies hidden beneath it. This venom is the deadliest poison of any fish, lethal enough to kill a swimmer or beachcomber in two hours.

There are about 60 species of rockfish, in the scorpionfish family, mostly found in the cool waters of the Pacific Ocean. Rockfish have a hard protective covering around their heads, as well as the needle-sharp spines common to all scorpionfish.

The most exotic of all the scorpionfish are the zebrafish, usually swimming in pairs in the open, marked with a striking pattern of stripes and feathery fins. Among those fins are 18 long, slender, pointed spines that deliver a venom that can cause a painful and swollen wound leading to gangrene, delirium, convulsions, cardiac failure and even death. The zebrafish is found in the Red Sea and the Indian Ocean, and in the waters surrounding China, Japan and Australia. Swimmers in these areas should avoid approaching a zebrafish, especially from the side, which irritates this fish. When frightened, it moves around so its spine is aimed directly at the intruder, stinging with a darting, lightning-fast jab.

Symptoms The sting of the scorpionfish causes an immediate severe stinging or throbbing pain, which may stay at the site of the wound or spread throughout the body and last for several hours or days. There may be redness and swelling at the site of the sting, and the area may become numb. The more dangerous varieties can cause loss of consciousness, paralysis, delirium and convulsions, leading to fatal cardiac arrest. The profound pain, convulsions, paralysis and unconsciousness—which can be immediate—can cause drowning. In addition, there is often a secondary infection and a fluctuating fever.

Treatment There is no known antidote, although stonefish antivenin may be administered. Contact medical help immediately; flush the wound with fresh or salt water and then soak the affected area in hot water or put hot compresses on it. The water should be very hot (120°F), so that the heat will deactivate the poison. Continue applying hot water for an hour. Recovery from a scorpionfish sting may take months and leave a permanent scar.

See also LIONFISH; STONEFISH.

sea cucumber (Holothurioidea class) Although sea cucumbers under most circumstances are safe to eat, there are toxic species that are difficult to identify. In addition, some species of sea cucumbers produce a poison that is quite toxic and can cause burning and inflammation on human skin and blindness if it comes in contact with the eyes.

The toxin is located in tubules within the creature's body, from which it can be excreted, forming long, sticky threads that can capture and trap an attacker.

Poisonous part   The toxin is called holothurin.

Symptoms   While little is known of the symptoms produced by poisonous sea cucumbers, eating those of the toxic species can be fatal. However, such intoxications are rare. Contact with liquid ejected from some sea cucumbers may cause rash or blindness.

Treatment   There is no known antidote. Treatment is symptomatic.

sea snake   (Hydrophidae) Considered by the *Guinness Book of World Records* to be the most venomous snake in the world, the sea snake has highly toxic venom—in some cases, more than 50 times as deadly as that of the king cobra. Of the 50 cataloged species of sea snakes, all are venomous, and as many as 25 percent of their victims will die.

Sea snakes inhabit the Pacific and Indian oceans and are widely found around the Ashmore Reef in the Timor Sea off the coast of northwestern Australia. None have ever been found in the Atlantic Ocean or the Mediterranean or Red seas. Huge clumps of many thousands of sea snakes may sometimes be found at sea; some experts believe this is because small fish often swim in shoals beneath floating debris.

True snakes, the Hydrophidae have lidless eyes and a forked tongue, growing an average of four feet long. They are very well adapted to life in the sea, with a streamlined body, nostrils on top of their heads and special glands that excrete salt. Reports conflict as to whether these snakes are considered to be docile or aggressive. They have long been killed for their leather.

Fortunately, however, the mechanism for injecting poison is not well developed in the sea snakes, and their fangs are very small. While it is often believed that these snakes have small mouths and can only bite a human's tender skin at the base of the thumb, this is not true. Many pearl divers in the Persian Gulf who weren't wearing goggles have died after accidentally grabbing sea snakes.

Poisonous sea snakes include the banded, or annulated, sea snake *(Hydrophis cyanocinctus)*; beaked sea snake *(Enhydrina schistosa)*; yellow-lipped sea krait *(Laticauda colubrina)*; olive-brown sea snake *(Aipysurus laevis)*; yellow sea snake *(Hydrophis spiralis)*; Hardwicke's sea snake *(Lapemis hardwickii)*; and the pelagic sea snake *(Pelamis platurus)*. The largest species is *Laticauda semifasciata*; the sea snakes of this species gather together in groups numbering in the thousands to breed in the large coastal caves of Gato north of Cebu. Some species, such as the *Laticauda colubrina*, live partly on land, entering the water occasionally, although they are well equipped for life in the sea.

Of all the sea snakes, the beaked sea snake is the most venomous and is responsible for more fatalities than all other sea snakes combined. The yellow sea snake and the Hardwicke's sea snake are not nearly as venomous, although both have caused several fatalities. The pelagic sea snake is the most common and least toxic, found on the west coast of the American tropics.

In general, however, sea snakes are fairly inoffensive and pose no great threat to humans, despite the toxicity of their venom.

Poisonous part The extremely toxic venom is a neurotoxin that affects the muscles and paralyzes the nervous system, causing the release of the protein myoglobin, which stains the urine red, damages the kidneys and affects the heart.

Symptoms Unlike the bite of many other poisonous sea creatures, the bite of a sea snake seems like a harmless pinprick. Because symptoms appear very slowly—between 20 minutes and eight hours—the victim often does not connect the snakebite with subsequent symptoms. First, the victim feels weakness and then pain in the skeletal muscles. Victims notice numbness and thickening of the tongue and mouth, blurred vision and difficulty in swallowing. Weakness increases, the eyelids droop, the jaws stiffen and the pulse weakens and becomes irregular. Sometimes, nausea and vomiting are present. In cases of severe poisoning, symptoms worsen and cyanosis appears, followed by breathing problems and convulsions. Death may come in a few hours to a few days.

Treatment Antivenin is available; the snake should be captured and identified to rule out the bite of a harmless water snake. Cortisone or epinephrine is sometimes given to prevent anaphylaxis, and fluids and electrolyte levels are monitored. If a person has not been severely bitten, recovery is rapid.

See also SNAKES, POISONOUS.

sea urchin *(Diadema setosum; Toxpneustes elegans; Asthenosoma jimoni)* Of all the sea urchins, the sting from the long-spined variety *(D. setosum)* is the most poisonous. Red sea urchins *T. elegans* and *A. jimoni* are less venomous. Sea urchins are commonly found in warm waters around rocks or wrecks, where they can sting swimmers or divers even through shoes and gloves. They are rounded, about the size of a golf or tennis ball, with sharp spines radiating outward.

Poisonous part Sea urchins have venomous spines with poisoned tips, and three pronged biting teeth that are extremely tenacious.

Symptoms Although death is rare, the sting of the sea urchin penetrates soft tissue, causing an immediate severe stinging or throbbing pain, which may stay at the site of the wound or spread throughout the body and last for several hours or days. There may be redness and swelling at the site of the sting, and the area may become numb, followed by muscle weakness and possible paralysis.

Treatment Contact medical help immediately. Remove spines; if the brittle tips break off and are not absorbed in two days, surgery may be required to remove them. Flush the wound with fresh or salt water, and then soak the affected area in hot water or put hot compresses on it. The water should be very hot (122°F), so that the heat will deactivate the poison. Continue applying hot water for 30 minutes to an hour. Have the victim lie still with the stung part immobile and lower than the heart. Tie a flat strip of cloth snugly around a stung arm or leg two to four inches above the sting, loose enough to allow a pulse farther out on the limb. Check periodically and loosen if necessary, but do not remove it. If swelling reaches the band, tie another band two to four inches higher up and remove the first one. There may be a purple stain on the skin around the wound, which is merely a pigment of the spine and not dangerous.

sea wasp (*Chironex fleckeri; Chiropsalmus quadrigatus*) One of the most venomous of the jellyfish, the sea wasp lives in warm water from Queensland northward to Malaya but also in cooler waters as far north as the central Atlantic seaboard; the Australian species is the most dangerous. Their tentacles may grow as long as 200 feet, although contact with only 20 feet of tentacle will be fatal. Sea wasps can be found close to shore, sometimes in only a few feet of water.

A moderate sting from a sea wasp can be fatal in a few minutes. The sea wasp is considered to be one of the most deadly organisms in the world, and in Australia alone it has caused more than 50 deaths in 20 years. In fact, the venom is so toxic that in laboratory experiments a solution diluted 10,000 times still killed the animal before the syringe could be extracted.

The only protection against the sting of a sea wasp is the wearing of tights, which the wasps cannot penetrate; all life-saving teams in Queensland are required to wear them for this reason.

Poisonous part The sea wasp's tentacles cluster at the corners of its body, and the stinging capsules within each contain a minute amount of one of the most deadly venoms ever discovered. The live nematocysts that contain the poison can live for months on the beach, if occasionally moistened with sea water, and are capable of injecting the poison; even nematocysts that have been dried on the beach for several weeks maintain potency.

Symptoms The sting of the sea wasp can be fatal within seconds. In general, there are painful swellings and purple-brown wheals at the site of the sting, which later necrose. Pain is said to be excruciating and can cause the victim to become distraught and irrational. Symptoms include muscular spasms, breathing problems, rapid and weak pulse, pulmonary edema, shock and respiratory failure followed almost always by death, within 30 seconds to three hours; in general, death occurs within 15 minutes. Even the mildest sting is not pleasant, with acute burning pain and a wheal that lasts for months.

Treatment There is not usually time to administer first aid or an antidote, although a sea wasp antivenin is available in Australia. Stings from the sea wasp do not occur in the United States.

See also JELLYFISH.

Seconal   See BARBITURATES.

selenium   A metallic element found normally in the soil, selenium is necessary for human health but is toxic in large amounts, although few cases of selenium poisoning in humans have been reported. Selenium poisoning is more of a problem for farm animals and birds, although it can be a problem for farm families with wells polluted by runoff from selenium-rich agricultural soil.

Selenium is used in a wide variety of products because of its ability to produce electricity when light is shined on it; it is widely used in photoelectric cells, light meters, photocopying machines and other electrical components. It is also used to create the red color in warning lights, traffic lights and brake lights.

A well-balanced diet is the best way to obtain selenium; about two-thirds of dietary selenium comes from meat, fish and dairy products, which provides enough selenium to satisfy daily requirements but not enough to be toxic.

Chronic poisoning may occur from numerous exposures during the manufacture of the wide range of products that use this element.

Symptoms   Chronic poisoning symptoms include pallor, garlicky odor to the breath, metallic taste, gastrointestinal disturbances, irritation of the nose, conjunctivitis, skin problems, drowsiness and chest constriction.

Treatment   Removal from the environment and a selenium-free diet.

shellfish poisoning   Shellfish are highly susceptible to bacterial and viral contamination because they live close to the shore, where pollution tends to be worst. Cooking usually destroys the microbes that infect shellfish—but eating raw clams, oysters and other shellfish is linked to nearly 1,000 cases of hepatitis alone each year.

There are three types of shellfish poisoning: gastrointestinal (or neurotoxic) shellfish poisoning, erythematous shellfish poisoning, and paralytic shellfish poisoning (PSP). Each has a quite different etiology, symptoms and prognosis for recovery, but of the three, PSP is by far the most serious.

While shellfish by themselves are not poisonous, they can become contaminated by bacteria and other organisms from their environment and pass them on to humans when the shellfish is eaten. Oysters, clams and mussels are particularly prone to becoming contaminated because of their metabolic system, which pumps water across the gills to isolate plankton for their food. This system makes them vulnerable to bacteria, viruses or other contaminants in the water. Lobsters and other crustacean shellfish only rarely become contaminated.

In mussels, toxins are concentrated in the digestive glands, and toxicity is usually lost within weeks. But the Alaskan butter clam can remain toxic for up to two years after accumulating the toxin. However, the part of the mollusk that humans generally eat—the white meat, without the digestive glands—stores fairly small amounts of toxin.

Some types of toxic plankton (dinoflagellates) multiply rapidly during the warm summer months; because their color is pink or red, this phenomenon has come to be called "red tide." Red tides are found in coastal waters (since waters offshore are not favorable to the growth of these plankton) in the Pacific from California to Alaska, in the Atlantic from New England to the St. Lawrence and across the west coast of Europe.

These plankton *(Gonyaulax)* produce the deadly poison saxitoxin, which blocks nerve impulses and causes paralytic shellfish poisoning; it is so toxic that even one contaminated shellfish can be fatal if eaten. This is why clams, oysters and mussels are not sold during months without an "R" (the summer months).

Red tides have been known since ancient times; it is believed that the name of the Red Sea was coined by ancient Greeks who were referring to red blooms off the Arabian coasts. It is believed that the first reference to red tide appears in the Bible: "And all the waters that were in the river were turned to blood. And the fish that was in the river died, and the river stank, and the Egyptians could not drink of the water of the rivers" (Exodus 7:20–21).

In addition, most cases of shellfish poisoning have occurred when people ate raw shellfish; cooking will kill bacteria (although the heat must be very high to kill the hepatitis A virus—and nothing will kill the toxins that cause PSP). Further, those with liver problems should never eat raw seafood, since one type of bacteria found in seafood can sicken those with liver problems.

PSP, gastrointestinal and erythematous shellfish poisoning are rarely fatal. Gastrointestinal poisoning is caused by various bacterial nonspecific pathogens; symptoms appear between 10 and 12 hours after ingestion. Recovery is rapid and death is rare. Erythematous shellfish poisoning is caused by a possible allergic response to decomposed shellfish.

Poisonous part The toxin saxitoxin and its analogues stop the flow of sodium, preventing nerve conductance. It is not possible to build up immunity by becoming exposed to sublethal doses.

Symptoms Symptoms of shellfish poisoning resemble those of curare poisoning and develop within five to 30 minutes after eating contaminated oysters, clams or mussels. Oral ingestion of as little as 0.5 to 1.0 mg of contaminated shellfish can be fatal, and a victim's survival depends on how much he has consumed. Symptoms are characterized by gradual paralysis and trembling. Other symptoms include nausea, vomiting and diarrhea. If the victim survives the first 12 hours, prognosis for complete recovery (within a few days to two weeks) is good. Between 8.5 and 23.2 percent of PSP poisonings are fatal.

In gastrointestinal shellfish poisoning, onset is within a few minutes to three hours, with gastroenteritis accompanied by muscular weakness and respiratory arrest. Paralytic shellfish symptoms include vomiting and diarrhea within 30 minutes of ingestion, followed by headache, weakness and, sometimes, respiratory arrest after one to 12 hours. Erythematous shellfish poisoning symptoms appear only a few hours after ingestion, including headache and rash. Recovery occurs in a few days; death is very rare.

   Treatment There is no known antidote to saxitoxin. As in any treatment of curarelike poisoning, administration of prostigmine may be effective, together with artificial respiration and oxygen as needed.

   See also CIGUATERA; DINOFLAGELLATE; FISH CONTAMINATION;FOOD POISONING; PARALYTIC SHELLFISH POISONING.

sick building syndrome   Symptoms experienced by people living in a building whose indoor air is heavily contaminated with toxic pollutants. Symptoms are believed to be caused by biological contamination, including bacteria, mold, pollen and viruses, which may breed in stagnant water collecting in air conditioners. Legionnaires' disease is the most famous example of this type of indoor contamination. Sick building syndrome may also be caused by the fact that since the 1973 oil embargo, many buildings have been made more airtight to improve their heating efficiency. Fresh air is slower to enter, and pollutants build up in the air.

   In addition, indoor pollutants such as adhesives, chemicals from carpet and tile, cleaning chemicals and pesticides may add to the problem. Formaldehyde, tobacco smoke and asbestos are some of the worst of the indoor pollutants. Finally, a building may be contaminated from outside sources, such as motor vehicle exhaust from garages and sewer gas from improperly vented drains.

   The most serious of the indoor air pollutants is carbon monoxide, which, according to the Consumer Products Safety Commission, causes about 200 deaths a year. Dangerous levels of the odorless gas may be caused by automobile exhaust and improperly installed or vented appliances. The CPSC now recommends that all homes be equipped with carbon monoxide detectors (similar to smoke alarms) that will sound a warning when the gas reaches dangerous levels. Although these detectors are not yet available, Underwriters Laboratories is in the process of evaluating the first ones under standards developed by UL and CPSC in the spring of 1992. These detectors, which should be installed outside the sleeping area, will be priced at less than $100.

sidewinder   *(Crotalus cerastes)*   Also known as the horned rattler, this is one of three rattlesnakes from the family Viperidae known for its quick sideways motion across the shifting desert floor. Its odd, sideways motion leaves a distinct trail of parallel J- shaped marks.

   The sidewinder has a distinctive look, with a prominent triangular, hornlike projection over each eye. The snake is found in arid deserts with mesquite-crowned sand hills throughout the southwestern United States and northeastern Mexico. It is most often encountered as it crosses roads at night in the spring; during the day, it usually hides in burrows or bushes.

Symptoms Symptoms appear within 15 minutes and include excessive thirst, nausea, vomiting, shock, paralysis, respiratory problems, anemia, necrosis, kidney problems and sometimes death. The bite of a rattlesnake is painful. Indications of a serious bite include swelling above the elbows or knees within two hours, hemorrhages, numbness at the puncture site, tingling around the mouth, yellow vision, vomiting and violent spasms.

Treatment Antivenin is available.

See also MASSASAUGA; PIT VIPERS; RATTLESNAKE, CANEBRAKE; RATTLE-SNAKE, CASCABEL; RATTLESNAKE, EASTERN DIAMONDBACK; RATTLE-SNAKE, MEXICAN WEST COAST; RATTLESNAKE, RED DIAMONDBACK; RATTLESNAKES; RATTLESNAKE, TIMBER; RATTLESNAKE, WESTERN DIA-MONDBACK; SNAKES, POISONOUS; VIPER, GABOON; VIPER, JUMPING; VIPER, MALAYAN PIT; VIPER, RUSSELL'S; VIPER, SAWSCALED; VIPER, WAGLER'S PIT; VIPERS; WATER MOCCASIN; WUTU.

silver nitrate   This astringent is used primarily to prevent a serious form of conjunctivitis in newborns and may also be used on burns and dressings. It dissolves readily in water and is fatal when ingested either in its salt form or as a liquid.

Symptoms Immediately upon ingestion, silver nitrate causes pain and burning in the mouth, blackened skin, mucous membranes, throat and abdomen, vomiting and diarrhea, collapse, shock, convulsions, coma and death. Repeated doses over a long period of time will cause a permanent blue-black color in the skin.

Treatment Give a mixture of water and table salt to dilute mixture in the stomach; administer a cathartic and give milk and painkillers to relieve stomach pain.

sleeping pills   There are a wide range of drugs used in the treatment of insomnia, including the benzodiazepines, barbiturates, antidepressants and chloral hydrate. Some antihistamines are also sold as nonprescription sleep aids to reestablish the habit of sleeping after self-help measures have failed. The drugs promote sleep by quieting nerve cell activity within the brain.

The smallest amount needed should be taken, and use of these drugs should be tapered off quickly, as they can become addictive. People who use sleeping pills over a period of time often develop tolerance and usually need more and more to achieve the desired effect.

Ethyl alcohol in combination with these drugs multiples the effects, and other drugs (such as those for the treatment of heart disease, depression and duodenal ulcers) adversely interact with sleeping pills.

Some common sleeping pills include Mogadon (nitrazepam); Soma (car-

isoprodol); Placidyl (ethychlorvynol); Valmid (ethinamate); Doriden (glutethimide); Restoril (temazepam); Halcion (triazolam); Noludar (methyprylon); Tegretol (carbamazepine); Ethotoin (peganone); Mesantoin
(mephenytoin); Milontin (phensuximide); Celotin (methsuximide); Zarotin
(ethosuximide); Phenurone (phenacemide); and Mysoline (primidone).

See also DALMANE; MEDICATIONS AS POISONS.

slug bait   See METALDEHYDE.

smooth-scaled snake   *(Parademansia microlepidotus)*   The most venomous
land snake in the world, according to the *Guinness Book of World Records*, this
snake is found in southwestern Queensland and northeastern South Australia and Tasmania. Until 1976, it was thought to be a Western form of the
taipan, but its venom is actually quite different. The smooth-scaled snake
grows to up to six feet six inches long, and its venom has been measured at
0.00385 oz. after milking—enough to kill 125,000 mice.

Symptoms   Pain and swelling within 30 minutes, dilated pupils and
low blood pressure followed by muscle weakness and paralysis of breathing
muscles.

Treatment   Antivenin is available.

See also SNAKES, POISONOUS; TAIPAN.

snakes, poisonous   There are about 3,000 species of snakes in the world,
but only about 10 percent of them are poisonous. Venomous snakes come
in all sizes, from the tiny desert vipers to the king cobra, growing up to 16
feet long; a king cobra, when angered, can rear up and stand as tall as a
person. While there are many old folk methods to quickly determine if a
snake is poisonous, such as counting the rows of scales, there is no practical
way to tell the poisonous from the harmless.

According to World Health Organization statistics, about 50,000 people
throughout the world die from snakebites each year—mostly in India; about
8,000 victims are treated each year in the United States. The highest death
rate from snakebite in the United States is reported from Arizona, Florida,
Georgia, Texas and Alabama, in that order. According to the *Guinness Book
of World Records*, Burma has the highest mortality rate—15.4 deaths per
100,000 population each year.

There are only four varieties of snakes in the United States that are
poisonous—the rattlesnake, copperhead, water moccasin and coral snake,
but they are widely distributed throughout the country. The water moccasin
is distributed over the Southwest, the Gulf states and the Mississippi Valley
as far north as southern Illinois. Of all poisonous snakes, the copperhead is
probably more commonly found throughout the country, especially in
North and South Carolina, West Virginia, Pennsylvania, Missouri, Okla-

homa, Arkansas and Illinois. Rattlesnakes are found throughout the continental United States.

The coral snake is usually associated with the southern United States. Of the 115 species in this country, only about 20 are dangerous, including 16 species of rattlesnakes. Generally, only the eastern and western diamondback, canebrake, timber and Mojave rattlers (and a few subspecies) could be considered life threatening. Of these, diamondbacks are considered to be the most dangerous, because of their large size, the length of their fangs, the large quantity of venom and the nature of their venom.

Rattlers account for about 65 percent of the venomous snakebites that occur in this country each year, and for nearly all of the nine to 15 deaths. A smaller fraction of bites comes from copperheads, fewer still from cottonmouths and only three or four bites a year from coral snakes. Many snakebite victims are children or members of religious sects that handle deadly snakes.

Poisonous part   Scientists have identified more than 100 proteins in rattlesnake venom, including deadly neurotoxic compounds that dissolve cells and damage blood vessels. Heart and kidney complications often follow. Most snakebite fatalities occur 18 to 32 hours after a bite, but death can occur within 60 minutes or after several days. Some snakes (such as cobras) lay eggs, while others (such as vipers) give birth to live young. Newly born venomous snakes are just as dangerous as their parents and can often be far more aggressive than the old folks; baby cobras, in particular, are vicious and will strike even while they are emerging from their eggs.

Symptoms   Fang marks and possibly teeth marks may be visible. Symptoms include an immediate, burning pain that spreads rapidly (especially with a pit viper's bite), and sudden swelling beginning soon after the bite in the bite area and then spreading throughout the body. (This is especially true for bites on the arm or leg.) Systemic symptoms include shock, nausea, weakness and numbness; muscles may twitch and skin may tingle. There are a number of factors that influence the severity of a snakebite: the amount of venom injected; the size and species of the individual snake; the age, size, health and sensitivity of the victim; the types of clothing worn; and the position and number of bites inflicted. If an hour passes after a snakebite and no symptoms appear, chances are not enough venom was injected and the danger is slight.

Treatment   Despite the long history of snakebites and their treatment, the problem of how to deal with snakebites remains controversial: ice or no ice? Tourniquet or constriction band? Cut and suck or not? More than 200 different first aid procedures for snakebite have been recommended by various experts, who even today do not agree.

The emphasis on treating a snakebite should be placed on getting prompt medical care, and first aid should never be considered to be a substitute for antivenin. Rapid treatment with an antivenin can help a snakebite victim regardless of whether or not the bite would have been fatal. Without antivenin treatment, hospital stays for venomous snake bites last about twice as long. The venom of all snakes in the Crotalidae family (rattlesnakes, copperheads and water moccasins) contains similar poisons, and all can be treated with antivenin. A bite from the eastern coral snake requires a separate antivenin, and there is no antivenin for the western coral snake.

In addition, there are different types of venom, and it is useless to treat a victim with an antivenin for viper bites if the injury was caused by a cobra. And venom even differs among specimens from different areas, even within the same species; for example, antivenin from an Indian member of a particular species will not be very helpful against bites of Thai cobras of the species.

Here are first aid suggestions based on the protocol of the American National Red Cross:

- Stop muscular activity at once. Immobilize victim to lessen the spread of venom.
- Apply a constriction band within 30 minutes of a bite (unless the snake is a coral snake, in which constriction will be ineffective). Place band above the bite area, making sure a finger can be inserted beneath the band. Don't apply a band around a bitten finger. Don't release the band if you are within 1 1/2 hours of medical care. As swelling appears, the band can be loosened but not released, because the band can stay on safely for up to an hour.
- Do not use ice, since the more toxic effects of the peptides in snake venom are not affected by cooling and the venom's enzymes are actually more active at cooler temperatures.
- Identify the snake species (since the amount of antivenin required varies with the venom toxicity of different species). If the snake is killed in order to bring it to the hospital for identification, the snake could still bite, even if the head is cut from the body, since head reactions persist for at least 20 minutes and sometimes up to an hour after death.

For all poisonous snakes EXCEPT coral snakes Cutting into a snakebite is controversial. If you are trained, have the right equipment and are far from medical help, you can incise a snakebite. Treat for shock and be prepared to give artificial respiration if breathing stops, if you are trained in CPR. Have someone phone ahead to alert the hospital, identifying the type of snake if possible (or take the dead snake with you).

Precautions When moving through a snake-infested area, hikers should watch the path and never put feet or hands where they can't be seen. If walking through tall grass or bushes, poke the clumps with a stick to warn snakes. Don't reach above your head or put hands into crevices. Since about half of all snake strikes are below the knee, wear heavy, leather, high-top shoes or boots and loose-fitting long pants, with cuffs reaching over the tops of the shoes. When camping, avoid areas near rocks, logs, burrows or caves.

Always wear heavy gloves when cleaning up debris—especially logs or old lumber, and use a crowbar to move them.

Snakes are more dangerous during early spring; they've been storing venom and the poison glands are full. If a snake is spotted, back away from it for at least two to three feet. Snakes can strike about half their body length (and most are less than five feet).

See also ADDER; ADDER, COMMON; ADDER, PUFF; BLACK SNAKE, AUSTRALIAN; BOOMSLANG; BROWN SNAKE; BUSHMASTER; CORAL SNAKE; CORAL SNAKE, ARIZONA; CORAL SNAKE, EASTERN; HABU, OKINAWA; KRAIT, BLUE; MAMBAS; MASSASAUGA; PIT VIPERS; RATTLESNAKE, CASCABEL; RATTLESNAKE, EASTERN DIAMONDBACK; RATTLESNAKE, MEXICAN WEST COAST; RATTLESNAKE, RED DIAMONDBACK; RATTLESNAKE, TIMBER; RATTLESNAKE, WESTERN DIAMONDBACK; RATTLESNAKES; SIDEWINDER; SMOOTH-SCALED SNAKE; VIPER, GABOON; VIPER, JUMPING; VIPER, MALAYAN PIT; VIPER, RUSSELL'S; VIPER, SAWSCALED; WATER MOCCASIN; WUTU.

sodium bicarbonate   This buffering agent is used in the treatment of poisoning by methanol, ethylene glycol or salicylate. It counteracts metabolic acidosis and enhances the elimination of salicylate or phenobarbital. It also helps to treat heart problems resulting from overdoses of cyclic antidepressants and some antiarrhythmic drugs. Used in gastric lavage solution, it can be helpful in the treatment of excessive iron ingestion.

sodium fluoroacetate   See COMPOUND 1080.

sodium hypochlorite   The most common form of the active ingredient in bleach.

See also ALKALINE CORROSIVES.

solvent abuse   Certain volatile liquids give off intoxicating fumes that, when sniffed, produce an effect similar to getting "high" on drugs or alcohol. Glue sniffing is the most common form of solvent abuse, but many other substances are used (especially those containing toluene or acetone).

The solvent is usually sniffed from a plastic bag containing the solvent, although sometimes aerosols are sprayed into the nose or mouth. The practice is often a group activity that usually lasts only for a few months at a time. However, solitary abuse is much more serious and may last for a much longer period of time.

Symptoms   Inhaling solvent fumes may cause hallucinations; chronic abuse may cause headache, vomiting, stupor, confusion and coma. Death may occur as the result of a direct toxic effect on the heart, from a fall, choking on vomit or asphyxiation due to the clinging bag around the nose and mouth. Other, long-term effects include damage to the membrane lining of the nose and throat, the kidneys, the liver and the nervous system. The signs of solvent abuse include intoxicated behavior, flushed face, mouth ulcers, solvent smell and personality changes.

Treatment Maintain airway, administer supplemental oxygen and monitor blood gases and chest X rays. Treat symptoms of coughing and coma and bronchospasm if they occur. Avoid the use of epinephrine because of the risk of aggravating arrhythmias.

See also TRICHLOROETHANE; TRICHLOROETHYLENE.

South American rattlesnake   See RATTLESNAKE, CASCABEL.

spathiphyllum *(Spathiphyllum)* Also known as the peace plant, this is an extremely common indoor potted plant popular as a commercial indoor landscape plant because of its limited light requirements. These plants, which can reach about two feet in height, produce a single white or greenish flower with a white spadix resembling a small ear of corn.

Poisonous part All parts of this plant are toxic and contain water-insoluble raphides of calcium oxalate.

Symptoms Upon ingestion, burning, swelling and pain of the lips, mouth, tongue and pharynx; because of this immediate pain, large amounts of this plant are not usually eaten. Contact dermatitis may be caused by the root juices.

Treatment Cool liquids, including milk, held in the mouth and analgesics may ease the pain.

spiders, poisonous Although most of the more than 50,000 species of spiders found in the United States actually possess poison glands connected to their fangs, only a very few are capable of piercing human skin. Those that can include the black widow *(Latrodectus)*, the brown recluse spider *(Loxosceles)*, the jumping spider *(Phidippus)* and the tarantula (a common name given to many large spiders).

In general, most spider attacks occur when someone disturbs a spider's nest while working outdoors or making house repairs. While tarantulas rarely cause problems, their bite is painful because of the size of their fangs.

See also BLACK WIDOW SPIDER; BROWN RECLUSE SPIDER; TARANTULA.

spindle tree *(Euonymus europaeus)* This small tree branches close to the ground and has thin gray bark, looking very similar to its close cousin burning bush *(E. atropurpureus)*, except that its flowers are yellow-green. Introduced from Europe, this tree spread from cultivation in Massachusetts to Wisconsin and south.

Poisonous part The leaves, seeds and bark of this tree contain the cardiac glycoside evomonoside, similar to digitalis; a group of alkaloids, including evonine, that have not been evaluated; and a protein that inhibits protein synthesis in intact cells.

Symptoms Within 10 to 12 hours, ingestion results in symptoms similar to those of meningitis: watery, bloody diarrhea; colic; vomiting; fever and convulsions; and liver damage that can be fatal within eight hours.

Treatment Recommendation for treatment is difficult, since the underlying toxin is unknown. Replace fluids and electrolytes.

See also CARDIAC GLYCOSIDES.

spurge nettle *(Jatropha stimulosus)* A plant found in North America, Europe and Asia that is poisonous by contact.

Poisonous part Its toxin is unknown.

Symptoms Contact produces instant, intense stinging and itching because of an irritating substance injected into the skin by the plant's stinging hairs, and causes a skin rash that disappears in about 30 minutes. A dull purple stain on the skin may linger for several weeks.

Treatment Symptomatic.

squill *(Scilla)* [Other names: Cuban lily, hyacinth-of-Peru, sea onion, star hyacinth.] This hyacinth look-alike is found as a hardy perennial in the north temperate zones to southern Canada. It is often grown for its attractive blue, purple or white flowers.

Poisonous part The whole squill plant is poisonous and contains digitalislike glycosides.

Symptoms There is a variable latency period between ingestion and symptoms, depending on the amount of the plant eaten. When they appear, symptoms include pain in the mouth, lips, tongue and throat, nausea and vomiting, abdominal pain, cramps and diarrhea, hyperkalemia and heart disturbances.

Treatment Gastric lavage followed by the administration of activated charcoal and saline cathartics. Monitoring of potassium levels and electrocardiogram should be performed. In the event of heart problems: administration of atropine for conduction defects; phenytoin for rhythm disturbances.

See also DIGITALIS.

staphylococcus enterotoxin One of the most common types of food poisoning in the United States, affecting almost everyone at least once. Although the bacteria are easily destroyed by high heat during cooking, they also produce a heat-resistant toxin. It is believed that only a few strains of staphylococci produce enterotoxins, which may occur in a wide variety of foods (such as milk, cheese, ice cream, cream-filled bakery goods, dried beef, sausage or chicken gravy). Poisoning with this type of bacteria most often occurs after eating food that has been kept warm for several hours before being served. In addition, food may be contaminated from infected food handlers.

Staphylococcus enterotoxin may be suspected when there has been only a brief interval between eating suspected tainted food and the onset of symptoms. It can be confirmed by bacteriological examination for the presence of staphylococci; enterotoxin may also be produced by staphylococci in persons treated with broad-spectrum antibiotics.

The best way to prevent this type of food poisoning is to refrigerate perishable foods adequately. While heat does destroy the bacteria, it does not destroy the enterotoxin.

Symptoms Symptoms usually appear within three hours of eating the tainted food; the incubation period depends on the amount of food eaten and the susceptibility of the consumer. (The aged, immunocompromised and the very young are the most vulnerable.) Symptoms begin with salivation, followed by nausea, vomiting, abdominal cramps, prostration and diarrhea; in severe poisoning, victims experience marked prostration together with vomiting, diarrhea and, sometimes, shock. Symptoms usually fade after five to six hours, although a few fatal cases have been reported among vulnerable populations.

Treatment Significant loss of fluids and disruption of electrolyte balance may require parenteral administration of fluids and electrolytes; treatment for shock may be required following significant loss of fluids.

See also, FOOD POISONING.

star of Bethlehem *(Ornithogalum umbellatum;* "wonder flower"—*O. thyrosides)* [Other names: African wonder flower, chincherinchee, dove's dung, nap at noon, summer snowflake, wonder flower.] Found in warm climates, the flower of the Bible has creamy white, starlike flowers on upright slender stems that may reach two feet in height, and long, narrow leaves with onion like bulbs. Found primarily in the Middle East, both species are also kept indoors and sold by florists as a cut flower. *O. umbellatum* has been naturalized in the southeastern United States, in Mississippi, Missouri, Kansas and eastward.

Poisonous part All parts of the star of Bethlehem plant are toxic, especially the onion like bulb; the poisons are convallatoxin and convalloside (the same as lily of the valley) plus cardiac glycosides.

Symptoms Immediately after ingestion, symptoms begin: shortness of breath, irritation of the mouth and throat, nausea, vomiting, abdominal pain, diarrhea and respiratory problems. Fatalities have been reported from ingesting this plant.

Treatment Gastric lavage and treatment of symptoms, followed by the administration of activated charcoal and saline cathartics. Electrocardiogram and potassium levels should be monitored repeatedly.

See also CARDIAC GLYCOSIDES; LILY OF THE VALLEY.

star-potato vine *(Solanum seaforthianum)* Also called the Brazilian night-shade, this South American plant is also cultivated in warmer areas in Florida and Hawaii. It is a member of a very large genus with 1,700 species, most of which have not been evaluated toxicologically.

Poisonous part Human poisoning is usually attributed to immature fruit, which contains the toxin solanine glycoalkaloid.

Symptoms While there is little danger of fatal poisoning in adults, children may ingest a fatal amount of this plant. Symptoms appear several hours after ingestion and include gastric irritation, scratchy throat, fever and diarrhea (solanine poisoning is often confused with bacterial gastroenteritis).

Treatment The same general supportive care that would be given in gastroenteritis cases; fluid replacement may be required.

Stelazine (trifluroperazine) This is one of the psychometric drugs used to treat psychotic anxiety and agitated depression. It is available as a tablet, liquid or injection and works by depressing the central nervous system.

Symptoms Within 20 minutes after an overdose, Stelazine causes agitation, convulsions, fever, low blood pressure, coma and cardiac arrest.

Treatment Perform gastric lavage and administer Cogentin; treat other symptoms as they appear.

See also ANTIDEPRESSANTS; MEDICATIONS AS POISONS.

stingray *(Urobatis halleri, Dasyatis longus* etc.) More than 1,500 cases of stingray attacks are reported in the United States each year, usually caused when a swimmer inadvertently steps on a stingray buried in the mud or sand. The *Dasyatis* stingrays are particularly noted for burying themselves in the mud or sand. When trod upon, the stingray flings its tail up and forward, burying the stinger in the victim's foot.

A stingray will never attack humans—fleeing if approached—unless it perceives itself under attack. When threatened, it can whip its tail around until it finds its attacker. It is possible to drive away stingrays by shuffling the feet in murky water.

Stingrays are found throughout the world and include the diamond, butterfly, European, eagle, California and South American freshwater sting-ray. All large varieties found in fresh water are dangerous. Many stingrays do not travel far from their own area, seeming to display a sense of territory.

Poisonous part The fearsome whiplike tail of the stingray is longer than its body, and near the base of its tail it has one, two or three flattened barbed spines with small, sharp teeth connected to a poison sac; the barbs point backward, making it difficult to remove the barb after penetration. The tail is coated with venomous slime that can cause serious injury or even death to humans. Often, the entire stinger is left embedded in the wound, and pulling it out may further damage surrounding skin. When the spine stabs into the skin, it tears the sheath around the spine, which releases the venom, producing a violent reaction in the skin tissue. Some varieties of stingrays can inflict such a deep wound that they can transmit the tetanus bacilli, causing tetanus in their victims. The stingray venom is one of the most powerful vasoconstrictors among all the animal toxins and is markedly unstable. It has caused coronary vessel and resultant heart damage in animal experiments.

Symptoms   While death is rare, the sting of the stingray causes an immediate severe stinging or throbbing pain, which may stay at the site of the wound or spread throughout the body and last for several hours or days. Most stingray wounds are found on the ankle or foot and may be more of a laceration than a wound. There may be redness and swelling at the site of the sting, and the area may become numb, followed by dizziness, weakness, cramps, sweating and falling blood pressure. Fatalities have been reported when the barb enters the chest or abdomen, but they are rare.

Treatment   There is no known antidote. Contact medical help immediately; flush the wound with salt water and then soak the affected area in hot water for one hour. The water should be very hot (122°F), so that the heat will deactivate the poison and also ease pain. Pain medication may be administered, and lacerations are surgically closed. Generally, victims recover within 48 hours, although hospitalization may be needed for those with persistent symptoms of chest pain, irregular pulse or hypotension. Victims who have been stung on the chest or abdomen may require exploratory surgery. Tetanus shots and antibiotics are also necessary.

stonefish   *(Synanceja horrida)*   One of the world's most virulent animals, this large, unattractive fish gets its name from its resemblance to a piece of dead coral, and it is found in coral reefs and mud flats in the Indo-Pacific and the waters around China, the Philippines and Australia. Closely related to the scorpionfish and several other poisonous fish of the Scorpaenidae family, the stonefish has well-developed jagged spines and venom glands along its back that can penetrate a flipper or thin canvas shoe. This rough covering allows it to envelope itself in slime, coral debris and algae, camouflaging itself and increasing its chances of being stepped on. Stonefish are most often found in the Australian waters, where they have reportedly killed swimmers within hours of being stepped on.

Poisonous part   The chemistry of the venom is unknown.

Symptoms   The sting from the back fin spines of the stonefish is extremely painful, causing swelling, discoloration, loss of consciousness and paralysis. The pain can be so severe that it may cause the victim to scream in agony. Victims who survive the first 24 hours usually will not die.

Treatment   Stonefish antivenin is available but difficult to find in remote areas. Otherwise, treatment is symptomatic and supportive. Irrigation and bleeding of the wound (to remove venom) should be followed by cleansing. Immerse the wound in hot water for one hour to deactivate the venom; administration of tetanus antitoxin and antibiotics is advised. Some researchers recommend the administration of emetine hydrochloride to alleviate pain and neutralize stonefish venom. Emetine is injected directly into the wound after the administration of a local anesthetic. Stonefish antivenin may also be used in other scorpionfish stings.

See also SCORPIONFISH.

Streunex   See BENZENE HEXACHLORIDE.

strychnine   This bitter-tasting, colorless, crystalline powder is an extremely deadly chemical found in the seeds of a species of tropical plants called *Strychnos*. Strychnine is normally used as a rat poison; its bitter taste and scarcity on store shelves, however, make poisoning from this substance a rare occurrence. Still, when it occurs, strychnine poisoning causes some of the most dramatic symptoms of any toxic substance; its explosive convulsions are responsible for its frequent use in literature and film. A victim can be poisoned by strychnine either by swallowing it, by absorbing it through the skin, by eye contact or by inhaling the dust. Once used therapeutically as a tonic and general stimulant, it is no longer used. Strychnine is found naturally in some seeds and plants, principally the tropical nux-vomica tree.

Symptoms   Strychnine attacks the central nervous system within 10 to 20 minutes, causing all the muscles to contract simultaneously, beginning with the victim's neck and face, and can be fatal if untreated. Arms and legs begin to spasm next, and the spasms become worse and worse until the victim's back arches almost continuously. The slightest sound or movement will bring on a fresh spate of spasms, and the strychnine victim dies from asphyxiation or exhaustion as a result of the spasms. Rigor mortis begins immediately, freezing the body in a spasm with the eyes wide open. The effects of strychnine are almost identical to those of tetanus.

Treatment   If treatment is begun before symptoms appear or after spasms have been controlled, physicians can pump the stomach and administer activated charcoal. Primary emphasis in treatment is to maintain breathing and to control spasms with a slow intravenous drip of succinylcholine or Valium. The victim may also be placed on a ventilator. The victim should be kept quiet during spasms, since any noise or light will worsen the symptoms. With prompt medical attention, victims will recover within 24 hours.

See also NUX-VOMICA; RAT POISON.

succinylcholine   See NEUROMUSCULAR BLOCKING AGENTS.

sulfites   Any of several sulfur-based preservatives added to food to retard the spoilage and discoloration. They are added to food to prevent browning of freshly cut fruits and vegetables when exposed to air, to control the growth of bacteria and molds, to prevent the breakdown of various oils that would lead to "off" flavors and to whiten potatoes.

It is impossible to tell by inspection or smell whether or not a food contains sulfites, but they are used in a wide variety of foods. Those that have been tested with the highest levels include dried fruits, dehydrated vegetables, dehydrated potatoes, wine and restaurant salad bars and potatoes (although the last two uses have now been banned). Other foods that may contain sulfites are baked goods and mixes, alcoholic and nonalcoholic beverages, coffee and tea, condiments and relishes, dairy product substitutes, fresh and prepared fish and shellfish, fresh and processed fruits and fruit juices, fresh and processed vegetables and vegetable juices, gelatins, grain products, gravies and sauces, jams and jellies, nuts and their products, snack foods, soups and mixes, sugar and sweet sauces, toppings and syrups. This does not mean, however, that all foods within these categories necessarily contain sulfites.

Sulfites are also used to preserve some prescription medications and drugs that are given intravenously; sensitive patients may react to either of these applications. Wine always contains sulfites because the yeasts that ferment the grapes unavoidably produce them.

All packaged foods now require labels that indicate the presence of sulfites, even if they are naturally present in detectable quantities. The chemical's GRAS rating (generally recognized as safe) was removed by the Food and Drug Administration in 1987, although it is still permitted to be used. Foods sold in bulk, or served in restaurants, are not allowed to contain detectable levels of sulfites.

Symptoms Sensitive individuals (especially asthmatics) experience a range of symptoms, usually involving the respiratory system, ranging from mild to severe—even life threatening. These symptoms include narrowing of the airways, wheezing, breathing problems, nausea, stomach cramps, diarrhea, hives, itching, swelling, tingling, flushing, low blood pressure, blue tinge to the skin, shock and loss of consciousness. It is estimated that as many as 10 percent of asthmatics may be sensitive to sulfites—especially those who take steroids for their condition. In addition, nonasthmatics can experience reactions as well. Chronic exposure to sulfites has not demonstrated health effects, and no evidence of cancer has been reported.

Treatment Supportive and symptomatic.

See also APPENDIX A.

superantigens Proteins that cause food poisoning and toxic shock by whipping the immune system into a destructive frenzy. Normally, when a person's immune system encounters a virus, only about one in 10,000 of the disease-fighting T lymphocytes react. These lymphocytes target the alien virus or protein, called an "antigen," and kill it. But some of these antigens, called superantigens, arouse not just a few lymphocytes but as many as one in every five, which can launch an autoimmune attack and actually hurt the individual they should protect. And sometimes, superantigens can trigger the death of the lymphocytes, punching holes in the body's immune system.

See also FOOD POISONING.

surgeonfish   A fish of tropical waters that is poisonous at certain times of the year because of contamination with poisonous dinoflagellates (plankton) often found in red tide. In addition, its sting causes severe pain.

Symptoms   While death is rare, the sting of the surgeonfish causes an immediate severe stinging or throbbing pain, which may stay at the site of the wound or spread throughout the body and last for several hours or days. There may be redness and swelling at the site of the sting, and the area may become numb.

Treatment   Contact medical help immediately; flush the wound with fresh or salt water, and then soak the affected area in hot water or put hot compresses on it. The water should be very hot (122°F) in order to deactivate the poison. Continue applying hot water for 30 minutes to an hour.

See also DINOFLAGELLATE; FISH CONTAMINATION; FOOD POISONING.

sushi   The popular Japanese dish made of raw fish that can cause a type of food poisoning. Raw fish may be tainted with a parasitic worm, *Anisakis marina*, that infests small crustaceans on which many kinds of fish feed.

Symptoms   Gastrointestinal distress with abdominal pain, nausea and vomiting.

Treatment   Symptomatic.

See also FOOD POISONING.

sweeteners, artificial   Compounds include saccharin (anhydro-o-sul-famine benzoic acid), sucaryl (sodium or calcium cyclamate) and aspartame (NutraSweet). These are all synthetic combinations of two amino acids used in the United States to artificially sweeten food. Artificial sweeteners are generally considered to be nontoxic except in very large doses.

Symptoms   Ingestion of very large amounts can produce symptoms including vomiting, diarrhea, abdominal pain, frothing at the mouth, muscle spasms, convulsions and stupor. While the United States announced a ban on saccharin on March 9, 1977 because it causes cancer in laboratory animals, it is still an ingredient in many packaged foods and almost all toothpastes in the United States. There is no evidence that cyclamates are toxic when ingested in large amounts, although they may cause soft stools. Cyclamates were removed from a list of substances recognized as safe in food and drink by the secretary of health, education and welfare on October 18, 1969 because of the carcinogenic effect on animals. Aspartame is now available in the United States for use as a food sweetener and in low-calorie soft drinks, and as a tablet or powder form. The long-term human safety of aspartame has not been determined.

Treatment In large doses of saccharin, perform gastric lavage or induce vomiting followed by the administration of a saline cathartic; cyclamate overdose should be treated with induced vomiting or gastric lavage; aspartame overdose requires only supportive symptomatic treatment.

swimming pool disinfectants Almost all of these products, used for keeping in-ground swimming pools free of contaminants, can be fire hazards and can cause gastric complaints if ingested. Most contain more than 70 percent calcium hypochlorite (70 percent available chlorine), which is a strong oxidant; exposure to high heat or contact with a range of household cleaning materials (such as mineral oils, kerosene, turpentine, lubricants, tobacco, etc.) can be a fire hazard.

Symptoms Ingestion causes severe gastric symptoms; skin contact can result in a local dermatitis. Inhaling the fumes from decomposition are very irritating to eyes and lungs.

Treatment If ingested, perform gastric lavage or induce vomiting. If eyes or skin have been contaminated, wash thoroughly with tap water immediately.

synthetic organic insecticides Compounds include chlorobenzene deriv atives such as DDT (dichlorodiphenyltrichloroethane), banned since 1973; TDE (tetrachlorodiphenylethane); DFDT (difluorodiphenyltrichloroethane); dimite dichlorodiphenylethanol; DMC (dichlorodiphenyl methyl carbinol); methoxychlor; neotrane; ovotran; dilan. Also, indane derivatives including chlordane (banned 1976); heptachlor (banned 1976); aldrin (banned 1974) dieldrin (banned 1974); endrin; kepone (chlordecone). Also, lindane (cyclohexane hexachloride) and toxaphene (chlorinated camphene). Finally, the phosphate esters which include chlorothion; diazinon; DFP (diisopropylfluorophosphate); EPN; leptophos; malathion; metacide; OMPA (octamethylpyrophosphoramide); para-oxon; parathion; potosan; systox; TEPP (tetraethyl pyrophosphate); and thio-TEPP.

See also BOTANIC INSECTICIDES; INSECTICIDES; ORGANOPHOSPHATE INSECTICIDES.

T

Tagamet See CIMETIDINE.

taipan *(Oxyuranus scutellatus)* One of the world's deadliest snakes, the taipan is the largest cobra found in Australia and can grow to almost 13 feet. Brown on its back with a yellow underbelly, the nonhooded snake has extremely long fangs whose venom is so poisonous that it is fatal in a few moments. However, the number of fatalities is not too high, since the species is rare and lives in fairly undisturbed parts of northeastern Australia.

Until 1976, the smooth-scaled or fierce snake *(Parademansia microlepidotus)* was considered to be a Western form of the taipan, but its venom is significantly different from that of the latter.

Symptoms Within 15 to 30 minutes symptoms appear: pain and swelling, a drop in blood pressure and confusion, slurring of speech, dilation of the pupils, strabismus (eye irregularities), drooping of the upper eyelids and muscle weakness. The respiratory muscles are affected last, and respiratory muscle paralysis is the most common cause of death.

Treatment Antiserum is available.

See also ADDER, DEATH; ANTIVENIN; BROWN SNAKE; COBRA; COBRA, SPITTING; COPPERHEAD, AUSTRALIAN; CORAL SNAKE; SNAKES, POISONOUS; TIGER SNAKE.

tansy *(Tanacetum vulgare)* This common perennial herb was once a popular plant in a witch's arsenal during the Middle Ages. It gets its name from the Greek word *athanasia,* meaning "immortality"—it was the main ingredient in a potion designed to give immortality to Ganymede, a handsome Greek boy who became the eternal cupbearer for Zeus. Tansy may have gotten its reputation for immortal powers because its flowers do not easily wilt or because it was often placed in coffins as an insect repellent.

Today it is considered to be a weed in many places throughout the eastern United States and Pacific Northwest, growing wild in pastures and fields, along roadsides and in waste areas. Introduced into America from the Old World, it has pretty, flat yellow or white flowers that bloom from July through September; they are often used decoratively and look very much like yarrow. The plant grows to three feet, with dark green, fernlike leaves, and spreads in an ever-widening mass through underground runners. When crushed, its flowers and leaves smell faintly of pine.

Native to Europe, tansy has been naturalized in North America from

Nova Scotia and Ontario to Minnesota, Missouri and North Carolina as well as in Oregon and Nevada.

The bitter oil of tansy has been used homeopathically to bring on menstruation, as an abortifacient by the American Indians and also as a treatment against intestinal worms.

Poisonous part   The leaves, flowers and stem contain the toxic oil tanacetin. Poisoning often occurs after drinking too much tea or taking too much oil for medicinal reasons. The leaves also contain thujone in amounts that vary from plant to plant; thujone is a relatively toxic substance also found in wormwood.

Symptoms   Touching the plant can cause dermatitis. Within several hours after ingestion, symptoms appear, including frothing at the mouth, rapid and weak pulse, kidney problems, violent spasms and convulsions followed by death.

Treatment   Perform gastric lavage and give symptomatic treatment. See also HERBS, UNSAFE.

tarantula   A common name given to many large, hairy spiders. The sight of one of these monsters might be enough to induce hysteria—but in fact tarantulas are fairly harmless. They are usually found in the Southwest, although they are also present in many other areas in the United States. While tarantulas do have venom, it is very mild and almost never causes a problem in humans, although sometimes an allergic response can occur. Captive tarantulas seldom try to bite. More and more popular in this country as pets, they are also sometimes used by jewelry stores to patrol window displays.

In the early days of the Old West, tarantulas were deeply feared, and their bite was believed to be fatal; it was thought that the only cure was whiskey, or "tarantula justice." True tarantulas (*Lycosa narbonensis*) originated in Europe, where they also have an unfounded reputation for being lethal. In fact, the superstition about the danger of a tarantula's bite originated in the Dark Ages when fears arose about the wolf spider (*Lycosa tarantula*).

During the Middle Ages in the town of Taranto, Italy, people claiming to have been bitten by this spider were seized with a dancing frenzy, born of the idea that the bite would be fatal if the victim did not dance hard and long enough to sweat the poison out of the system. The dance and the music to which it was performed were called "tarantellas" after the spider. The whole episode evolved into a popular fad involving a mass delusion—that these spiders bit people intentionally and that the venom was fatal.

In truth, the European spider is no more venomous and no more likely to bite than its American wolf spider relative. Still, historians are not sure what started the outbreak of biting and dancing. One theory suggests that the dances, which were community affairs rather than individual performances, were actually pagan religious festivals masquerading as medical procedures to fool the clergy.

Symptoms Although tarantulas rarely cause serious poisonings, their bite produces a painful skin reaction, with itching, swelling, redness and, on rare occasions, soreness and fever for several days. The pain from the bite results from the puncture wound of the fangs, not from any toxin, which is comparatively mild and intended to paralyze animals smaller than the tarantula itself. Of course, it is still possible to sustain an allergic reaction, in much the same way that some people are overly sensitive to a bee sting. Even more common is an allergy to tarantula hairs, which can cause a rash on some people. These hairs are used by the spider as a defense; when irritated, the tarantulas comb the hairs off their abdomens with their hind legs and throw them at the enemy. These flying hairs can actually divert an attack of a lizard or mouse if they land in the attacker's nose or eyes.

Treatment Wash the wound and treat if infection occurs; give tetanus shot if necessary.

See also SPIDERS, POISONOUS.

taxine A plant alkaloid found in the common yew *(Taxus)* that can cause irregular or slow heartbeat and heart failure, and respiratory problems or failure. Ingestion of taxine can lead quickly to coma and death.

See also YEW.

tear gas The most commonly used tear gases are chloroacetophenone (CN), ethylbromoacetate, bromoacetone, bromomethylethylketone and orthochlorobenzylidene malononitril (CS). Tear gases can cause extreme irritation and swelling of the mucous membranes of the nose and eyes if discharged into the face and can even cause a temporary blindness.

Tear gas is usually expelled as a vapor that condenses to liquid droplets that are intensely irritating.

Symptoms Exposure causes severe tearing and sneezing, chest tightness, coughing, nausea and vomiting.

Treatment Remove victim to fresh air—separate from other sufferers—face into the wind with eyes open, and have him or her breathe deeply. Tear gas should be washed off the skin with soap and water; eyes should be washed with saline or water. Thoroughly decontaminate the victim, including clothing, by washing with soap and water.

TEPP (tetraethylpyrophosphate) A highly toxic insecticide derived from phosphoric acid, TEPP is a colorless liquid with an agreeable odor that can be inhaled, absorbed through unbroken skin or ingested. It is poisonous in all cases.

Symptoms This central nervous system poison causes symptoms to appear within 15 minutes to four hours, including vision problems, headache, loss of depth perception, cramps, sweating, chest pain, cyanosis, anorexia, vomiting and diarrhea, paralysis, convulsions, low blood pressure and death. Skin absorption irreversibly inhibits nerve signals.

Treatment Administration of extremely large doses of atropine, plus treatment of symptoms.

See also ORGANOPHOSPHATE INSECTICIDES.

teratogen Any toxic substance (such as aspirin and caffeine) that can cause birth defects; teratogenicity is the ability to cause birth defects.

tetrachloroethane This industrial solvent is the most toxic of all the chlorinated hydrocarbons. It causes prolonged narcosis, liver damage and severe toxic hepatitis, with acute yellow atrophy of the liver.

Symptoms Contact causes irritation of the eyes, skin and mucous membranes; inhalation causes cough, salivation, perspiration, confusion, vertigo and intoxication, with headache, excitement, weakness, nausea and vomiting, weak pulse and stupor. Ingestion causes severe gastrointestinal irritation with abdominal cramps, diarrhea and bloody stool. There may be kidney and liver damage.

Treatment Remove victim from exposure immediately and maintain breathing. Induce vomiting or perform gastric lavage if ingested, and follow with a saline cathartic. For skin or eye contact, wash with water (using soap for skin)and remove contaminated clothing. Hemodialysis for kidney problems may reverse damage.

See also CHLORINATED HYDROCARBON PESTICIDES.

tetrodotoxin Toxin produced in the skin of pufferfish, California newts, sun fish, porcupine fish, and some South American frogs that is similar to saxitoxin and interferes with the transfer of salt and neuronal transmission in muscles.

Symptoms Symptoms occur within 30 to 40 minutes after ingestion, with vomiting, salivation, twitching, weakness, low blood pressure, slow heartbeat and respiratory arrest from six to 24 hours after ingestion.

Treatment Replace fluid and electrolytes; induce vomiting or perform gastric lavage if ingestion occurred within the preceding hour.

See also FISH CONTAMINATION; SAXITOXIN.

thallium This soft metal is a minor constituent in ores and is commonly found in flue dusts; thallium salts are used in industry and chemical analysis, including the manufacture of optical lenses, photoelectric cells and costume jewelry.

As a rodenticide, it is a tasteless, odorless inorganic chemical pesticide banned for household use in the United States since 1965. However, poison control centers still report cases of thallium poisoning, primarily from old products still found on home and store shelves. Before it was banned for such use, thallium was contained in a wide range of pesticide products designed to control roaches, ants, silverfish, water bugs, moles, mice and rats. Poisoning most often occurs by accidentally ingesting rat or ant bait; chronic poisoning can also occur from skin absorption.

The minimum lethal dose of thallium salts is between 12 and 15 mg/kg, although its toxicity varies depending on the compound. There are reports of fatalities following adult ingestion of as little as 200 mg, and only one ounce of a 1 percent concentration can kill a 55-pound child.

Symptoms   Thallium acts by breaking down all cells in the body, especially hair follicles and the central nervous system. From one to three weeks after ingestion, hair begins to fall out, followed by pain in the extremities, fever, conjunctivitis, abdominal pain and nausea, bloody diarrhea, lethargy, tremors, convulsions and cyanosis. In severe poisonings, pulmonary edema and pneumonia may be followed by death from respiratory failure. There may also be organic brain damage, causing personality changes, anxiety or depression and even psychotic behavior.

Treatment   There is no recommended specific treatment in the United States. Prussian blue is believed to enhance removal of thallium from tissues and increases kidney and fecal elimination, but it is not available for use in the United States. Activated charcoal is probably just as good at enhancing fecal elimination. Induce vomiting or perform gastric lavage, followed by the administration of activated charcoal for at least five days with potassium chloride, plus symptomatic treatment. For skin contamination, all thallium should be washed off the skin with soap and water.

See also RAT POISON.

theophylline   This bronchodilator is widely used in the treatment of asthma and to prevent attacks of apnea (cessation of breathing) in premature infants. The drug is also used to treat heart failure, since it stimulates heart rate. Most common brands include Theo-Dur, Slo-Phyllin and Theobid.

Poisoning by theophylline may either be chronic or acute, with different symptoms in each case.

Symptoms   Poisoning by an acute single dose is usually the result of a suicide attempt or accidental child poisoning, although it may be caused by an accidental therapeutic overdose. In these cases, symptoms include vomiting, tremors, anxiety and rapid heartbeat, with high blood sugar and metabolic acidosis. With severe overdose, there may be irregular heartbeat and seizures that may not appear until 12 or 16 hours following ingestion.

Chronic poisoning occurs when excessive doses are given over at least a 24-hour period, or when another drug interferes with its metabolism. Victims of chronic poisoning are usually the very old and the very young. Symptoms include vomiting and rapid heart rate without accompanying metabolic effects. Seizures are common in higher doses.

Treatment Give propranolol to offset low blood pressure and irregular heartbeat, but beta blockers should be used cautiously in those with a history of asthma. Treat symptoms and monitor vital signs and electrocardiogram. Induce vomiting with syrup of ipecac, which may be more effective than gastric lavage, followed by the administration of activated charcoal and a cathartic. For large ingestions, administer repeat doses of activated charcoal and cathartic.

See also MEDICATIONS AS POISONS.

thermometers Despite frequent calls to poison control centers by desperate parents whose child has broken a thermometer and swallowed the mercury, this type of accident actually represents very little danger. Ingestion of the free metal from the thermometer does no harm, since in this state mercury is not absorbed from the gastrointestinal tract. Still, parents may wish to rinse the child's mouth with water.

Provided that the child has not cut the lip from the glass, has no embedded glass in the mouth or throat and can freely breathe and swallow, the glass should not pose a threat to the child's health, either.

Likewise, outdoor thermometers (which contain only small amounts of xylene, toluene, alcohol or other chemicals) are harmless.

It is important to clean up mercury spills. A filter tip from a cigarette may be helpful. After the mercury is removed, wash the area with a phosphate detergent.

See also MERCURY.

thiamine (vitamin B_1) This B-complex vitamin is used as part of the treatment in persons poisoned with ethylene glycol.

Thorazine (chlorpromazine) This synthetic chemical is derived from phenothiazine and is used primarily to treat manic-depression, although it can also be used to treat hiccups, tetanus and severe behavior problems in children and adults. It is available as a tablet, syrup, suppository or injection. First used in 1952, it is one of the most common psychiatric drugs available today.

Combining Thorazine with barbiturates or alcohol can be dangerous.

Symptoms When taken in large doses, Thorazine can cause drowsiness, fainting, low blood pressure, fast heartbeat, tremor, dizziness, electrocardiogram changes, convulsions and coma. Since Thorazine suppresses the cough reflex, a person can aspirate vomitus while under the influence of this drug. Thorazine has also been linked to "phenothiazine sudden death" among psychiatric patients who take the drug in large doses. Patients who are receiving an overdose will also often exhibit balance problems, slobbering, stuttering, restlessness, hand tremors and contraction of the face and neck muscles.

Treatment   Perform gastric lavage; treat symptoms, and give fluids to offset severe low blood pressure.

See also ANTIDEPRESSANTS; MEDICATIONS AS POISONS.

thrombolytics   See ANTICOAGULANTS.

tiger snake   *(Notechis scutatus)*   Considered to be the most dangerous snake of southern Australia, this relatively small member of the cobra family has no hood and is colored with yellow and brown bands. It is commonly found in wet areas of Australia and Tasmania. The snake is only about four feet long, and when about to strike, it flattens its head and appears to jump.

Symptoms   Beginning 15 to 30 minutes after a bite, symptoms include pain, swelling, falling blood pressure and convulsions and, quite often, death, which is caused by respiratory failure. Symptoms resemble poisoning from the deadly nightshade alkaloids. The respiratory muscles are affected last, and respiratory muscle paralysis is the most common cause of death.

Treatment   The specific antivenin should be used.

See also ANTIVENIN; COBRA; SNAKES, POISONOUS.

TNT   See TRINITROLUENE.

toad, Bufo   Under stress, all toads of this genus secrete venom contained in glands behind their eyes at the base of the skull. There are many different species of *Bufo* found throughout the world; the biggest one is the marine toad *(Bufo marinus)*, which can grow bigger than a dinner plate. The marine toad originated in South America but has been introduced all over the world because of its penchant for eating rodents and insects. It has been introduced in the United States in southern Florida, where dogs may occasionally bite one; while technically capable of killing a small dog who eats a toad, in fact the *Bufo* has such a terrible taste that dogs immediately spit it out; no cases of canine deaths from *Bufo* poisoning have been reported.

Poisonous part   Toads of the *Bufo* genus have venom containing bufonin and bufogin and bufotalin compounds (called *Bufo* toxin), whose action is similar to that of digitalis.

Symptoms   Untreated skin contact may cause a generalized skin irritation.

Treatment   Upon skin contact, immediately wash with water and soap. Eye contact may be extremely painful; affected eyes should be washed out with copious amounts of water of saline solution.

tobacco   *(Nicotiana)*   A member of the nightshade family, tobacco is responsible for one of the most widespread narcotic habits in the world and has been used by the Central and South American Indians since prehistoric times. It was popularized in Europe by the French Ambassador Jean Nicot de Villemain, who introduced Catherine de' Medici to tobacco chewing.

The plant may be an annual or perennial; if perennial, it usually grows into a large shrub or small tree. Its tubular flowers may be white, yellow or red, and its fruit contains tiny seeds. *N. tabacum* is the most common species used for smoking tobacco; several species are grown in the United States.

Poisonous part The whole plant is poisonous, although the most dangerous poisoning results from eating the large, fresh leaves in a salad, using infusions for enemas or absorbing the alkaloid through the skin during harvest. Other ways of obtaining the nicotine are also dangerous, in descending order: chewing without spitting; inhaling the smoke; chewing and spitting; inhaling as snuff; and smoking without inhaling.

In addition, the smoke of tobacco neutralizes 500 mg of vitamin C in the body for every pack of cigarettes smoked. Although the specific toxin varies depending on the species, all include nicotine and related alkaloids, including anabasine; nicotine is so potent it is sometimes used as an insecticide. Tobacco is also a botanical cousin to the heart regulator digitalis.

Symptoms Ingestion can produce anxiety, irritability, confusion, halting speech, dizziness, sleepiness, stupor, nausea, vomiting, appetite loss, tinnitus (ringing in the ears), cough, trembling, heart palpitations and irregular pulse. Reports in the literature include one death of a child from blowing soap bubbles through a tobacco pipe and another from accidentally swallowing snuff.

Treatment Gastric lavage followed by administration of activated charcoal.

See also NICOTINE; NICOTINE GUM; NICOTINE PATCH.

toilet cleaners See ALKALINE CORROSIVES.

toxalbumins See PHYTOTOXINS.

toxaphene The chemical name of this synthetic organic pesticide is chlorinated camphene, which can be used as a spray, a wettable powder or a dust to combat a range of insects, ticks and mites. This tasteless, pleasant-smelling insecticide is fat soluble but does not dissolve in water.

Symptoms When accidentally ingested or absorbed into the skin, toxaphene can cause symptoms similar to those caused by DDT, including a range of neurological symptoms and convulsions. Lethal doses result in a series of convulsions followed by anoxia (absence of oxygen supply to tissue) and respiratory failure. While there have been no adverse reports of chronic, low-level cases of poisoning, toxaphene is carcinogenic in animals. Fatal dose is estimated to be 5 g/70 kg.

Treatment Gastric lavage followed by saline, cathartics. Early administration of barbiturates to prevent convulsions. Following the onset of convulsions, administration of faster-acting intravenous barbiturates (even to the point of sedation).

See also DDT; SYNTHETIC ORGANIC INSECTICIDES.

toxin A poisonous protein that is produced by some bacteria, animals, insects and plants; a toxin is less complex than a poison or a venom but not as identifiable as a chemical compound. Occasionally, bacterial toxins are subdivided into endotoxins (released from dead bacteria), exotoxins (released from living bacteria) and enterotoxins (intestinal inflammators). Sometimes, the term "toxin" is restricted to poisons spontaneously produced by a living organism ("biotoxin"). Toxins produced by fungi are called mycotoxins; higher plants produce phytotoxins, and animal toxins are called zootoxins.

While some biotoxins seem to have little benefit to the organism that produces them, they may be involved in some unknown way in metabolism. However, many other biotoxins are noticeably helpful to their organism, primarily by inhibiting predators—especially insects.

toxoid A bacterial toxin that has been deactivated by either heat or chemicals, which removes its toxicity but maintains its ability to stimulate antibody production by the immune system. Certain types of toxoids are used in immunizations against specific diseases, such as diphtheria or tetanus.

See also EXOTOXIN.

tranquilizers See ANTIANXIETY DRUGS.

trichloroethane Also known as methyl chloroform, this common household solvent is found as an ingredient in a wide range of products, including fabric cleaners, spot removers, insecticides and paint removers. Together with trichloroethylene, it is used in most typewriter correction fluids, a form in which it can be abused by those who sniff it for its euphoric effects. It is available in two forms: 1,1,2 and (more commonly) 1,1,1-. A colorless, heavy liquid, it is considered by the National Institute of Occupational Safety and Health (NIOSH) to be a possible carcinogen. There is potential for abuse in those who have access to the substance and sniff the vapors.

Because of several deaths resulting from intentionally sniffing typewriter correction fluid, manufacturers have added oil of mustard as a deterrent, in both Liquid Paper and Liquid Paper Thinner (which contains more trichloroethane than the correctional fluid).

Symptoms Trichloroethane is a central nervous system depressant, but it also affects the heart, liver and kidneys and can reach toxic levels as a result of inhalation, skin contact or ingestion. It has a rapid anesthetic action and was used for this purpose prior to the 1960s, until safer agents were developed. Symptoms depend on the concentration and type of exposure but generally include headache, eye irritation, vertigo, sleepiness, visual disturbances, nausea, stupor, unconsciousness and coma. In extreme cases, inhaling these fumes can be fatal. Skin contact causes severe swelling followed by sloughing of the skin.

Ingestion causes symptoms including burning mouth, nausea, vomiting, abdominal pain and heart irregularities. Chronic abuse by sniffing produces weight loss, nausea, fatigue, visual problems, dermatitis and jaundice. The lethal dose in humans is reportedly between 0.5 and 5 ml/kg.

Treatment Move victim to a well-ventilated area and remove contaminated clothing; management is mainly supportive. Oxygen and artificial respiration should be used in the event of respiratory failure. Give supplemental oxygen and treat hydrocarbon aspiration pneumonitis if it occurs. Treat seizures, coma and arrhythmias if they occur, but do not use epinephrine because of a risk of inducing or worsening cardiac arrhythmias. There is no specific antidote. If ingested, do NOT induce vomiting; perform gastric lavage if the patient is seen within an hour of ingestion or has taken a large overdose. This is followed by the administration of activated charcoal and a cathartic.

See also TRICHLOROETHYLENE.

trichloroethylene This common household solvent is used as an inhalation anesthetic, a metal degreaser, a solvent for oils and greases and a paint remover. Together with trichloroethane, it is used in most typewriter correction fluids, a form in which it can be abused by those who sniff it for its euphoric effects. A colorless, heavy liquid, it was formerly popular as an anesthetic during labor prior to 1965. There is potential for abuse in those who have access to the substance and sniff the vapors.

Symptoms Trichloroethylene is a central nervous system depressant, but it also affects the heart, liver and kidneys. Symptoms depend on the concentration and type of exposure but generally include headache, eye irritation, vertigo, sleepiness, visual disturbances, nausea, stupor, unconsciousness and coma. In extreme cases, inhaling these fumes can be fatal.

Skin contact causes severe erythema followed by sloughing of the skin. Ingestion causes symptoms including burning mouth, nausea, vomiting, abdominal pain and heart irregularities. Chronic abuse by sniffing produces weight loss, nausea, fatigue, visual problems, dermatitis and jaundice.

Treatment Move victim to a well-ventilated area and remove contaminated clothing; management is mainly supportive. Oxygen and artificial respiration should be used in the event of respiratory failure. If ingested, perform gastric lavage followed by the administration of a saline cathartic.

See also TRICHLOROETHANE.

trihexyphenidyl (Artane) An anticholinergic drug used together with other drugs to relieve the symptoms of Parkinson's disease (rigidity and tremors); it is also used to treat symptoms of excessive use of Haldol (haloperidol) and Thorazine. These symptoms (unsteady gait, slobbering, slurring words, shuffling feet) are similar to those of Parkinson's disease.

trinitrotoluene (TNT) This solid, colorless to pale yellow explosive blows up when heated to 240° (or when shocked); it becomes even more explosive when combined with oxidizers. Prolonged skin contact will cause a type of skin rash; inhalation and ingestion of TNT are far more toxic.

Until industry tightened safety practices in the 1950s, TNT exposure was responsible for fatal cases of aplastic anemia and toxic hepatitis.

Symptoms The principal symptom of inhalation of TNT dust or vapor is jaundice of the skin, nails and hair. Other symptoms include sneezing, coughing, sore throat, yellow stain on skin, hair or nails, rash, blue color, pallor, nausea, anorexia, anemia, kidney failure, delirium, convulsions and coma. Chronic poisoning causes stomach disorders with heart irregularities and kidney failure. Fatal toxic dose is between one and two grams.

Treatment Ingested TNT should be removed by induced vomiting or gastric lavage, followed by the administration of a cathartic. For skin contamination, thoroughly wash with soap and water. Soap with 10 percent potassium sulfite will turn red in contact with TNT and can be used to determine thorough cleansing. Observe victim for possible liver damage.

tropical rattlesnake See RATTLESNAKE, CASCABEL.

trumpet plant (*Solandra*) Also known as chalice vine, this climbing woody vine has large, showy yellow trumpet-shaped flowers with fleshy berries. It is found in tropical America and Mexico and is cultivated outdoors in Florida, the West Indies and Hawaii.

Poisonous part All parts of the plant are toxic, including the nectar, and contain atropine alkaloids.

Symptoms Following ingestion, symptoms include dry mouth, fast heartbeat, dry, hot flushed skin, fever and blurred vision. Children are particularly prone to excitement, headache, delirium and hallucinations.

Treatment If poisoning is severe enough to cause high fever or delirium, administer slow intravenous drip of physostigmine until symptoms disappear; repeated administration may be required.

See also ATROPINE.

trunkfish (*Lactoria cornutus*) A fish of tropical oceans that is poisonous at certain times of the year because of feeding on poisonous plankton. Symptoms may develop quickly or slowly and involve tingling sensations in the lips and mouth followed by numbness, nausea, vomiting, abdominal cramps, weakness, paralysis, convulsions, skin rash, coma and death in about 12 percent of cases.

See also CIGUATERA; DINOFLAGELLATES; FISH CONTAMINATION.

tuna, bluefin One of a group of scombroid fishes (including mackerel, swordfish and others) that contain a chemical in the flesh called histidine. When these fish are allowed to stand at room temperature for several hours, histidine interacts with bacteria to form a histaminelike substance called saurine. Scombroid fish are more susceptible to the development of saurine poison than most other kinds of fish. All of the species that are potentially toxic live in temperate or tropical waters, especially around California and Hawaii; even commercially canned tuna can become toxic, although the most common fish responsible is mahimahi.

Scombroid poisoning can be prevented simply by adequately refrigerating fish.

Symptoms Symptoms of saurine poisoning resemble those of a severe allergy: Soon after eating the affected fish (which is said to have a sharp, pungent taste), the victim begins to experience headache, throbbing blood vessels in the neck, nausea, vomiting, burning throat, massive welts and itching. Recovery occurs after eight to 12 hours.

Treatment Gastric lavage; administration of antihistamines or the histamine blocker cimetidine (Tagamet).

See also FISH CONTAMINATION; FOOD POISONING; SCROMBROID POISONING.

tuna, skipjack *(Euthynnus pelamis)* One of a group of scrombroid fishes (including mackerel, swordfish and allies) that contain a chemical in the flesh called histidine. When these fish are allowed to stand at room temperature for several hours, histidine forms a histaminelike substance called saurine. Scrombroid fish are more susceptible to the development of saurine poison than most other kinds of fish.

See also FISH CONTAMINATION; FOOD POISONING; SCOMBROID POISONING; TUNA, BLUEFIN.

turbantop *(Gyromitra esculenta)* Also called false morel *(G. infula)*, this mushroom varies in toxicity from variety to variety and individual to individual. Those found in North America are almost all poisonous, but a few of the European varieties are extremely tasty and harmless. The turbantop is brown with a thick, hollow stem.

Poisonous part The poisonous compound is monomethylhydrazine (mmh), found in all Gyromitra mushrooms. It destroys the red blood cells and affects the kidneys and central nervous system. Some of the toxins in these mushrooms may be removed by drying, boiling, rinsing and reboiling.

Symptoms Symptoms begin between two hours and a day after ingestion and can include severe liver damage, vomiting, diarrhea, jaundice, convulsions, destruction of the red blood cells and coma. Fatality rate from liver failure ranges from 15 to 40 percent. Toxicity in humans varies from one individual to the next. Overall fatality rate is about 15 percent.

Treatment Give pyridoxine for seizures; treat methemoglobinemia with methylene blue.

See also GYROMITRA; MUSHROOM POISONING; MUSHROOM TOXINS.

turpentine This common household solvent is used as a thinner for paint, varnish and lacquer. A volatile oil, turpentine is derived from sapwood of cone-bearing trees like pines and firs and has been used medically as a skin irritant. Still, it is not usually fatal, since its fumes make it too painful to swallow or inhale for any appreciable length of time.

Symptoms Breathing these solvent fumes can cause headache, eye irritation, dizziness, visual disturbances, nausea, unconsciousness and convulsions. With skin contact, it causes local irritation and immediate reddening. Ingestion can result in abdominal pain, nausea, vomiting, diarrhea, urinary problems, unconsciousness, shallow breathing and convulsions. In extreme cases, kidney failure and pulmonary edema can be fatal.

Treatment Avoid vomiting. Gastric lavage followed by the administration of demulcents, such as milk. For skin contamination, wash thoroughly with soap and water.

See also PETROLEUM DISTILLATES; VOLATILE OILS.

2,4-D [Trade names: Agrotect, Lawn-keep, Rider, Super D Weedone, Weed-B-Gone, Weedone.] This herbicide was introduced in 1944 as the first hormonelike weed killer and has grown to become the most extensively used herbicide in the world. In 1985, agriculture and forestry applications in the United States accounted for nearly 40 million pounds of 2,4-D. As an herbicide, it is fairly selective; it is toxic to many broad-leaved plants but does not affect grasses (such as cereal crops, ornamental lawns or pastures). It works by interfering with normal plant growth processes, and it is also used to control ripening of fruit and root development.

This corrosive white powder is widely used in agriculture to control weeds in corn, wheat, sorghum, oats, barley and sugarcane, with considerable chance for widespread exposure. It is available as an aerial or ground spray, or by direct injection into plants.

Studies suggest that normal exposure levels of 2,4-D for agricultural and forestry workers and animals such as deer, rabbits and fish are considerably lower than those levels producing toxic effects. Protective clothing should be worn when applying the herbicide. It is uncertain to what extent the public is exposed, but it is possible that some residue remains on food; therefore, experts suggest washing all fresh produce.

Symptoms When ingested in large doses, 2,4-D causes gastrointestinal irritation, spasms of the heart and central nervous system depression. It is also a skin and eye irritant, and prolonged inhalation causes coughing, dizziness and temporary loss of coordination. Prolonged exposure to low levels can produce a variety of responses ranging from a reversible loss of coordination to stomach ulcers—and sometimes death.

A review by the International Agency for Cancer Research concluded there were insufficient data to assess the carcinogenicity of 2,4-D.

Treatment Induce vomiting or perform gastric lavage, followed by the administration of activated charcoal and a saline cathartic. Quinidine may be necessary if ventricular fibrillation occurs. Chronic exposure can produce aplastic anemia.

U

universal antidote Although milk is most popularly considered to be the universal antidote, there is really no such thing, according to most toxicologists. Milk is actually used to dilute poison, not combat its effects, and it is only useful with some toxic substances. Another so-called universal antidote—two parts activated charcoal, one part milk of magnesia and one part strong tea solution—is also ineffective, despite its popularity in the press. According to toxicology experts, the use of activated charcoal alone would be much more effective, and some evidence suggests that the addition of milk of magnesia and tea actually interferes with the absorptive activity of the charcoal.

Salt water, which at one time was considered to be a universal antidote because of its ability to absorb poison in the stomach, can be harmful and actually cause cardiac arrest. Because many antidotes are dangerous in and of themselves, no treatment should be considered before talking with a physician or poison control center. Using an antidote depends on the type and amount of substance ingested, and how long it has been between ingestion and treatment.

urushiol A resin contained in the sap of poison oak, poison ivy and poison sumac that causes contact dermatitis in seven out of 10 Americans who come in contact with it. About five out of 10 Americans are extremely sensitive to urushiol.

See also POISON IVY; POISON OAK; POISON SUMAC.

V

Vacor (PNU, or 2 percent *N*-3-pyridylmethyl-*N'p*-nitrophenylurea) This yellow or green rat killer causes irreversible insulin-dependent diabetes and autonomic nervous system injury. Fatal poisonings are usually the result of suicide, since ingestion of a small amount will not usually be fatal. Vacor was banned for household sale in 1979, but it is still found in some homes and is available to professional exterminators.

Ingestion of one packet of Vacor (39 g) has caused acute toxicity.

Symptoms Because Vacor destroys the insulin-producing cells in the pancreas, symptoms include twitching, low blood pressure, thirst, diabetes, nausea and vomiting, abdominal and chest pain, weakness, blurred vision, lethargy, impaired mental function, delirium, collapse, coma and respiratory failure ending in death.

Treatment Administer nicotinamide within 30 minutes, followed by symptomatic treatment; although its success has not been proven in humans, its use can prevent PNU-induced diabetes in rats. Induce vomiting or perform gastric lavage, followed by the administration of activated charcoal and a cathartic. Treat coma and give intravenous fluids for low blood pressure; chronic therapy includes a high-salt diet and fluorocortisone. Treat diabetes as usual.

See also NICOTINAMIDE; RAT POISON.

Valium See DIAZEPAM.

venin de crapaud An ancient poison popular throughout Europe during the 15th century, it was made by feeding arsenic to toads and distilling the juices from their bodies after their death.

See also ARSENIC.

viper, gaboon *(Bitis gabonica)* This close relative of the puff adder is found in African rain forests and remnant forest and thickets, although it is not arboreal. One of the largest and heaviest Old World vipers, it is usually placid but capable of lightning strikes and is considered to be one of the most dangerous snakes.

The gaboon viper is easily concealed by its colors: purple, crimson, rose, pale blue, silver, yellow russet and black, arranged in complex geometrical patterns. It has the longest fangs of any snake in the world (almost two inches) and has enough venom to kill 200 people. Yet it is so placid that small children can pick one up by the tail and carry it.

Symptoms A bite from the gaboon viper may pass unnoticed until the pain begins—and when it may be too late to administer antivenin. Although less toxic than that of its puff adder cousin, gaboon viper venom can still be fatal. Without treatment, victims begin bleeding from the gums, nose and eyes and experience chills, fever, sweating, falling blood pressure, convulsions and death. In cases of a severe bite, the victim will also experience swelling above the elbows or knees within two hours.

Treatment Antivenin is available.

See also MASSASAUGA; PIT VIPERS; RATTLESNAKE, CANEBRAKE; RATTLE-SNAKE; CASCABEL; RATTLESNAKE, EASTERN DIAMONDBACK; RATTLE-SNAKE, MEXICAN WEST COAST; RATTLESNAKE, RED DIAMONDBACK; RATTLESNAKE, TIMBER; RATTLESNAKE, WESTERN DIAMONDBACK; RAT-TLESNAKES; SIDEWINDER; SNAKES, POISONOUS; VIPER, JUMPING; VIPER, MALAYAN PIT; VIPER, RUSSELL'S; VIPER, SAWSCALED; VIPER, WAGLER'S PIT; WATER MOCCASIN; WUTU.

viper, horned   See SIDEWINDER.

viper, jumping *(Bothrops)* Also known as the tommygoff, this aggressive relative of the fer-de-lance is found throughout Central and South America. Brown or gray with diamond-shaped crosswise marks, it can grow to about two feet long and can strike with such force that it can lift itself off the ground. Its venom is not as dangerous as that of others in the fer-de-lance group.

Symptoms Because the venom interferes with the coagulation of the blood, it hemorrhages into muscles and the nervous system and results in bleeding from the gums, nose, mouth and rectum. It is possible to assess the seriousness of the bite by checking the level of swelling or hemorrhages that appear above the elbows or knees two hours after the bite. After a person is bitten, the area above the bite quickly swells and turns purple. The victim vomits blood, perspires and collapses within an hour, with blood flowing from the nose and eyes, followed by unconsciousness and death if no antivenin is administered. In fact, absent antivenin, death from cardiorespiratory failure is unavoidable.

Treatment Antivenin is available.

See also MASSASAUGA; PIT VIPERS; RATTLESNAKE, CANEBRAKE; RATTLE-SNAKE, CASCABEL; RATTLESNAKE, EASTERN DIAMONDBACK; RATTLE-SNAKE, MEXICAN WEST COAST; RATTLESNAKE, RED DIAMONDBACK; RATTLESNAKE, TIMBER; RATTLESNAKE, WESTERN DIAMONDBACK; RAT-TLESNAKES; SIDEWINDER; SNAKES, POISONOUS; VIPER, GABOON; VIPER, MALAYAN PIT; VIPER, RUSSELL'S; VIPER, SAWSCALED; VIPER, WAGLER'S PIT; VIPERS; WATER MOCCASIN; WUTU.

viper, Malayan pit *(Agkistrodon rhodostoma)* Found in forests, plantations and other cultivated areas, this snake (also known as the Malayan moccasin) is often quick to strike. Its long, tubular fangs are located in a maxillary bone that can be rotated 90 degrees, effectively swinging the fangs from a vertical to a horizontal position. The head is triangular with large scales, and the small eyes have vertical pupils; its snout is pointed and upturned, and the sturdy body is reddish brown with a series of dark brown crossbands that narrow along the back's midline. A light stripe extends from the eye to the nape of neck, and there is a wide light-colored band on the lip.

This snake is normally found in forested areas, where it stays coiled up under rocks or dense vegetation; at twilight it hunts for food. Fairly aggressive, when molested it assumes a threatening posture, curling up its body and vibrating the tip of its tail.

Symptoms Those who have been bitten by vipers show much the same symptoms as victims of cobra bites, plus bleeding from the gums, chills and fever. It is possible to assess the seriousness of the bite by checking the level of swelling or hemorrhages that appear above the elbows or knees two hours after the bite. After a person is bitten, the area above the bite quickly swells and turns purple. The victim vomits blood, perspires and collapses within an hour, with blood flowing from the nose and eyes, followed by unconsciousness and death if no antivenin is administered. In fact, absent antivenin, death from cardiorespiratory failure is unavoidable.

Treatment Antivenin is available.

viper, Palestine *(Vipera palestinae)* This member of the viper family is a considerable threat in the Middle East and causes more cases of snakebite in Palestine than any other venomous snake.

See also MASSASAUGA; PIT VIPERS; RATTLESNAKE, CANEBRAKE; RATTLESNAKE, CASCABEL; RATTLESNAKE, EASTERN DIAMONDBACK; RATTLESNAKE, MEXICAN WEST COAST; RATTLESNAKE, RED DIAMONDBACK; RATTLESNAKE, TIMBER; RATTLESNAKE, WESTERN DIAMONDBACK; RATTLESNAKES; SIDEWINDER; SNAKES, POISONOUS; VIPER, GABOON; VIPER, JUMPING; VIPER, RUSSELL'S; VIPER, SAWSCALED; VIPER, WAGLER'S PIT; VIPERS; WATER MOCCASIN; WUTU.

viper, Russell's *(Vipera russelli)* Also called the tic polonga or daboia, the Russell's viper is found in both forests and open occupied areas from the Himalayas and southern China to Sri Lanka and Indonesia. This snake is very aggressive and is one of the most deadly in the world. Growing up to five feet long, it has rows of reddish brown spots circled by black and white lines, with a wide head and a square snout.

Aggressive and assertive, it is normally found on margins of woods and forests, brushy fields, mountain meadows, cultivated lands and thickets near villages, usually on the ground—but it is also capable of climbing fences to find prey.

This viper is active mainly at twilight and during the night, coiling up under stones and brushy places during the day. It is generally lazy and slow, but when irritated it becomes aggressive, hissing loudly and striking with force and speed.

Symptoms Those who have been bitten by vipers show much the same symptoms as victims of cobra bites, plus bleeding from the gums, chills and fever. It is possible to assess the seriousness of the bite by checking the level of swelling or hemorrhages that appear above the elbows or knees two hours after the bite. After a person is bitten, the area above the bite quickly swells and turns purple. The victim vomits blood, perspires and collapses within an hour, with blood flowing from the nose and eyes, followed by unconsciousness and death if no antivenin is administered. In fact, absent antivenin, death from cardiorespiratory failure is unavoidable.

Treatment Antivenin is available.

See also MASSASAUGA; PIT VIPERS; RATTLESNAKE, CANEBRAKE; RATTLE-SNAKE, CASCABEL; RATTLESNAKE, EASTERN DIAMONDBACK; RATTLE-SNAKE, MEXICAN WEST COAST; RATTLESNAKE, RED DIAMONDBACK; RATTLESNAKE, TIMBER; RATTLESNAKE, WESTERN DIAMONDBACK; RAT-TLESNAKES; SIDEWINDER; SNAKES, POISONOUS; VIPER, GABOON; VIPER, JUMPING; VIPER, MALAYAN PIT; VIPER, SAWSCALED; VIPER, WAGLER'S PIT; VIPERS; WATER MOCCASIN; WUTU.

viper, sawscaled *(Echis carinatus)* The most venomous of the Viperidae vipers, the sawscaled viper is found in semidesert and dry, arid regions in the Afro-Asian deserts, India and Sri Lanka. This alert and vicious snake is known for its irritability and aggressiveness; its bite is usually fatal. A small snake no longer than two feet, it has a gray sandy color with rows of white spots and zigzag lines.

Active at night, this snake is easily disguised and can be very dangerous in a land where most of the people don't wear shoes. Even a newborn snake can kill a person and will bite with very little provocation. When disturbed, this snake moves itself into an S shape, rubbing its scales together to produce a hissing sound. It moves in a peculiar sidewise motion known as sidewinding.

While there is a solid market for the sale of these snakes, the 200,000 animals brought in over a period of six years have done little to decimate the population.

Symptoms The venom of the sawscaled viper is unusually toxic; it causes both internal and external hemorrhages and is fatal within 12 to 16 days after the bite. Those who have been bitten by vipers show much the same symptoms as victims of cobra bites, plus bleeding from the gums, chills and fever. It is possible to assess the seriousness of the bite by checking the level of swelling or hemorrhages that appear above the elbows or knees two hours after the bite. After a person is bitten, the area above the bite quickly swells and turns purple. The victim vomits blood, perspires and collapses within an hour, with blood flowing from the nose and eyes, followed by unconsciousness and death if no antivenin is administered. In fact, absent antivenin, death from cardiorespiratory failure is unavoidable.

Treatment Antivenin is available.

See also MASSASAUGA; PIT VIPERS; RATTLESNAKE, CANEBRAKE; RATTLE-SNAKE, CASCABEL; RATTLESNAKE, EASTERN DIAMONDBACK; RATTLE-SNAKE, MEXICAN WEST COAST; RATTLESNAKE, RED DIAMONDBACK; RATTLESNAKE, TIMBER; RATTLESNAKE, WESTERN DIAMONDBACK; RAT-TLESNAKES; SIDEWINDER; SNAKES, POISONOUS; VIPER, GABOON; VIPER, JUMPING; VIPER, MALAYAN PIT; VIPER, RUSSELL'S; VIPER, WAGLER'S PIT; VIPERS; WATER MOCCASIN; WUTU.

viper, Wagler's pit *(Trimeresurus Wagleri)* A species of snake found in Asia and one of a group collectively known as fer-de-lance. The venom of this snake remains almost completely poisonous even after being in a sterilizer. It causes extremely fast collapse and death, without local swelling.

Symptoms With a bite from this viper, blood cannot coagulate and hemorrhages into muscles and the central nervous system. There is local pain, bleeding from the bite, gums, nose, mouth and rectum. Those who have been bitten by vipers show much the same symptoms as victims of cobra bites, plus bleeding from the gums, chills and fever. It is possible to assess the seriousness of the bite by checking the level of swelling or hemorrhages that appear above the elbows or knees two hours after the bite. After a person is bitten, the area above the bite quickly swells and turns purple. The victim vomits blood, perspires and collapses within an hour, with blood flowing from the nose and eyes, followed by unconsciousness and death if no antivenin is administered. In fact, absent antivenin, death from cardiorespiratory failure is unavoidable.

Treatment Antivenin is available.

See also MASSASAUGA; PIT VIPERS; RATTLESNAKE, CANEBRAKE; RATTLE-SNAKE, CASCABEL; RATTLESNAKE, EASTERN DIAMONDBACK; RATTLE-SNAKE, MEXICAN WEST COAST; RATTLESNAKE, RED DIAMONDBACK; RATTLESNAKE, TIMBER; RATTLESNAKE, WESTERN DIAMONDBACK; RAT-TLESNAKES; SIDEWINDER; SNAKES, POISONOUS; VIPER, GABOON; VIPER, JUMPING; VIPER, MALAYAN PIT; VIPER, RUSSELL'S; VIPER, SAWSCALED; VIPERS; WATER MOCCASIN; WUTU.

vipers (Viperidae) This major family of poisonous snakes includes some 160 species found in most parts of the world; they possess the most efficient way of injecting venom of all snakes. The Viperidae family consists primarily of two subfamilies: the pit vipers (Crotalinae), found throughout the Americas and southeastern Asia, numbering about 120 species; and the Viperinae, numbering 39 species, including the European adder, the sawscaled viper and the puff adder found throughout Europe, Africa and Asia.

In general, vipers share many of the same characteristics; for example, the head is triangular or spade shaped, distinct from the body. Because they are so different from other groups, the vipers are the most easily identified of all poisonous snakes. Their long, tubular fangs are located in a maxillary bone that can be rotated 90 degrees, effectively swinging the fangs from a vertical to a horizontal position.

The true vipers (Viperinae) differ from the pit vipers in internal anatomy, and they also lack the temperature-sensitive pit organs. The pit vipers (Crotalinae) are characterized by a unique sense organ on each side of the head between the nostril and the eye. As the snake moves its head, it can ascertain the direction of objects by sensing heat; if the object is directly in front of the snake, the heat radiation will enter both the left and right pit organs at the same time, which indicates distance as well as direction.

The bites of even the smallest European vipers are always potentially dangerous. The Russell's viper (one of the largest members of the subfamily) is one of the deadliest snakes in the world.

Symptoms   Those who have been bitten by vipers show much the same symptoms as victims of cobra bites, plus bleeding from the gums, chills and fever. It is possible to assess the seriousness of the bite by checking the level of swelling or hemorrhages that appear above the elbows or knees two hours after the bite. After a person is bitten, the area above the bite quickly swells and turns purple. The victim vomits blood, perspires and collapses within an hour, with blood flowing from the nose and eyes, followed by unconsciousness and death if no antivenin is administered. In fact, absent antivenin, death from cardiorespiratory failure is unavoidable.

Treatment   Antivenin is available.

See also MASSASAUGA; PIT VIPERS; RATTLESNAKE, CANEBRAKE; RATTLE-SNAKE, CASCABEL; RATTLESNAKE, EASTERN DIAMONDBACK; RATTLE-SNAKE, MEXICAN WEST COAST; RATTLESNAKE, RED DIAMONDBACK; RATTLESNAKE, TIMBER; RATTLESNAKE, WESTERN DIAMONDBACK; RAT-TLESNAKES; SIDEWINDER; SNAKES, POISONOUS; VIPER, GABOON; VIPER, JUMPING; VIPER, MALAYAN PIT; VIPER, RUSSELL'S; VIPER, SAWSCALED; VIPER WAGLER'S PIT; WATER MOCCASIN; WUTU.

vitamins   Sales of vitamin supplements in the United States are a $450 million-a-year business, with more than 40 percent of the population over age 16 taking at least one tablet every day. Some Americans, however, take many more than one tablet, and it is these megadoses of certain vitamins that can be toxic. Whether a vitamin is sold as "natural" or "synthetic," it has the same basic molecular structure and has the same potential for toxicity. It is utilized by the body in exactly the same way. The "natural" vitamins have been extracted from a substance found in nature (such as vitamins A and D extracted from cod liver oil, vitamin E from wheat germ oil, etc.). It is, however, quite expensive to extract these vitamins, and therefore most available today are synthetic, which have been manufactured by a drug company.

There remains some controversy about the correct safe dosage of vitamins. For more than 50 years, Americans have been guided by the Recommended Daily Allowance (RDA) introduced during World War II as a way to make sure recruits didn't suffer from malnutrition. Technically, the National Academy of Sciences sets different RDAs for people based on age and sex, but since 1968 the Food and Drug Administration has taken the highest RDAs (suitable for teenage boys) and made them the national standard. In 1990, the FDA announced it would average the RDAs for all age groups; the new figures are considerably lower and, according to the agency, a better measurement of a typical American's vitamin needs.

The FDA would like to cut the RDAs for many vitamins and nutrients (including A, B, C, E and iron) from 10 to 80 percent and rename the RDA as the Reference Daily Intake (or RDI). Scheduled to go into effect in 1993, the new levels are controversial. The current RDA for vitamin C, for example, is 60 mg—but research suggests that protection against cancer or cataracts may require 100 mg. What are really needed, according to vitamin advocates, are guidelines for optimal consumption depending on age, sex and life-style.

Vitamins are either soluble in water or oil; those that dissolve easily in water are passed out of the body in the urine and don't usually cause toxicity. These water-soluble vitamins include ascorbic acid, thiamine, riboflavin, niacin, pantotheate, pyridoxine, cobalamin, folate and biotin. The fat-soluble vitamins (A, D, E and K) are not so easily excreted.

Multiple-vitamin products usually contain a variety of vitamins, minerals and trace elements, including the water-soluble vitamins, and pose little toxicity problems. However, routinely taking large doses of these multiple-vitamin supplements can be toxic, especially in preparations containing iron that are given to children.

VITAMIN A

Excessive use of vitamin A (either as a daily supplement or as an acne treatment) can cause liver and kidney problems. Megadoses of this vitamin have also been used (more than 50,000 International Units (IU) daily for months) to treat children with learning disabilities or as an "anticancer" treatment for adults. Reports indicate that doses over 40,000 IU per day for several months have resulted in hypervitaminosis A in adults; acute ingestion of more than 12,000 IU/kg may lead to stomach problems. Other studies suggest that doses in excess of 25,000 IUs (five times the recommended daily allowance) can lead to liver damage, hair loss, blurred vision and headaches.

Symptoms In children, symptoms of vitamin A toxicity include irritability, anorexia, skin problems, swollen legs and forearms, hair loss, bleeding lips, severe headache and a craving for butter. Massive doses of vitamin A may also increase pressure within the skull. Symptoms in adults are much the same, only not so serious. In adults, changes in menstruation and skin pigmentation have been reported.

Treatment Withdrawal from the vitamin. According to experts, treating vitamin A overdose with vitamin E is controversial. Steroids may relieve intracranial pressure in children. The symptoms will disappear in a few weeks after the megadoses have stopped.

VITAMIN B$_6$ (pyridoxine)

This B-complex vitamin is used to manage seizures caused by poisoning by the Gyromitra mushrooms, hydrazine (rocket fuel) or isoniazid. It is also given as part of the therapy for ethylene glycol poisoning.

VITAMIN D

Vitamin D is essential for the formation of strong bones and has been added to milk since the 1930s as a way to reduce the incidence of rickets. Toxicity with vitamins D$_3$ or D$_4$ is rare and would require between 5,000 and 10,000 IU daily for several months, although some sensitive people experience symptoms at lower doses. In daily doses of 50,000 IUs (125 times the U.S. RDA) this vitamin can cause the buildup of calcium deposits in the blood that can interfere with the functioning of muscles, including the heart. Sunbathing, which stimulates the body's production of vitamin D, will not create an overdose, however.

Recently, a spate of vitamin D poisonings were linked to accidental overdoses in milk fortification at one dairy in Boston, in dosages ranging up to 232,565 IUs. Normally, milk contains 400 IUs of vitamin D per quart. In testing across the country, milk and formula were found to rarely contain the amount of vitamin D as stated on the label; most dairies, however, add too little rather than too much.

Symptoms Anorexia, nausea, vomiting, fatigue, weakness, headache, diarrhea and weight loss. Kidney problems, excess calcium in the blood (hypercalcemia) and osteoporosis may also occur. Megadoses of vitamin D during pregnancy are implicated in a variety of fetal abnormalities, including mental retardation and supravalvular aortic stenosis. In severe cases, overdoses of vitamin D can cause irreversible kidney and cardiovascular damage.

Treatment Withdrawal from the vitamin. The excess levels of calcium in the blood may continue for a few weeks, which may require a restriction in the amount of calcium intake, plenty of fluids and the administration of glucocorticoids. Vitamin D can also be removed with dialysis.

VITAMIN E

Acute poisoning with vitamin E is rare, although chronic use of extreme megadoses of this vitamin (more than 600 IU per day) could cause headaches, dizziness, fatigue, stomach problems, swollen lips and muscle weakness.

VITAMIN K (phytonadione)

This vitamin is used to reverse the excessive anticoagulation following overdose of coumarin and indanedione derivatives and is also used in the treatment of salicylate poisoning.

WATER-SOLUBLE VITAMINS

Probably the most popular vitamin to be taken in very large doses is vitamin C, which very rarely causes toxic symptoms beyond stomach irritation and diarrhea after very large doses. However, it can result in scurvy in those who abruptly discontinue taking megadoses, and there have been reports that chewable tablets have eroded teeth if taken daily for more than three years. Earlier reports of vitamin C causing kidney stones is unsupported by research.

Thiamine (vitamin B_1) toxicity has been reported in doses of 5 mg per day for about a month and can cause headaches, irritability, sleeplessness, tachycardia and weakness.

Toxicity with vitamin B_6 has been reported in doses of two per day for four months, or more quickly at higher doses, causing symptoms including unsteadiness and numb hands and feet. Symptoms disappear after stopping the vitamin; also, some reports indicate that numbness lingers for up to six months.

Niacin in doses of 2,000 IUs (more than 100 times the RDA) may help lower cholesterol, but people who take this much should watch for possible symptoms of jaundice and liver damage.

volatile oils   Also known as essential oils, these are colorless liquids that evaporate quickly and are often used as skin irritants; many have reputations as abortifacients. One of the best-known essential oils is camphor, found in many over-the-counter products including Campho-Phenique, Vicks Vaporub, camphorated oil and Mentholatum. Topical application of these products leads to inflammation followed by a feeling of comfort, but if ingested they can be fatal.

Plants that contain volatile oils include nutmeg, pine, absinthe, pennyroyal, juniper, savin, rue, citronella, sassafras, hemlock, anise, cinnamon, pepper, clove, rape, tansy, eucalyptus, turpentine and menthol.

Symptoms   Acute ingestion of 15 ml of a volatile oil can be fatal, since it irritates all tissues, damages the kidneys and causes swelling in the lungs, brain and lining of the stomach. Symptoms include nausea, vomiting, diarrhea, unconsciousness, shallow breathing and convulsions. Inhaling the volatile oils causes dizziness, rapid and shallow breathing, rapid heartbeat, unconsciousness or convulsions. Further, volatile oils in amounts large enough to cause an abortion are also large enough to cause irreversible kidney and liver damage.

Treatment   There are no specific antidotes. Administer liquid

VOLATILE OILS

Birch oil	Contains 98% methyl salicylate
Camphor oil	FDA banned in 1980 as liniment; causes fetal deaths
Clove oil	Contains 80–90% eugenol
Cinnamon oil	Can burn skin after prolonged contact; potent antigen and smoked as a hallucinogen
Eugenol	Phenol derived from clove oil
Eucalyptus oil	Contains 70% eucalyptol; toxic
Gualacol	Nontoxic
Lavender oil	Contains coumarin
Menthol	Alcohol derived from various mint oils; toxic
Myristica oil	Nutmeg oil, used as a hallucinogen
Pennyroyal oil	Can be fatal
Peppermint oil	Contains 50% menthol; toxic
Thymol	Antiseptic
Turpentine oil	Toxic
Wintergreen oil	Contains methyl salicylate, toxic

petrolatum or castor oil and then perform gastric lavage, followed immediately by the administration of activated charcoal. Give milk or mineral oil to ease stomach irritation, give plenty of fluids and keep the victim warm and quiet. Convulsions can be controlled with diazepam or barbiturates.

See also CAMPHOR.

W

warfarin   A derivative of the anticoagulant coumarin, warfarin is used to interfere with the body's ability to clot blood. Many other drugs interact with warfarin, strengthening its action. Warfarin is also used as a rat poison.

Symptoms   An overdose seriously interferes with clotting ability, so a victim could bleed to death from a cut. Other symptoms include hemoptysis (a sudden hemorrhage of the larynx, trachea or lungs, bringing up bright red blood and a salty taste into the mouth); bloody stools; hemorrhages in various organs; widespread bruising; skin rash; fever; and vomiting. Kidney and liver damage are often fatal, and repeated daily doses of anticoagulants have led to death, even two weeks after the drug has been discontinued.

Treatment   Bed rest together with the administration of mephenytoin; therapy with vitamin K will normalize plasma proteins affecting blood clotting within 48 hours.

See also ANTICOAGULANTS; RAT POISON.

water arum   (*Calla palustris* L.) [Other names: female water dragon, water dragon, wild calla.] This small, water-loving plant has heart-shaped leaves on 10-inch stems, with thick clusters of red berries, and grows in swampy areas in parts of Canada, Colorado, Texas and Florida.

Poisonous part   The whole plant—especially the root—is toxic and contains calcium oxalate raphides.

Symptoms   Chewing any part of this plant almost immediately causes burning of the lips, mouth, tongue and throat; therefore, large amounts of the poison are rarely swallowed. Contact dermatitis is also common.

Treatment   Pain and swelling fade by themselves; keeping cold liquids or demulcents (such as milk) in the mouth may ease the pain. The oxalates are insoluble and do not cause systemic poisoning.

See also OXALATES.

water dropwort (*Oenanthe crocata*) [Other names: dead men's fingers, hemlock water dropwort.] This European perennial has been accidentally naturalized into marshy areas in Washington, D.C.; it grows to five feet tall with a bundle of long, thin roots containing latex, which turns to orange when exposed to air. Its white flowers appear in ball clusters. Its cousin, *O. sarmentosa*, grows on the west coast from southwest Alaska to central California and is not toxic.

Poisonous part   The entire plant is toxic, especially the roots, which contain an unsaturated aliphatic compound called oenanthotoxin, closely related to the poisons contained in water hemlocks.

Symptoms After ingesting the root, the victim experiences salivation followed within minutes by convulsions.

Treatment Assist breathing; convulsions respond to intravenous diazepam.

water lily See DEATH CAMAS.

water moccasin *(Agkistrodon piscivorus)* This aquatic pit viper (also known as "cottonmouth" because of the color of the inside of its mouth) is found throughout the southeastern United States and is particularly dangerous because it won't move away if disturbed. It does give a warning before striking, however; when bothered, it stands its ground and repeatedly opens its mouth wide, showing the white interior of its mouth. Unlike other water snakes, the water moccasin swims with its head well out of the water, and its eyes are not visible from directly above.

Usually more than three feet long, with a heavy body and broad head, it has a black, olive or brown body with dark crossbands. Young snakes have strong pattern colors and bright, yellow-tipped tails.

The water moccasin is never far from water and is found in swamps, lakes, rivers, irrigation ditches, canals, rice fields and clear, rocky mountain streams of the southeastern United States, from Virginia to the upper Florida Keys, west to Illinois, southern Missouri, Oklahoma and Texas. There is also an isolated population in north central Missouri.

While this snake may be seen sunning itself during the day, it is more often active at night, when it preys on frogs, fishes, other snakes and birds. The water moccasin is one of the very few snakes that feeds on carrion; in the wild, it has been seen eating fish heads and entrails thrown away by fishermen.

The shoes of the North American Indians—called moccasins—got their name from the skins of the water moccasins, from which they were made.

Symptoms The bite of the water moccasin is far more venomous than that of the copperhead and can be fatal. Its venom dissolves whatever tissue it touches, and the victim dies from bleeding to death within the body's tissues. The wound site darkens and oozes fluid while swelling spreads, with an extensive hemorrhage beneath the wound area and hemorrhages in the heart, lungs and other organs. Symptoms may begin within 10 minutes and alternate between hyperactivity and quietness, culminating in death because the veins that carry blood to and from the heart have been destroyed.

Treatment Antivenin is available.

See also MASSASAUGA; PIT VIPERS; RATTLESNAKE, CANEBRAKE; RATTLE-SNAKE, CASCABEL; RATTLESNAKE, EASTERN DIAMONDBACK; RATTLE-SNAKE, MEXICAN WEST COAST; RATTLESNAKE, RED DIAMONDBACK;

RATTLESNAKE, TIMBER; RATTLESNAKE, WESTERN DIAMONDBACK; RAT-
TLESNAKES; SIDEWINDER; SNAKES, POISONOUS; VIPER, GABOON; VIPER,
JUMPING; VIPER, MALAYAN PIT; VIPER, RUSSELL'S; VIPER, SAWSCALED;
VIPER, WAGLER'S PIT; VIPERS; WUTU.

weever fish *(Trachinus)* While most fish are not particularly poisonous,
the weever is another matter. Found in the British Isles and continental
Europe as far south as Morocco, it lives in water up to 160 feet deep,
although it is most at home in less than 20 feet of water with clean sand on
the bottom.

Weevers are particularly abundant in the Mediterranean Sea, where it is
possible to find several varieties, including the spotted weever *(Trachinus
araneus)* and the greater weever *(T. draco)*, which is sold for food throughout
Europe.

The fish lies buried just below the sand's surface, where it can sting anyone
who steps on it with its first dorsal fin and the spines on the gill covers.
Weevers hunt at night, catching and eating small crustaceans and fish, but
they do not use their poisonous spines for anything other than defense.

Symptoms While death is rare, the sting from the back fin spines of
the weaver fish causes an immediate severe stinging or throbbing pain,
which may stay at the site of the wound or spread throughout the body and
last for several hours or days. Pain can be so severe that the victim loses
consciousness. There may be redness and swelling at the site of the sting,
and the area may become numb.

Treatment There is no known antidote. Contact medical help
immediately; flush the wound with fresh or salt water and then soak the
affected area in hot water or put hot compresses on it. The water should be
very hot (122°F), so that the heat will deactivate the poison. Continue
applying hot water for 30 minutes to an hour. Folk wisdom also advocates
applying urine to the sting site.

white snakeroot *(Eupatorium rugosum* or *Ageratine altissima)* This eastern North American herb causes "milk sickness," which occurs after consuming dairy products from livestock poisoned by the plant. The milk of
cows that feed on the plant becomes poisoned by tremetol, an unstable
alcohol that occurs together with an incomplete resin acid.

Milk sickness was common in the United States from North Carolina to
the Midwest until the late 19th century, until milk processing methods
improved. In fact, it spread like wildfire throughout the western pioneers in
the early 19th century; Abraham Lincoln's mother Nancy Hanks Lincoln
died of the disease when he was only seven. In Dubois County, Indiana at
that time, the death toll was as high as one out of every two people.

Although physicians often confused the illness with other diseases and
had little time to publicize information about the strange new symptoms,

settlers realized that the sickness seemed to be associated with drinking milk from cows with "trembles," a disease they got by grazing on woodland plants. Soon, they had narrowed their suspicions to poison ivy and white snakeroot, and in 1821 the Tennessee legislature required fencing around certain forested areas to "prevent animals from eating an unknown vegetable, thereby imparting to their milk and flesh qualities highly deleterious."

The mystery was finally solved by two women: Anna Pierce, an Illinois doctor who had taken midwife and nursing courses at a time when women were not accepted in medical school, and a fugitive Shawnee woman. When milk sickness arrived in Anna Pierce's town, killing her mother and sister-in-law and sickening her father, Pierce made a series of critical observations about the disease and campaigned to prevent drinking milk during the summer.

Then she befriended a Shawnee woman known as Aunt Shawnee, a fugitive from an area of forced relocations of Native Americans, Aunt Shawnee showed Anna the white snakeroot, explaining that it caused both trembles and milk sickness and was used by the Shawnee as a treatment for snakebite. When Pierce fed snakeroot to a calf, it developed trembles; in 1928, scientists isolated tremetol, an alcohol similar to rotenone, from the white snakeroot; in 1987, scientists discovered that the constituents of snakeroot are not in themselves toxic but are converted to toxic substances by the body's own metabolic processes.

White snakeroot belongs to the family of medicinally active plants including joe-pye weed (used to cool fevers), boneset (similar to aspirin) and dog fennel (used to treat insect bites). It thrives in deep, rich, loamy soil that is often found in woods, and its toxicity varies from region to region, being least dangerous in the East and the South.

Today snakeroot only occasionally kills livestock, and milk sickness is almost nonexistent because of the improvement of eastern pastures, clearing of woodlots and the mixing of milk from many cows in commercial dairy operations. It remains a possibility for those who drink milk or eat cheese from their own cows, or who buy dairy products directly from farmers whose cows browse in rich woods.

Symptoms   Anyone who consumes milk or other dairy products from cows that have eaten the plant will become weak, nauseated, constipated, prostrate and delirious; between 10 and 25 percent of victims will die. There is a latency period ranging from several hours to several days. Milk sickness also causes a sickly sweet breath, a product of acidosis due to a buildup of lactic acid in the muscles, and thirst, with a burning sensation in the stomach.

Treatment   Treat liver damage and anuria; other treatment is symptomatic.

wintergreen, oil of   See SALICYLATES.

wintersweet *(Acokanthera oblongifolia)* This dense evergreen shrub is native of Africa, with large leathery leaves and fragrant flowers. The fruit resembles a reddish purple plum with two seeds. Wintersweet is often found as a hedge in California, Florida and Hawaii and as a greenhouse plant.

Poisonous part The fruit pulp is considered to be edible in some areas, although it contains small amount of a cardiac glycoside similar to ouabain; the seeds contain the greatest amount, although the toxin is distributed throughout the plant (including the wood).

Symptoms Mouth pain, nausea, vomiting, abdominal pain, cramps, diarrhea, and possible heart rhythm disturbances.

Treatment Induce vomiting or perform gastric lavage, followed by the administration of activated charcoal and saline cathartics. Electrocardiogram and potassium levels should be monitored. Phenytoin or atropine may be required to treat seizures.

wonder flower *(Ornithogalum thyrsoides)* A lily plant of Old World origin, the wonder flower is a common garden plant with an oniony bulb and grasslike leaves, with white flowers borne in a cluster on an upright spike; seeds are contained in a capsule.

Poisonous part All parts of the plant are poisonous, especially the bulb, and contain convallatoxin and convalloside, a digitalislike glycoside identical to those of the toxic lily of the valley.

Symptoms Digitalis glycoside toxicity has a variable latency period depending on how much was ingested; symptoms include pain in the mouth, nausea, vomiting, abdominal pain, cramps and diarrhea, with heart problems and rhythm disturbances.

Treatment Perform gastric lavage or induce vomiting, followed by the administration of activated charcoal and saline cathartics. Monitor electrocardiogram and blood levels of potassium, Administration of atropine or phenytoin may be required to prevent seizures.

See also LILY OF THE VALLEY.

wood alcohol See METHYL ALCOHOL.

wood preservative See PETROLEUM DISTILLATES.

wutu *(Bothrops alternus)* A dangerous South American pit viper and cousin of the fer-de-lance.

Symptoms With a bite from this viper, blood cannot coagulate and hemorrhages into muscles and the nervous system. There is local pain, bleeding from the bite, gums, nose, mouth and rectum. Shock and respiratory arrest are followed by death.

Treatment Antivenin is available.

See also ADDER; MASSASAUGA; PIT VIPERS; RATTLESNAKE, CANEBRAKE;

RATTLESNAKE, CASCABEL; RATTLESNAKE, EASTERN DIAMONDBACK; RATTLESNAKE, MEXICAN WEST COAST; RATTLESNAKE, RED DIAMONDBACK; RATTLESNAKE, TIMBER; RATTLESNAKE, WESTERN DIAMONDBACK; RATTLESNAKES; SIDEWINDER; SNAKES, POISONOUS; VIPER, GABOON; VIPER, JUMPING; VIPER, MALAYAN PIT; VIPER, RUSSELL'S; VIPER, SAWSCALED; VIPER, WAGLER'S PIT; WATER MOCCASIN; VIPERS.

Y

yew *(Taxus)* The poisonous yews include the English yew *(T. baccata)*, Pacific or western yew *(T. brevifolia)*, American yew or ground hemlock *(T. canadensis)* and Japanese yew *(T. cuspidata)*. Yew trees are found throughout the Northern Hemisphere and in ancient times were used as an abortifacient—often with deadly consequences. Survival after yew poisoning is uncommon.

Yew trees are evergreen, with reddish brown scaly bark and needlelike leaves; the hard seeds are green or black. English yew grows in the southern United States; western yew is found from Alaska south along British Columbia's coast, to western Washington, Oregon, California, Idaho and Montana. Canada yew is found in Pennsylvania, West Virginia to Iowa and north. Japanese yew is found throughout the northern temperate zone.

Poisonous part All parts of this evergreen shrub except the red berries contain the poison taxine—especially the wood bark, leaves and seeds. While the red berries are not poisonous, the small black seeds inside the berries may be toxic.

Symptoms Symptoms appear after about an hour and include dizziness, dry mouth, nausea, vomiting, diarrhea, stomach pain, difficulty in breathing, muscle weakness, slow heartbeat, rash and blue lips. Convulsions, shock and coma are followed by death from heart or respiratory failure. Chewing the needles can also cause an anaphylactic reaction. Ingestion of English or Japanese yew foliage may cause sudden death, as the alkaloid weakens and eventually stops the heart.

Treatment Gastric lavage followed by activated charcoal; a temporary pacemaker may be necessary; oxygen given as needed. Epinephrine is given in the treatment of anaphylactic shock.

yew, Canadian See YEW.

yew, English See YEW.

yew, Japanese See YEW.

yew, western See YEW.

APPENDIXES

Every effort has been made to ensure the accuracy of phone numbers, addresses, etc. in the following sections. However, certain errors are unavoidable because of the relocation of organizations and other factors. If you have difficulty tracking down any of the institutions or other groups listed here, contact one of the national associations (such as the National Center for Toxicological Research). Please refer to the beginning sections ("If You Must Call a Poison Control Center" and "Rescue and Treatment") for information on handling an emergency.

APPENDIX A
HOME TESTING KITS FOR
TOXIC SUBSTANCES

There are a range of kits consumers can purchase to test their homes for toxic environments. Some, like radon kits, have been on the market for many years; others (such as lead kits) are fairly new; still others—like many of the microwave test kits—have been taken off the market.

Asbestos
Contact your state department of environmental protection for a list of state-approved asbestos contractors.

Combination kits
DSK Safer Home Test Kit
Available through 22 mail-order catalogs, including:
Swanson's Health Shopper
(800) 437-4148
About $50 for a box containing Frandon lead test for 40 pieces, plus tests for radon, carbon monoxide, microwave and UV.

Formaldehyde
Air Technology Corp.
815 Harbour Way South
Richmond, CA

Dosimeter Corp.
6106 Interstate Circle
Cincinnati, OH 45242

AirCheck
Box 2000
Arden, NC 28704
(800) 247-2435

Eco-Check Healthy House Testing Kit
555 Fulton St., Suite 212
San Francisco, CA 94102
(800) 862-4325

John Banta's Healthful Hardware
PO Box 3217

Prescott, AZ 86302
(602) 445-8225

Hair test for metals and minerals
American Mineral Society
PO Box 35249
Phoenix, AZ 85069

AirCheck
Box 2000
Arden, NC 28704
(800) 247-2435

Lead
DSK Safer Home Test Kit
Available through 22 mail-order
catalogs, including:
Swanson's Health Shopper
(800) 437-4148

LaMotte Chemical Products Co.
PO Box 329
Chestertown, MD 21620
(800) 344-3100
Lead in solder ($36)

LeadCheck Swabs
HybriVet Systems
PO Box 1210
Framingham, MA 01701
(800) 262-LEAD
One glass vial and swab tests one or two pieces; two swabs, $5; four swabs, $10–11.

Leadcheck II
Michigan Ceramic Supplies
4048 Seventh St.

PO Box 342
Wyandotte, MI 48192
(313) 281-2300
A liquid test for lead in ceramics, paint and other substances. A kit costs $24.95 and can test up to 60 pieces.

AirCheck
Box 2000
Arden, NC 28704
(800) 247-2435

Eco-Check Healthy House Testing Kit
555 Fulton St., Suite 212
San Francisco, CA 94102
(800) 862-4325
Six LeadCheck swabs packaged together, $50; also sells separately LeadCheck and Frandon lead tests.

Enzone
110–19 15th Ave.
PO Box 92
College Point, NY 11356
(800) 448-0535

Misc.
AirCheck
Box 2000
Arden, NC 28704
(800) 247-2435
Tests for carbon monoxide, soil, paint, etc.

Eco-Check Healthy House Testing Kit
555 Fulton St., Suite 212
San Francisco, CA 94102
(800) 862-4325
Tests for carbon monoxide

Enzone
110–19 15th Ave.
PO Box 92
College Point, NY 11356
(800) 448-0535
Tests for carbon monoxide and a variety of other toxic substances.

John Banta's Healthful Hardware
PO Box 3217
Prescott, AZ 86302
(602) 445-8225
Tests for carbon monoxide, molds

RCI Environmental, Inc.
17772 Preston Rd.,
Suite 202

Dallas, TX 75252
(214) 250-6608
Kits to test for pesticides, volatile organic compounds, mold, dust mites.

Radon
AirCheck
Box 2000
Arden, NC 28704
(800) 247-2435

Eco-Check Healthy House Testing Kit
555 Fulton St., Suite 212
San Francisco, CA 94102
(800) 862-4325

John Banta's Healthful Hardware
PO Box 3217
Prescott, AZ 86302
(602) 445-8225

RCI Environmental, Inc.
17772 Preston Rd.,
Suite 202
Dallas, TX 75252
(214) 250-6608

Sulfites
For a portable kit to use in restaurants:
Center Laboratories
35 Channel Drive
Port Washington, NY 11050

Water quality
For a list of local testing labs, look in the yellow pages for state-certified water testing labs.
Or, for a mail-in kit, contact:
Water Test
33 S. Commercial St.
Manchester, NH 03130
(800) 426-8378

National Testing Labs
6151 Wilson Mills Rd.
Cleveland, OH 44143
(800) 458-3330

Suburban Water Testing Labs
4600 Kutztown Road
Temple, PA 19560
(800) 433-6595

John Banta's Healthful Hardware
PO Box 3217
Prescott, AZ 86302
(602) 445-8225

APPENDIX B
HOTLINES

Art materials
Arts and Crafts Theatre Safety
(212) 777-0062
Answers questions regarding toxic properties
of arts and crafts materials.

Food poisoning
Food Safety and Inspection Service Meat and
Poultry Hotline
(800) 535-4555
FDA-operated hotline answers questions
about meat and poultry contamination,
grading and proper storage procedures.

Pesticides
National Pesticide Telecommunications
Network
(800) 858-7378
(806) 743-3091 in Texas
Responds to nonemergency questions
concerning the effects of pesticides, toxicology
and symptoms, environmental effects, waste
disposal and cleanup and safe use of pesticides.
The National Pesticide Telecommunications
Network is a service of the Environmental
Protection Agency and Texas Tech University.

Pet poisoning
National Animal Poison Control Center
(900) 680-0000 ($2.95 per minute)
(800) 548-2423 ($30 per call)
A 24-hour-a-day emergency center dealing
with pet poisons, staffed by veterinary health
specialists.

Toxic chemicals
Community Right to Know
(800) 535-0202
EPA group answers questions about chemical
accidents, how to get more information on
toxic chemical releases in your community.

RCRA Superfund Hotline
(800) 424-9346
Answers questions and provides
documentation related to Superfund
regulations and cleanup operations. Call
between 8:30 A.M. and 4:30 P.M. Eastern
Standard Time.

Toxic Substances Hotline
(202) 554-1404; Fax (202) 554-5603
EPA group answers questions about toxic
substances.

APPENDIX C
NEWSLETTERS

Air/Water Pollution Report or Clean
  Water Report
BPI
951 Pershing Dr.
Silver Spring, MD 20910
(301) 587-6300
An environmental newsletter covering environmental legislation, regulations and litigation from Washington, with special reports on state and local activities, pollution control industry news and research and development.

CLIS Lifelines
National Research Council
2010 Constitution Ave. NW
Washington, DC 20418
(202) 334-2000
Covers environmental health, nutrition, radiation effects and toxicology.

Hazardous Materials Control Research
  Institute FOCUS
Hazardous Materials Research Institute
7237 Hanover Parkway
Greenbelt, MD 20770
(301) 982-9500
Covers control, management and cleanup of hazardous waste and hazardous chemicals in the environment.

Hazardous Substances Advisor
J. J. Keller and Associates, Inc.
145 West Wisconsin Ave.
Neenah, WI 54956
(414) 722-2848
Monthly information report on congressional and regulatory activity to control, monitor or eliminate hazards created by hazardous and toxic substances.

Hazchem Alert
VNR Information Services
115 Fifth Ave.

New York, NY 10003
(212) 254-3232
Information from more than 100 domestic and international sources is monitored to produce this biweekly newsletter on chemical hazards.

Inside EPA Weekly Report
Inside Washington Publishers
PO Box 7167
Ben Franklin Station
Washington, DC 20044
(202) 296-2925
Reports on policy and news of the EPA.

Pesticide and Toxic Chemical News
Food Chemical News
1101 Pennsylvania Ave. SE
Washington, DC 20003
(202) 544-1980
Weekly reports on hazardous wastes, pesticides, toxic substances and general issues of regulation and legislation.

Toxic Exposure Bulletin
Thompson Publishing Group
1725 K St. NW, Suite 200
Washington, DC 20006
(202) 872-1766 or (800) 424-2959
Current information on federal, state and community notice and disclosure requirements, community emergency response programs and needs, industry emergency response programs, liability and litigation.

World Environment Report
BPI
951 Pershing Dr.
Silver Spring, MD 20910
(301) 587-6300
Reports on environmental problems and solutions in other countries, offering coverage of international air and water pollution control, waste management and toxic substances, energy and natural resources and other environmental protection issues.

APPENDIX D
ORGANIZATIONS

Academy of Toxicological Sciences
  Dept. of Pharmacology and
  Toxicology
Medical College of Virginia
Box 613
Richmond, VA 23298
(804) 786-0329
Recognizes and certifies currently active tox-icologists who have demonstrated certain lev-els of knowledge and experience in toxicology.

American Academy of Clinical
  Toxicology
(913) 532-4334
Kansas State University
Comparative Toxicology Laboratories
Manhattan, KS 66506

American Academy of Environmental
  Medicine
PO Box 16106
Denver, CO 80216
(303) 622-9755; Fax (303) 622-4224
Can provide more information about envi-ronmental irritants.

American Academy of Veterinary and
  Comparative Toxicology
College of Veterinary Medicine
  University of Tennessee
Box 1071
Knoxville, TN 39701
(615) 546-9243
Fosters and encourages education, training and research in veterinary toxicology. Pub-lishes *Veterinary and Human Toxicology.*

American Association of Poison Control
  Centers
Arizona Poison and Drug Information Center
Health Sciences Center, Rm. 3204K
1501 N. Campbell
Tucson, AZ 85725
(602) 626-7899
Procures information on the ingredients and

potential acute toxicity of substances that may cause accidental poisonings and establishes standards for poison information and control centers.

American Board of Toxicology
PO Box 76422
Washington, DC 20003
(202) 544-5533
Certifies toxicologists and encourages the study of toxicology, establishes standards for the profession and administers tests for the implementation of these standards.

American College of Toxicology
9650 Rockville Pike
Bethesda, MD 20814
(301) 571-1840
Membership includes those interested in tox-icology or related fields; disseminates infor-mation, provides discussions and publishes journals and newsletters.

Chemical Industry Institute of Toxicology
PO Box 12137
Research Triangle Park, NC 27709
(919) 541-2070
A nonprofit toxicological research institute supported by 33 chemical companies to seek new knowledge about the toxicity and mech-anisms of toxicity of basic industrial chemicals and to train scientists in toxicology.

Citizens' Clearinghouse for Hazardous
  Wastes
PO Box 926
Arlington, VA 22216
(703) 237-2249
A nonprofit organization providing informa-tion to manage chemical waste problems.

Conservation Foundation
1250 24th St. NW
Washington, DC 20037
(202) 429-5660
Nonprofit organization specializing in re-

search on environmental and resource issues; its Toxic Substances Project advises the EPA on implementing the Toxic Substances Control Act and helps the agency inform the public about programs to control chemical hazards.

Genetic Toxicology Association
1725 N St. NW
Washington, DC 20036
Members exchange information related to recent developments in genetic toxicology.

Hazardous Materials Control Research
  Institute
7237 Hanover Pkwy
Greenbelt, MD 20770-3602
(301) 982-9500
This institute is interested in hazardous and toxic materials and their control, risk assessment, spills and uncontrolled hazardous waste sites.

National Animal Poison Control Center
2001 S. Lincoln St, Urbana, IL, 61801
(900) 680-0000 ($2.95 per minute)
(800) 548-2423 ($30 per call)
A 24-hour-a-day emergency center dealing with pet poisons, staffed by veterinary health specialists.

National Pesticide Telecommunications
  Network
Texas Tech University Health Sciences
  Center
School of Medicine
Dept. of Preventive Medicine
4th and Indiana
Lubbock, TX 79430
(806) 743-3096; (800) 858-7378
Serves as information clearinghouse on pesticides and poisonings.

Society of Toxicology
1133 15th St. NW, Suite 620
Washington, DC 20005
(202) 293-5935
Established in 1961, this group is a professional organization of scientists from academic institutions, government and industry. The society promotes information about toxicology and has a strong commitment to education in this field.

Toxicology Information Center
National Academy of Science
2600 Virginia Ave.

Washington, DC 20418
(202) 334-2000

Toxicology Information Program
Division of Specialized Information
  Services
National Library of Medicine
8600 Rockville Pike
Bethesda, MD 20209
(301) 496-6095

Toxicology Information Response Center
PO Box X
Bldg. 2024, Rm. 53
Oak Ridge, TN 37830

Women's Occupational Health
  Resource Center
School of Public Health
Columbia University
600 West 168 St.
New York, NY 10032
(718) 857-7669
Collects and disseminates information on occupational health and safety issues confronting women.

GOVERNMENTAL ORGANIZATIONS

Agency for Toxic Substances and
  Disease Registry
1600 Clinton Road NE
Atlanta, GA 30333
(404) 452-4113
An operating agency within the Public Health Service since 1983 (as required by the Comprehensive Environmental Response, Compensation and Liability Act of 1980). The agency, in collaboration with other agencies, collects, analyzes and provides information about human exposure to toxic or hazardous substances, establishes registries for long-term follow-up and is involved in a wide range of programs designed to protect the public health and workers.

Centers for Disease Control
1600 Clinton Road NE
Atlanta, GA 30333
(404) 639-3311
This agency within the Public Health Service, among its many activities, develops programs to deal with environmental health problems

(including responding to environmental, chemical and radiation emergencies).

Chemical Hazard Response
   Information System
U.S. Coast Guard
Office of Marine Safety
2100 Second St. SW
Washington, DC 20593
(202) 267-2200
Using a hazard assessment computer system, this organization provides information during emergencies involving the water transport of hazardous chemicals.

Consumer Product Safety Commission
5401 Westbard Ave.
Bethesda, MD 20816
(301) 504-0580; hotline (800) 638-CPSC
Among other responsibilities, the CPSC supports the System for Tracking the Inventory of Chemicals, a computerized data base and management tool used to review and select chemical substances that may pose a chronic chemical hazard to consumers from their presence in consumer products.

Division of Poison Prevention and
   Scientific Coordination
(Same as Consumer Product Safety Commission)

Council on Environmental Quality
722 Jackson Place NW
Washington, DC 20006
(202) 395-5750
Established by the National Environmental Policy Act of 1969 to recommend national policies to promote the improvement of the quality of the environment.

Department of Agriculture
14th St. and Independence Ave. SW
Washington, DC 20250
(202) 720-8732
USDA has a wide range of responsibilities and is involved in several areas of toxicology. Its programs include the Food Safety and Inspection Service, the Animal and Plant Health Inspection Service, the Food Quality Assurance Program and the Food and Nutrition Service. USDA also encourages the safe use of pesticides.

Toxicology and Biological Constituents
   Research Unit
PO Box 5677

Athens, GA 30613
(706) 546-3158
Investigates the toxicological and pharmacological properties of natural toxicants.

Veterinary Toxicology and Entomology
   Research Laboratory
PO Drawer GE
F&B Rd.
College Station, TX 77841
(409) 260-9372
Protects livestock and poultry from toxic effects of pesticides and conducts basic and applied research.

Department of Energy
1000 Independence Ave. SW
Washington, DC 20585
(202) 727-1800
The Office of Health and Environmental Research conducts major research to identify the health and environmental problems associated with energy technologies.

Department of the Interior
Fish and Wildlife Service
18th and C Sts. NW
Washington, DC 20240
(202) 208-5634
This agency conserves and protects fish and wildlife; activities include biological monitoring and the surveillance of pesticides, heavy metals and thermal pollution, etc.

Department of Transportation
400 Seventh St.
Washington, DC 20590
(202) 366-4000
DOT regulates the transportation of hazardous materials in commerce and publishes the *Emergency Response Guidebook*, which provides direction in the actions required to handle hazardous incidents.

Environmental Protection Agency
401 M St. SW
Washington, DC 20460
(202) 260-7400 (air and radiation programs)
5700 (water programs)
4610 (solid waste and emergency response programs)
2902 (pesticides and toxic substances program)
7676 (research and development)
The EPA is the principal federal agency responsible for identifying and controlling environmental pollutants of air and water, solid

waste, pesticides, toxic substances, radiation and energy.

Food and Drug Administration
5600 Fishers Lane
Rockville, MD 20857
(301) 443-3380
The FDA is the primary consumer health protection agency of the federal government responsible for ensuring that food is safe; biological products (such as vaccines, human and vet drugs and medical devices) are safe; cosmetics are safe; use of radiological products doesn't result in unsafe exposure to radiation. Toxicology research is designed to provide data to strengthen the scientific base for assessing risk or safety. The Poisoning Surveillance and Epidemiology Branch of the Center for Drugs and Biologics within the FDA assists poison control centers throughout the country and has developed a standard for reporting poisoning incidents. It also stimulates research and development of antidotes.

Poisoning Surveillance and
   Epidemiology Branch
5600 Fishers Lane
Rockville, MD 20857
(301) 443-6260

Hazardous Materials Technical Center
PO Box 8168
Rockville, MD 20856
Established in 1982, this center provides the most up-to-date information and regulations for those involved with the handling, storage, transportation and disposal of hazardous substances. It operates its own database and prepares handbooks, monographs and reports.

National Center for Toxicological Research
National Institute of Environmental
   Health Sciences
PO Box 12233
Research Triangle Park, NC 27709
(919) 541-3212
This agency has the broadest responsibility to

support research and training in the effects of chemical environmental agents on human health.

National Institute of Neurological and
   Communicative Disorders and Stroke
9000 Rockville Pike
Bethesda, MD 20205
(800) 352-9424
Among its wide research interests are the drug-induced adverse reactions and neurotoxic substances.

Toxicology Information Program
8600 Rockville Pike
Bethesda, MD 20209
(301) 496-1131
The TIP was created in 1967; its objectives include managing computer-based toxicology data banks from scientific literature and the files of collaborating industrial, academic and governmental agencies and providing toxicology information services for the scientific community. TIP provides information and publications to the public. It developed a range of online services available on the library's MEDLARS system: CHEMLINE, TOXLINE, RTECS and DIRLINE. Also available on the TOXNET system are HSDB and CCRIS.

Natural Toxins Research Center
Food and Drug Administration
4928 Elysian Fields Ave.
New Orleans, LA 70122
(504) 589-2471
Develops methods to be used to analyze natural toxins and poisons; research also involves determination of mycotoxins and other natural poisons in food.

Seafood Products Research Center
5009 Federal Office Building
Seattle, WA 98174
(206) 442-5302
Researches the chemical and microbiological indexes of decomposition in seafood products and determines potentially hazardous contamination in seafood.

APPENDIX E
POISON EDUCATION AND
INFORMATION MATERIALS

1. CHILDREN AND POISONING

Your Child and Household Safety
Monograph by poison expert and pediatrician Jay Arena, M.D., discussing need to protect children from harmful substances. 75 cents each; special rate is available for orders of 1,000 or more.

Chemical Specialties Manufacturers
  Association, Inc.
1001 Connecticut Ave. NW, Suite 1120
Washington, DC 20036

We Want You to Know About Preventing Childhood Poisonings
Leaflet explaining some of the hazards of accidental poisonings and how to prevent them; how to get help if a child is poisoned. Available in English and Spanish. Limited quantities available.

U.S. Food and Drug Administration
HFE-88
5600 Fishers Lane
Rockville, MD 20857

"Dear Mom and Dad": Lead Poisoning Prevention
Pamphlet explaining dangers of old lead paint; Spanish editions available. 1–99 copies, 12 cents each.

National Paint and Coatings Association
1500 Rhode Island Ave. NW
Washington, DC 20005

Common Poisonous and Injurious Plants
Information on emergency care of a child who has eaten a plant; $3.25 per copy. Stock #017-012-00196-0.

Superintendent of Documents

U.S. Government Printing Office
Washington, DC 20402

Home Safe Home
Tips for parents on protecting young children in the environment; English or Spanish. Up to 100 copies free.

The Soap and Detergent Association
475 Park Ave. South at 32d St.
New York, NY 10016

Perils of Pip—Preventing Poisoning
Comic book about an elephant who teaches poison prevention. $2.75 for single copies; stock #052-011-00176-7.

Superintendent of Documents
U.S. Government Printing Office
Washington, DC 20402

Legend of Happy the Poison Prevention Dog
Brochure introducing the SIOP Poison Prevention Program to kids. 1–10 copies, 50 cents each.

Happy's Poison Prevention Activity Book
A 44-page children's activity book to teach children to avoid items that have a SIOP sticker. 1–10 copies, $1 each.

Order either brochure from:
Human Action for Poison Prevention in
  Youth
236 E. Front St.
Bloomington, IN 61701

The Poison Safety Game
Game for older elementary children to help them protect younger siblings from poisoning. Free.

Food and Drug Administration
HFE-88

5600 Fishers Lane
Rockville, MD 20857

***A Guide to Teaching Poison Prevention in
Kindergarten and Primary Grades***
A 68-page manual with games, pictures and
work sheets designed to help teach poison
prevention to children. Single copy $4.75.
Stock #052-003-00257-4.

Superintendent of Documents
U.S. Government Printing Office
Washington, DC 20402
(202) 783-3238

***Poison Awareness: Resource Book for
Teachers, Grades 7–9***
Activities and guide for teaching seventh
through ninth grades about poison prevention,
especially the use, storage and disposal of four
types of poisons. Stock # 052-011-00201-1,
single copy $5.

Superintendent of Documents
U.S. Government Printing Office
Washington, DC 20402
(202) 783-3238

2. SAFE MEDICINE USE

The Medicines Your Doctor Prescribes
Tips on ensuring safe use of prescribed drugs,
up to 50 copies free.

Pharmaceutical Manufacturers Association
1155 15th St. NW
Washington, DC 20005

Medicine Labels and You
Large-print brochure explaining labels of
nonprescription medicines and how to use
them safely. Free.

The Proprietary Association
Public Affairs
1700 Pennsylvania Ave. NW
Washington, DC 20006

Ten Guides to Proper Medicine Use
Brochure describing steps to follow when
buying and taking drugs. One copy free;
larger quantities 50 cents each.

Council on Family Health
420 Lexington Ave.
New York, NY 10017

Danger Lurks
Medicine cabinet chart with information on

what to do in case of accidental poisoning. Up
to 99 copies, $1 each.

American Medical Association
Order Dept.
PO Box 821
Monroe, WI 53566

Medicines and How to Use Them
Explains the function and need of
prescriptions, with 10 tips on the safe way to
take medicine. Up to 99 copies, 30 cents
each; 100–499, 20 cents each; 500 or more,
18 cents each.

American Medical Association
Order Dept.
PO Box 821
Monroe, WI 53566

Tips Against Tampering
Tips to protect yourself against criminal
tampering with over-the-counter
medicine. Free.

The Proprietary Association
Public Affairs
1700 Pennsylvania Ave. NW
Washington, DC 20006

3. HOME SAFETY AND POISONS

Poison Perils in the Home
12-page booklet explaining everyday
household poisons that might be toxic. Less
than 50, free.

National Safety Council
444 N. Michigan Ave.
Chicago, IL 60611

Solid and Liquid Poisons
Data sheet (six pages) with practical
information on poisons in and around the
home, highlighting special dangers to
children. 10–99, 38 cents each.

National Safety Council
444 N. Michigan Ave.
Chicago, IL 60611

Safe Use of Aerosols Around the House
Information on safe use and storage of
these products, how they work and how to

understand directions and cautions. Up to 10 copies free.

Chemical Specialties Manufacturers
  Association
1001 Connecticut Ave. NW
Suite 1120
Washington, DC 20036

Formaldehyde: Everything You Wanted to Know but Were Afraid to Ask
Send a self-addressed stamped envelope for a copy of this booklet.

Consumer Federation of America
1424 16th St. NW, Suite 604
Washington, DC 20036

For information on wood preservatives, mildewcides:
National Pesticides Telecommunications
  Network
Texas Tech Pesticide Laboratory
PO Box 2031
San Benito, TX 78586

The Inside Story: A Guide to Indoor Air Quality (Item 433)
A 32-page booklet; costs 50 cents. Include booklet name and item number.

R. Woods
Consumer Information Center—2A
PO Box 100
Pueblo, CO 81002

4. FIRST AID FOR POISONING

General Approach to the Emergency Management of Poisonings
Large wall chart displaying poisoning information designed for medical, nursing and allied health personnel. $5 per copy.

American College of Emergency Physicians
PO Box 61911
Dallas, TX 75261

First Aid for Poisoning
Three-fold card on first aid instructions for poisoning. Up to 200 free.

Secretary, Poison Prevention Week Council
PO Box 1543
Washington, DC 20013

SIOP's Poison First Aid Chart
Colored chart (9 x 12) listing various

categories of poisons with general first aid instructions. 1–10 copies, 50 cents each.

Human Action for Poison Prevention in
  Youth
236 E. Front St.
Bloomington, IL 61701

First Aid for Poisoning
A 16-page booklet in emergency care techniques written by authorized American Red Cross first aid instructors. ARC stock #32081; also, a two-color flyer/poster, ARC stock #320800.

Contact local Red Cross chapter.

Emergency Action for Poisoning
Card outlining first aid steps for poisoning, up to five copies free.

American Association of Poison Control
  Centers
University of California Medical Center
Regional Poison Center
225 Dickinson St.
San Diego, CA 92103

First Aid for Poisoning Chart
An 11 x 17 chart with first aid for poisoning. Singe copy free.

American Academy of Pediatrics
Publication Dept.
PO Box 927
Elk Grove Village, IN 60007

5. FOOD POISONING

Who, Why, When and Where of Food Poisons
Chart identifying more common sources of food poisoning and how to prevent food contamination. Free in single quantities.

Food and Drug Administration
HFE-88
5600 Fishers Lane
Rockville, MD 20857

6. SAFE USE OF PESTICIDES

Guide to Safe Pest Management Around the House
Available for $3.90 postpaid.

Distribution Center
7 Research Park

Cornell University
Ithaca, NY 14850

For information on insecticides:

National Pesticides Telecommunications
  Network
Texas Tech Pesticide Laboratory
PO Box 2031
San Benito, TX 78586

Pesticide information available from:

County Agent
U.S. Department of Agriculture
  Extension Service
(check local phone directory for address)
or
Regional Office
U.S. Environmental Protection Agency
(check local phone directory for address)

For information on pesticide residue on
  food:

Regional Office
Food and Drug Administration
(check local phone directory for address)

7. MISCELLANEOUS POISON INFORMATION

For information on toxins:

Chemtrec
Chemical Manufacturers Assoc.
Chemical Referral Center
2501 M St. NW

Washington, DC 20037
(800) 262-8200

National Campaign Against Toxic
  Hazards
Henry S. Cole
317 Pennsylvania Ave. SE
Washington, DC 20003
Offers copies of EPA study providing
complete state-by-state listing of accidents
and toxic spills available for $25.

Toxic Substances Information Line
(800) 648-6732

Plants That Poison
Illustrated chart of common poisonous plants
indicating size, toxic parts and symptoms of
poisoning. Also has information on
preventing plant poisoning and emergency
treatment. Single copy free with SASE.

The Kalamazoo Poison Prevention Council
PO Box 2261
Kalamazoo, MI 49003

National Poison Prevention Week Packet
Annually the third week in March; folder has
list of available material, fact sheet, state and
local officials' proclamations, other
promotional material.

Secretary
Poison Prevention Week Council
PO Box 1543
Washington, DC 20013

APPENDIX F
POISONS BY SYMPTOM

Poisons are listed here by symptom and grouped by body organ or major symptom category. It is important to understand that most poisons cause several symptoms, which can vary in severity depending on the type of poison ingested.

BLOOD

Anemia Dilantin, pathalene, rattlesnake, trinitrotoluene

Bleeding aspirin, atophan, Depakene, warfarin

Blood sugar—high Lasix, Vacor

Blood sugar—low akee, *Amanita* mushroom, Dilantin, Inderal, insulin, phosphorus

Hemorrhage adder, aspirin, atophan, castor bean, chlordane, cinchona bark, cottonmouth, Depakene, fer-de-lance, isopropanol, paternoster pea, potassium permanganate, rhubarb, savin, Vacor, warfarin

Low red blood count carbon monoxide, ethinamate, warfarin

BRAIN

Coma akee, aldrin, amphetamines, aniline, antimony, arsenic, aspirin, atropine, barbiturates, belladonna, boric acid, bromates, bryony, cantharidin, cassava, castor bean, Catapres, celandine, chloral hydrate, cinchona bark, cinchophen, cocaine, codeine, columbine, corn cockle, *Cortinarius* mushroom, croton oil, daphne, death camas, dieldrin, Elavil, epinephrine, ergot, ethyl alcohol, *Gyromitra* mushroom, Haldol, heroin, hydrogen sulfide, Inderal, Indian tobacco, insulin, isopropanol, jimsonweed, lead, lithium, Lomotil, LSD, mandrake, marijuana, morphine, nicotine, nitroglycerin, opium, panther mushroom, paral, paternoster pea, PCP, Percodan, Permitil, petroleum distillates, phenol, potato, procaine, rhododendron, savin, silver nitrate, Sinequan, sodium fluoroacetate, Stelazine, tetrachloroethane, Thorazine, toxaphene, Vacor, Valium, yew

Headache Aldomet, aldrin, aniline, arsenic, barbiturates, benzene, bronchial tube relaxers, cadmium, camphor, carbon monoxide, corn cockle, DDT, dieldrin, dyphylline, elderberry, ergot, ethylene chlorohydrin, foxglove, galerina mushrooms, hydrogen sulfide, Inderal, jimsonweed, Lasix, lily of the valley, malathion, methyl alcohol, Minipress, naphthalene, nicotine, nitroglycerin, nitrous oxide, panther mushroom, parathion, persantine, potato, Preludin, quinidine, stibine, Tagamet, TEPP, tetrachloroethane, Thyrolar, trichloroethane, yellow jessamine

Swelling aspirin, dimethyl sulfate, methanol, nitrous oxide, potato

COLLAPSE

adder, ammonia, bromates, cantharidin, castor bean, cationic detergents, chloramine-T, cinchona bark, cottonmouth, ethylene chlorohydrin, formaldehyde, Haldol, Indian tobacco, ipecac, lead, narcissus, nicotine, nitroglycerin, privet, procaine, silver nitrate, stingray, Vacor

CONVULSIONS/SEIZURES

akee, aldrin, amphetamines, aniline, arsenic, aspirin, atropine, barium, belladonna, benzene, benzene hexachloride, betel nut seed, boric acid, bromates, bronchial tube relaxers, bryony, caffeine, calcium, camphor, cassava, castor bean, cationic detergents, cinchophen, cobra, cocaine, columbine, *Cortinarius* mushroom, cyanide, daphne, DDT, dieldrin, dyphylline, Elavil, elderberry, endrin, epinephrine, ethyl alcohol, fool's parsley, grounsel, *Gyromitra* mushroom, hydrangea, Inderal, Indian tobacco, ipecac, jimsonweed, oleander, Lomotil, LSD, meadow saffron, monkshood, monoamine oxidase (MAO) inhibitors, moonseed, mountain laurel, narcissus, nicotine, panther mushroom, parathion, paternoster pea, PCP, Permitil, Phenergan, physostigmine, pokeweed, potato, procainamide, procaine, pyrethrum, quaalude, Ritalin, rhododendron, rotenone, scorpionfish, scorpions, silver nitrate, sodium fluoroacetate, sodium thiocyanate, spindle tree, Stelazine, stingray, stonefish, strychnine, tansy, TEPP, Thorazine, toxaphene, turpentine, water hemlock, yellow jessamine, yew

DEHYDRATION

Amanita mushroom, antimony, aspirin, laxatives, opium

DIZZINESS/VERTIGO

acid, Aldomet, aldrin, amphetamines, aniline, arsenic, aspirin, baneberry, Barbados nut, barbiturates, benzene, bloodroot, bronchial tube relaxers, camphor, carbon tetrachloride, chloral hydrate, codeine, *Cortinarius* mushroom, dieldrin, Dilantin, elderberry, ethylene chlorohydrin, fly agaric, geography cone, Gila monster, hydrogen sulfide, jimsonweed, Lasix, methanol, monkshood, morphine, nicotine, nitroglycerin, Norflex, panther mushroom, Percodan, Persantine, petroleum distillates, Phenergan, phenol, Preludin, procaine, propane, quinidine, Sinequan, sodium fluoroacetate, stingray, Tagamet, Thorazine, toxaphene, trichloroethane, turpentine, Vacor, Valium

EMOTIONAL PROBLEMS

Aggression   atropine, belladonna, PCP, Preludin

Anxiety   amphetamines, barium, bronchial tube relaxers, camphor, carbon monoxide, mercury, Minipress, PCP, potassium, sodium fluoroacetate, Thyrolar, water hemlock, yellow jessamine

Confusion   amphetamines, aniline, atropine, barbiturates, carbon monoxide, carbon tetrachloride, chloral hydrate, DDT, Dilantin, endrin, Inderal, lithium, nicotine, opium, Preludin, sodium thiocyanate, Tagamet, Tylenol

Delirium   atropine, benzene, brown recluse spider, cinchophen, corn cockle, ethylene chlorohydrin, foxglove, henbane, horse chestnut, Inderal, iodine, jimsonweed, lead, meadow saffron, panther mushroom, Tagamet, tetrachlorethane, Vacor, white snakeroot

Depression   amphetamines, mountain laurel

Euphoria   amphetamines, benzene, Halcion, heroin, LSD, marijuana, nitrous oxide, opium, Preludin

Excitement   benzene, boric acid, cinchona bark, codeine, corn cockle, cottonmouth, DDT, dieldrin, endrin, epinephrine, ethylene chlorohydrin, insulin, jimsonweed, LSD, morphine, naphthalene, phenol, procaine, pyrethrum, Stelazine, Valium, yellow jessamine, yew

Hallucinations   amphetamines, atropine, belladonna, betel nut seed, bronchial tube relaxers, cocaine, Elavil, ethyl alcohol, Haldol, Inderal, lily of the valley, LSD, marijuana, mercury, PCP, Preludin, toxaphene, Valium

Hyperactivity   cocaine, cottonmouth, PCP, Preludin, Thyrolar

Irritability   barbiturates, carbon monoxide, cottonmouth, dieldrin, lily of the valley, propane

Psychosis   atropine, camphor, cocaine, Depakene, Dilantin, epinephrine, ergot, ethyl alcohol, Halcion, Haldol, LSD, marijuana, mercury, Preludin

Restlessness   amphetamines, aspirin, black widow spider, heroin, horse chestnut, LSD, Preludin, water hemlock

EYES

Dilation   atropine, belladonna, bloodroot, cocaine, Elavil, epinephrine, ethyl alcohol, heroin, horse chestnut, Indian tobacco, jimsonweed, lily of the valley, marijuana, parathion, tansy, water hemlock, yellow jessamine, yew

Pinpoint pupils   morphine, opium, physostigmine, TEPP

Reddening   dimethyl sulfate, hydrogen sulfide, marijuana

Tearing   dimethyl sulfate, fly agaric, formaldehyde, malathion, mountain laurel, panther mushroom, rhododendron, TEPP

GASTROINTESTINAL TRACT

Abdominal pain   alkalies, *Amanita* mushroom, ammonia, arsenic, aspirin, baneberry, barium, bloodroot, bromates, cantharidin, carbon tetrachloride, cassava, cinchophen, cocaine, colocynth, corn cockle, daphne, fool's parsley, formaldehyde, hydrangea, iodine, isopropanol, jellyfish, lead, lily of the valley, meadow saffron, mercury, methanol, Minipress, mountain laurel, paraquat, parathion, Portuguese man-of-war, potato, privet, rhubarb, rotenone, scorpions, spindle tree, stibine, stingray, tetrachloroethane, Thyrolar, turpentine, Vacor, water hemlock, yew

Appetite loss   Preludin

Bloating   Barbados nut

Constipation   opium, Percodan, Vacor, white snakeroot

Cramps   arsenic, castor bean, colocynth, elderberry, heroin, panther mushroom, pokeweed, scorpions, stingray, TEPP

Diarrhea (bloody)   acid, *Amanita* mushroom, antimony, baneberry, colocynth, croton oil, daphne, fool's parsley, meadow saffron, mercury, moonseed, oleander, tetrachloroethane, warfarin

Diarrhea   alkalies, amphetamines, arsenic, Barbados nut, barium, benzene hexachloride, betel nut seed, black hellebore, boric acid, bromates, bryony, cadmium, cantharidin, cinchophen, digitoxin, false hellebore, fly agaric, formaldehyde, foxglove, *Gyromitra* mushroom, hemlock, horse chestnut, Inderal, iodine, lead, malathion, mandrake, Minipress, naphthalene, nicotine, panther mushroom, paraquat, parathion, paternoster pea, phosphorus, poinsettia, pokeweed, potato, privet, pyrethrum, quinidine, rhododendron, silver nitrate, spindle tree, Tagamet, TEPP, Thyrolar, turpentine, water hemlock, yew

Nausea   akee, aldrin, *Amanita* mushroom, amphetamines, antimony, arsenic, baneberry, barium, benzene, black locust, black widow spider, botulism, brown recluse spider, bryony, cadmium, camphor, cantharidin, carbon monoxide, carbon tetrachloride, cassava, castor bean, Catapres, cationic detergents, celandine, cinchona bark, cobra, columbine, corn cockle, *Cortinarius* mushroom, daphne, Depakene, dieldrin, digitoxin, dyphylline, elderberry, endrin, epinephrine, ergot, ethyl alcohol, ethylene chlorohydrin, false hellebore, fly agaric, foxglove, Gila monster, grounsel, Halcion, hydrangea, hydrogen sulfide, Inderal, Indian tobacco, insulin, ipecac, isopropanol, larkspur, Lasix, lily of the valley, malathion, mercury, methanol, Minipress, monkshood, monoamine oxidase (MAO) inhibitors, morphine, mountain laurel, naphthalene, narcissus, nicotine, Norflex, opium, panther mushroom, parathion, paternoster pea, Percodan, Permitil, Persantine, phosphorus, pokeweed, privet, pyrethrum, quaalude, quinidine, rattlesnake, Reglan, rhododendron, rhubarb, Ritalin, rotenone, shellfish poisoning, stibine, stingray, Talwin, tanghin, tetrachloroethane, trichloroethane, trinitrotoluene, turpentine, Tylenol, Vacor, water hemlock, white snakeroot

Stool (dark) lead

Vomiting acid, akee, aldrin, alkalies, *Amanita* mushroom, ammonia, amphetamines, antimony, arsenic, atophan, baneberry, Barbados nut, barium, benzene, benzene hexachloride, betel nut seed, black locust, black widow spider, bloodroot, blue ringed octopus, boric acid, bromates, bronchial tube relaxers, brown recluse spider, bryony, cadmium, caffeine, camphor, cantharidin, carbon tetrachloride, cassava, castor bean, celandine, cinchona bark, cocaine, columbine, *Cortinarius* mushroom, croton oil, daphne, DDT, dieldrin, digitoxin, dog mercury, dyphylline, epinephrine, ergot, ethyl alcohol, ethylene chlorohydrin, false hellebore, formaldehyde, foxglove, grounsel, *Gyromitras* mushroom, Halcion, hemlock, horse chestnut, Inderal, Indian tobacco, insulin, iodine, ipecac, larkspur, Lasix, lead, lily of the valley, malathion, mandrake, meadow saffron, mercury, Minipress, monkshood, monoamine oxidase (MAO) inhibitors, mountain laurel, naphthalene, narcissus, nicotine, nitroglycerine, Norflex, oleander, opium, paraquat, Percodan petroleum distillates, phosphorus, physostigmine, poinsettia, pokeweed, potato, privet, pyrethrum, quaalude, rattlesnake, rhododendron, rhubarb, Ritalin, rotenone, savin, shellfish poisoning, silver nitrate, sodium fluoroacetate, spindle tree, stingray, Tanghin, TEPP, toxaphene, turpentine, Tylenol, Vacor, water hemlock, white snakeroot, yew

GENITOURINARY TRACT

Membrane swelling potassium permanganate

Menstrual problems Librax, pennyroyal

Sexual dysfunction Aldomet, Elavil

Testicular degeneration   phosphorus

HEART

Cardiac arrest   bloodroot, calcium, Catapres, cocaine, Elavil, ergot, insulin, oleander, Percodan, potassium, sodium, Stelazine, Valium

Chest pain   cadmium, carbon monoxide, ergot, foxglove, jellyfish, monkshood, Portuguese man-of-war, sea anemone, TEPP, turpentine, Vacor

High blood pressure   amphetamines, bronchial tube dilators, cadmium, Demerol, monoamine oxidase (MAO) inhibitors, PCP, Preludin, scorpion, Sinequan, Thyrolar, yellow jessamine

Irregular heartbeat   barbiturates, black hellebore, bloodroot, caffeine, Dilantin, Elavil, epinephrine, ether, formaldehyde, foxglove, *Inocybe* mushroom, ipecac, nitrous oxide, phosphorus, Portuguese man-of-war, sodium fluoroacetate, stingray, Tylenol

Low blood pressure   acid, alkalies, aniline, arsenic, barbiturates, boric acid, bromates, cantharidin, carbon tetrachloride, Catapres, chloral hydrate, cobra, curare, cyanide, dyphylline, Elavil, ethylene chlorohydrin, false hellebore, fly agaric, Haldol, heroin, Inderal, insulin, ipecac, Lasix, monkshood, monoamine oxidase (MAO) inhibitors, nitroglycerin, opium, panther mushroom, Percodan, Permitil, Phenergan, physostigmine, procainamide, procaine, quinidine, rhododendron, scorpions, sodium azide, sodium thiocyanate, Stelazine, stingray, Tagamet, TEPP, Thorazine, trichloroethane, Tylenol, Vacor

Rapid heartbeat   acid, amphetamines, atropine, baneberry, belladonna, bromates, caffeine, camphor, cocaine, *Cortinarius* mushroom, croton oil, cyanide, digitoxin, dyphylline, elderberry, epinephrine, fool's parsley, foxglove, Halcion, Haldol, hemlock, insulin, ipecac, marijuana, Minipress, monoamine oxidase (MAO) inhibitors, morphine, nicotine, paral, paraquat, paternoster pea, Phenergan, Sinequan, tansy, Thorazine, turpentine

Slow heartbeat/pulse   black locust, bloodroot, carbon tetrachloride, Catapres, codeine, curare, dog mercury, false hellebore, fly agaric, foxglove, Inderal, larkspur, lily of the valley, monkshood, morphine, panther mushroom, physostigmine, rhododendron, yellow jessamine

Weak, irregular pulse   black locust, hemlock, *Inocybe* mushroom, monkshood

KIDNEYS

Damage   botulism, daphne, Dilantin, galerina mushrooms, methanol, naphthalene, phenol, potassium permanganate, privet, rhubarb, tansy, Tylenol

Failure cadmium, colocynth, excessive fluid intake, mercury, mountain laurel, PCP, sodium, turpentine

LIVER

Damage arsenic, botulism, Catapres, chlordane, Depakene, Dilantin, formaldehyde, methanol, monoamine oxidase (MAO) inhibitors, potassium permanganate

LUNGS

Breathing problems aldrin, anaphylaxis, aniline, antimony, atropine, Barbados nut, barbiturates, barium, belladonna, benzene, betel nut seed, bloodroot, bronchial tube relaxers, cadmium, calcium, camphor, carbon monoxide, carbon tetrachloride, cassava, Catapres, chloral hydrate, cobra, cocaine, codeine, curare, death camas, dimethyl sulfate, Elavil, elderberry, ergot, fer-de-lance, geography cone, Gila monster, hemlock, heroin, horse chestnut, Inderal, insulin, ipecac, isopropanol, jellyfish, larkspur, Lasix, Lomotil, malathion, meadow saffron, mercury, Minipress, morphine, mountain laurel, nicotine, opium, paral, parathion, PCP, percodan, petroleum distillates, Phenergan, phosgene, pokeweed, potassium, pufferfish, physostigmine, rattlesnake, rhubarb, scorpion, shellfish poisoning, sodium, sodium fluoroacetate, stibine, TEPP, trichloroethane, turpentine, Valium, water hemlock, yellow jessamine

Bronchitis dimethyl sulfate, lead dust, malathion

Cough acid, ammonia, cadmium, hydrogen sulfide, mercury, paral, petroleum distillates, potassium permanganate, trinitrotoluene, turpentine

Coughing blood aspirin, castor bean, warfarin

Pulmonary edema ammonia, aspirin, antimony, bronchial tube relaxers, cadmium, epinephrine, formaldehyde, hydrogen sulfide, isopropanol, malathion, methanol, parathion, petroleum distillates, phosgene, quaalude, scorpion, sodium fluoracetate, turpentine

Respiratory failure anectine, blue-ringed octopus, bryony, cantharidin, cinchona bark, corn cockle, ether, fool's parsley, geography cone, Gila monster, heroin, meadow saffron, monkshood, nicotine, nitroglycerin, oleander, opium, Pavulon, procaine, star of Bethlehem, strychnine, Thorazine, toxaphene, tubarine, Vacor, water hemlock

MOUTH

Drooling cadmium, columbine, death camas, fly agaric, Haldol, *Inocybe* mushroom, lily of the valley, malathion, mercury, mountain laurel, panther mushroom, PCP, Phenergan, rhododendron, silver nitrate

Foaming acid, ammonia, chloramine-T, phenol, tansy, water hemlock

Gum problems adder, cobra, Dilantin, fer-de-lance, lead, mercury

Swelling black hellebore, dimethyl sulfate, *Inocybe* mushroom, potassium permanganate

MUSCLES

Cramps (leg) Barbados nut, potassium

Flaccidity calcium, chloral hydrate, marijuana, potassium, Percodan, Valium

Rigidity ammonia, black widow spider, camphor, Haldol, PCP

Spasms aldrin, amphetamines, benzene, boric acid, caffeine, camphor, cocaine, DDT, dieldrin, Dilantin, Elavil, epinephrine, Lasix, lithium, LSD, mercury, nicotine, parathion, physostigmine, pokeweed, Preludin, procaine, pyrethrum, Reglan, rotenone, scorpion, sodium fluoroacetate, sodium thiocyanate, strychnine, tansy, TEPP, Thorazine, Thyrolar, Vacor, white snakeroot, yellow jessamine

Stiffness atropine, black widow spider, marijuana, Permitil, strychnine

Weakness acid, Aldomet, aldrin, barium, beaked sea snake, benzene, bloodroot, cadmium, corn cockle, *Cortinarius* mushroom, daphne, death camas, dieldrin, endrin, false hellebore, Gila monster, hemlock, Indian tobacco, Lasix, lead, meadow saffron, Minipress, morphine, Norflex, parathion, Persantine, petroleum distillates, potassium, phenol, pokeweed, rhubarb, sodium thiocyanate, stibine, stingray, Thyrolar, Vacor, Valium, white snakeroot, yellow jessamine, yew

NOSE

Bloody nose malathion, parathion

Congestion Permitil

OTHER

Hair Loss arsenic, boric acid, Depakene, Minipress

PARALYSIS

atropine, benzene, blue-ringed octopus, botulism, bryony, calcium, cobra, croton oil, curare, geography cone, hemlock, jimsonweed, monkshood, mountain laurel, narcissus, parathion, Pavulon, potassium, pufferfish, pyrethrum, rattlesnake, rhododendron, scorpionfish, sea anemone, sodium, stonefish, TEPP

SENSORY PROBLEMS

Blindness ammonia, atropine, hemlock, jimsonweed, methanol, phenol, propane

Blurred/double vision alkalies, atropine, beaked sea snake, belladonna, benzene, betel nut seed, botulism, cinchona bark, digitoxin, dimethyl sulfate, Elavil, epinephrine, ethyl alcohol, false hellebore, fool's parsley, foxglove, Haldol, hemlock, henbane, heroin, hydrogen sulfide, jimsonweed, Lasix, Librax, malathion, methanol, Minipress, monkshood, nicotine, Norflex, panther mushroom, Permitil, Tanghin, TEPP, Vacor

Deafness/hearing loss aspirin, bromates, quinine

Sensitivity to light atropine, Lasix, parathion

Tingling calcium, Elavil, Lasix, Lomotil, Minipress, monkshood

Tinnitus aspirin, cinchona bark, Elavil, endrin, Gila monster, nicotine

SHOCK

ammonia, baneberry, cadmium, fer-de-lance, insulin, iodine, Lasix, malathion, moonseed, phenol, Portuguese man-of-war, potassium permanganate, rattlesnake, sea anemone, silver nitrate, stingray, yew

SKIN

Bleeding adder, black widow spider, brown recluse spider, cobra, rattlesnake

Bruises aspirin, Depakene, Lasix, warfarin

Discoloration—black silver nitrate

Discoloration—blue (cyanosis) acid, *Amanita* mushroom, amphetamines, aniline, aspirin, boric acid, brown recluse spider, castor bean, chloral hydrate, chloramine-T, curare, cyanide, dimethyl sulfate, epinephrine, ether, ethinamate, Gila monster, heroin, hydrangea, *Inocybe* mushroom, jellyfish, larkspur, nitroglycerin, paral, paraquat, phenol, phosgene, procaine, TEPP, tetrachloroethane, trinitrotoluene

Discoloration—brown acid, potassium permanganate

Discoloration—red ammonia, atropine, belladonna, bronchial tube relaxers, brown recluse spider, cyanide, *Inocybe* mushroom, insulin, lily of the valley, nitroglycerin, persantine, procaine, pufferfish, turpentine

Discoloration—yellow Indian tobacco, nicotine, trinitrotoluene

Irritation acid, Aldomet, antimony, arsenic, atropine, belladonna, benzene hexachloride, boric acid, brown recluse spider, cadmium, cantharidin, Catapres, croton oil, DDT, dog mercury, ethylene chlorohydrin, formaldehyde, hydrogen sulfide, larkspur, Librax, malathion, Minipress, narcissus, paraquat, parathion, phosphorus, pyrethrum, sodium azide, Tagamet, tansy, tetrachloroethane, trinitrotoluene

Itching larkspur, opium

Necrotic tissue acid, alkalies, aniline, benzene, brown recluse spider, cantharidin, cobra, cottonmouth, ergot, ether-chloroform, iodine, jellyfish, mercury, phenol, phosphorus, potassium permanganate, rattlesnake, sea anemone, Tylenol

Paleness malathion, phenol, trinitrotoluene, yew

Swelling adder, anaphylaxis, blue-ringed octopus, brown recluse spider, cobra, jellyfish, rattlesnake, scorpionfish

SLEEP

Insomnia amphetamines, bronchial tube relaxers, caffeine, dyphylline, Elavil, endrin, Inderal, Phenergan, Preludin, Reglan

Nightmares Aldomet

Sleep-inducing Aldomet, Barbados nut, barbiturates, boric acid, castor bean, Catapres, chloral hydrate, codeine, Dalmane, Demerol, dimethyl sulfate, dog mercury, Elavil, Haldol, hydrogen sulfide, jimsonweed, mandrake, marijuana, Minipress, morphine, Percodan, Permitil, Reglan, Stelazine, tetrachloroethane, Thorazine, Tylenol, Valium

SPEECH PROBLEMS

blue-ringed octopus, chloral hydrate, codeine, curare, ethyl alcohol, Haldol, lithium, marijuana, pufferfish, Thorazine, yellow jessamine

STUPOR

aniline, black locust, castor bean, Indian tobacco, *Inocybe* mushroom, iodine, monoamine oxidase (MAO) inhibitors, PCP, Percodan, potato, rotenone

UNCONSCIOUSNESS

benzene, camphor, carbon fumes, carbon monoxide, carbon tetrachloride, chloral hydrate, cocaine, codeine, cyanide, Dalmane, endrin, ether, ethyl alcohol, ethylene chlorohydrin, formaldehyde, heroin, hydrangea, hydrogen sulfide, *Inocibe* mushroom, marijuana, Minipress, morphine, oleander, opium, petroleum distillates, stonefish, trichloroethane, turpentine, Valium

URINARY TRACT

Anuria (lack of urine) atropine, belladonna, black widow spider, bromates, colocynth, cort mushrooms, Elavil, ergot, iodine, meadow saffron, rhubarb, savin, silver nitrate, tansy, trinitrotoluene

Dark color flagyl, phenol

Dysuria (painful urination) Barbados nut, naphthalene, turpentine

Frequent urine Lasix, Vacor

Oliguria (urinary retention) aspirin, atropine, belladonna, black widow spider, bromates, colocynth, isopropanol, lead, naphthalene, paraquat, savin, trinitrotoluene

Uremia aldrin, aspirin, brown recluse spider, cantharidin, carbon tetrachloride, castor bean, cort mushrooms, dieldrin, iodine, mercury, naphthalene, savin, turpentine, warfarin

Yellow urine atophan

APPENDIX G
REGIONAL POISON
CONTROL CENTERS

For cases of pet poisonings, dial 900-680-0000 ($2.95 per minute) or 800-548-2423 ($30 per call).

* Indicates certified by American Association of Poison Control Centers

ALABAMA
Alabama Poison Center*
809 University Blvd. East
Tuscaloosa, AL 35401
(205) 345-0600
(800) 462-0800 (Alabama only)

The Children's Hospital of Alabama Poison
  Control Center
1600 Seventh Ave. S.
Birmingham, AL 35233
(800) 292-6678 (statewide)
(205) 933-4050 (local)
939-9201 (local)
939-9202 (local)

ALASKA
Anchorage Poison Center
Providence Hospital
PO Box 196604
3200 Providence Dr.
Anchorage, AL 99519
(800) 478-3193
(907) 261-3193

Fairbanks Poison Control Center
Fairbanks Memorial Hospital
1650 Cowles St.
Fairbanks, AL 99701
(907) 456-7182

ARIZONA
Arizona Regional Poison Control System*
Arizona Health Sciences Center
Room 3204K
University of Arizona

Tucson, AZ, 85724
(800) 362-0101

Central Arizona Regional Poison
  Management Center
St. Luke's Hospital Medical Center
1800 E. Van Buren St.
Phoenix, AZ 85006
(602) 253-3334

ARKANSAS
Statewide Poison Control Drug Information
  Center
University of Arkansas Center for Medical
  Sciences
College of Pharmacy
4301 W. Markham St.
Little Rock, AK 72205
(800) 482-8948 (statewide);
(501) 666-5532 (Pulaski County)

CALIFORNIA
Los Angeles County Medical Assn. Regional
  Poison Control Center
1925 Wilshire Blvd.
Los Angeles, CA 90057
(213) 484-5151 (for public)
(213) 664-2121 (for physicians)
(800) 825-2722 (for physicians)

Fresno Regional Poison Control Center of
  Fresno Community Hospital and Medical
  Center
Fresno and R Sts.
Fresno, CA 93715
(800) 346-5922; (209) 445-1222

San Diego Regional Poison Center*
University of California, San Diego
  Medical Center
225 Dickson St.
San Diego, CA 92103
(800) 876-4766 (CA only);
(619) 294-6000

San Francisco Bay Area Regional Poison
  Center*
San Francisco General Hospital
R. 1-E-86
1001 Potrero Ave.
San Francisco, CA 94110
(800) 523-2222 (CA only);
(415) 476-6600

UC Davis Medical Center Regional
  Poison Center*
2315 Stockton Blvd.
Sacramento, CA 95817
(800) 342-9293 (CA only);
(916) 453-3692 (emergency poison
information);
(916) 453-3414 (nonemergency business
information)

Children's Hospital Medical Center
  of Northern California
747 52nd St.
Oakland, CA 94609
(415) 428-3248

University of California Poison Control
  Center
Irvine Medical Center
101 City Drive S., Rte. 78
Orange, CA 92668
(714) 634-5988

Central-Coast Counties Regional
  Poison Control Center
Santa Clara Valley Medical Center
751 Bascom Ave.
San Jose, CA 95128
(800) 662-9886; (408) 299-5112

COLORADO (Also Montana and
Wyoming)
Rocky Mountain Poison Control
  Center*
645 Bannock St.
Denver, CO 80204
(303) 629-1123; (800) 332-3073 (Colorado
only); (800) 525-5042 (Montana only); (800)
442-2702 (Wyoming only)

CONNECTICUT
Connecticut Poison Control Center
University of Connecticut Health
  Center
Farmington, CT 06032
(203) 674-3456; 674-3457

St. Vincent's Medical Center
2800 Main St.
Bridgeport, CT 06606
(203) 576-5178

DELAWARE
Poison Information Center
Medical Center of Delaware
Wilmington Division
501 W. 14th St.
Wilmington, DE 19899
(302) 655-3389

FLORIDA
Tampa Bay Regional Poison Control
  Center*
Tampa General Hospital
Davis Island, FL 33606
(813) 253-4444; (800) 282-3171 (FLA only)

St. Vincent's Medical Center
1800 Barrs St.
Jacksonville, FL 32202
(904) 378-7500; 378-7499 (TDD)

GEORGIA
Georgia Poison Control Center*
Grady Memorial Hospital
80 Butler St. SE
Atlanta, GA 30335
(404) 589-4400; (800) 282-5846 (GA only);
(404) 525-3323 (TDD)

Regional Poison Control Center
Medical Center of Central Georgia
777 Hemlock St.
Macon, GA 31202
(912) 744-1427; 744-1146; 744-1000

Savannah Regional Poison Control
  Center
Dept. of Emergency Medicine
Memorial Medical Center
Savannah, GA 31403
(912) 355-5228

HAWAII
Hawaii Poison Center
Kapiolani-Children's Medical Center
1319 Punahou St.

Honolulu, HI 96826
(800) 362-3585; (808) 941-4411

IDAHO
Idaho Emergency Medical Poison Center
St. Alphonsus Regional Medical Center
1055 N. Curtis Rd.
Boise, ID 83704
(800) 632-8000; (208) 334-2241

ILLINOIS
Chicago and Northeastern Illinois
  Regional Poison Control Center*
Rush-Presbyterian–St. Luke's Medical
  Center
1753 W. Congress Pkwy.
Chicago, IL 60612
(800) 942-5969; (217) 753-3330

INDIANA
Indiana Poison Center*
Wishard Memorial Hospital
1001 W. Tenth St.
Indianapolis, IN 46202
(317) 630-7351
(800) 382-9097 (Indiana only);
(317) 630-6666 (TDD)

Parkview Memorial Hospital
2200 Randalia Dr.
Ft. Wayne, IN 46805
(219) 484-6636

IOWA
University of Iowa Hospitals and Clinic
  Poison Control Center*
Iowa City, IA 52242
(800) 272-6477; (319) 356-2922

Variety Club Poison and Drug
  Information Center
Iowa Methodist Medical Center
1200 Pleasant St.
Des Moines, IA 50309
(800) 362-2327; (515) 283-6254

KANSAS
Mid-America Poison Center
University of Kansas Medical Center
39th and Rainbow Blvd.
Kansas City, KN 66103
(800) 332-6633; (913) 588-6633

Mid-Plains Poison Control Center*
(See Nebraska)
(800) 228-9515

Wesley Medical Center
550 N. Hillside Ave.

Wichita, KN 67214
(316) 688-2277

KENTUCKY
Kentucky Regional Poison Control
  Center of Kosair Children's Hospital*
PO Box 35070
Louisville, KY 40232
(800) 722-5725 (KY only); (502) 589-8222
(metropolitan Louisville)

St. Luke Hospital of Campbell County
Northern Kentucky Poison Center
85 N. Grand Ave.
Ft. Thomas, KY 41075
(800) 352-9900; (606) 572-3215

LOUISIANA
Louisiana Regional Poison Control
  Center*
Louisiana State University School of
  Medicine
1501 Kings Hwy.
Shreveport, LA 71130
(318) 425-1524;
(800) 535-0525 (Louisiana only)

MAINE
Maine Poison Control Center at Maine
  Medical Center
22 Bramhall St.
Portland, ME 04102
(800) 442-6305 (Maine only);
(207) 871-2381 (ER)

MARYLAND
Maryland Poison Center*
University of Maryland School of
  Pharmacy
20 N. Pine St.
Baltimore, MD 21201
(410) 528-7701;
(800) 492-2414 (Maryland only)

MASSACHUSETTS
Massachusetts Poison Control System*
300 Longwood Ave.
Boston, MA 02115
(617) 232-2120; (800) 682-9211;
(617) 277-3323 (TDD)

MICHIGAN
Blodgett Regional Poison Center*
Blodgett Memorial Medical Center
1840 Wealthy St. SE
Grand Rapids, MI 49506
(800) 442-4112 (for area code 616 only);

(800) 632-2727 (Michigan only)
Great Lakes Poison Center
Bronson Methodist Hospital
252 E. Lovell St.
Kalamazoo, MI 49001
(800) 442-4112 (only in area code 616);
(616) 383-6409

Poison Control Center*
Children's Hospital of Michigan
3901 Beaubien Blvd.
Detroit, MI 48201
(313) 745-5711; (800) 462-6642 (area code
313 only); (800) 572-1655 (rest of Michigan)

MINNESOTA
Hennepin Regional Poison Center*
Hennepin County Medical Center
701 Park Ave.
Minneapolis, MN 55415
(612) 347-3141;
(612) 347-6219 (TDD)

Minnesota Poison Control System*
St. Paul Ramsey Medical Center
640 Jackson St.
St. Paul, MN 55101
(612) 221-2113;
(800) 222-1222 (Minnesota only)

MISSISSIPPI
Regional Poison Control Center
University Medical Center
2500 N. State St.
Jackson, MS 39216
(601) 354-7660

MISSOURI
Cardinal Glennon Children's
    HospitalRegional Poison Center*
1465 S. Grand Blvd.
St. Louis, MO 63104
(314) 772-5200;
(800) 392-9111 (MO only)

The Children's Mercy Hospital
24th and Gillham Rd.
Kansas City, MO 64108
(816) 234-3000

MONTANA
(See COLORADO: Rocky Mountain Poison
    Control Center)

NEBRASKA
Mid-Plains Poison Control Center*
8301 Dodge St.
Omaha, NE 68114

(402) 390-5400 (Omaha); (800) 642-9999
(Nebraska only); (800) 228-9515 (CO, IA;
KN; MO; SD; WY)

NEW HAMPSHIRE
New Hampshire Poison Information
    Center
2 Maynard St.
Hanover, NH 03756
(800) 562-8236 (NH only); (603) 646-5000
(outside NH)

NEW JERSEY
New Jersey Poison Information
    and Education System*
201 Lyons Ave.
Newark, NJ 07112
(201) 923-0764; (800) 962-1253 (New Jersey
only); (201) 926-8008 (TDD)

NEW MEXICO
New Mexico Poison and Drug
    Information Center*
University of New Mexico
Albuquerque, NM 87131
(505) 843-2551; (800) 432-6866
(New Mexico)

NEW YORK
Long Island Regional Poison Control
    Center*
Nassau County Medical Center
2201 Hempstead Turnpike
East Meadow, NY 11554
(516) 542-2323 (TDD);
(516) 542-2324, 2325

New York City Poison Control Center*
455 1st Ave., Rm 123
New York, NY 10016
(212) 340-4494; (212) 764-7667;
(800) 225-0658 (outside New York only)

Southern Tier Poison Center
Binghamton General Hospital
Mitchell Ave.
Binghamton, NY 13903
(607) 723-8929

Western New York Poison Control
    Center at Children's Hospital of Buffalo
219 Bryant St.
Buffalo, NY 14222
(716) 878-7654; (716) 878-7655

Hudson Valley Regional Poison Center
Nyack Hospital
N. Midland Ave.

Nyack, NY 10960
(914) 353-1000

Finger Lakes Poison Center
LIFE LINE
University of Rochester Medical Center
Box 777
Rochester, NY 14620
(716) 275-5152; 275-2700 (TDD)

Central New York Poison Control
  Center
Upstate Medical Center
750 E. Adams St.
Syracuse, NY 13210
(315) 476-4766; (800) 252-5655 (outside
Onandaga County)

NORTH CAROLINA
Duke University Poison Control
  Center*
Duke University Medical Center
Box 3007
Durham, NC 27710
(919) 684-8111;
(800) 672-1697 (North Carolina only)

NORTH DAKOTA
North Dakota Poison Information Center
St. Luke's Hospital
Fifth St. N. and Mills Ave.
Fargo, ND 58122
(800) 732-2200 (ND only);
(800) 280-5575

OHIO
Central Ohio Poison Center*
Columbus Children's Hospital
700 Children's Dr.
Columbus, OH 43205
(614) 228-1323;
(800) 682-7625 (Ohio only)

Cincinnati Regional Poison Control
  System and Drug and Poison
  Information Center*
University of Cincinnati Medical Center
231 Bethesda Ave., M.L. #144
Cincinnati, OH 45267
(513) 872-5111; (800) 872-5111

Greater Cleveland Poison Control
  Center
2101 Aldelbert Rd.
Cleveland, OH 44106
216 231-4455

OKLAHOMA
Oklahoma Poison Control Center
Oklahoma Children's Memorial
  Hospital
PO Box 26307
940 N.E. 10th
Oklahoma City, OK 73126
(800) 522-4611 (OK only);
(405) 271-5454

OREGON
Oregon Poison Control and Drug
  Information Center
Oregon Health Sciences University
3181 SW Sam Jackson Park Rd.
Portland, OR 97201
(800) 452-7165; (503) 225-8968

PENNSYLVANIA
Delaware Valley Regional Poison
  Control Center*
One Children's Center
34th and Civic Center Blvd.
Philadelphia, PA 19104
(215) 386-2100

Pittsburgh Poison Center*
One Children's Place
3705 5th Ave. at DeSota St.
Pittsburgh, PA 15213
(412) 647-5600; (administration);
(412) 681-6669 (emergency)

RHODE ISLAND
Rhode Island Poison Center
Rhode Island Hospital
593 Eddy St.
Providence, RI 02902
(401) 277-5727; (401) 277-8062 (TDD)

SOUTH CAROLINA
Palmetto Poison Center
University of South Carolina
College of Pharmacy
Columbia, SC 29208
(800) 922-1117; (800) 765-7359

SOUTH DAKOTA
Mid-Plains Poison Control Center*
(See Nebraska)

TENNESSEE
T. C. Thompson Children's Hospital
910 Blackford St.
Chattanooga, TN 37403
(615) 778-6100

TEXAS
North Central Texas Poison Center
PO Box 35926
Dallas, TX 75235
(214) 920-2400;
(800) 441-0040 (Texas only)

Texas State Poison Center
University of Texas Medical Branch
Galveston, TX 77550
(409) 765-1420; (713) 654-1701 (Houston);
(516) 478-4490 (Austin); (800) 392-8548 (TX only)

UTAH
Intermountain Regional Poison Control
  Center*
50 N. Medical Dr., Bldg. 428
Salt Lake City, UT 84132
(801) 581-2151;
(800) 662-0062 (Utah only)

VERMONT
Vermont Poison Center
Medical Center Hospital of Vermont
Colchester Ave.
Burlington, VT 05401
(802) 658-3456 (poison information); (802)
656-2721 (education programs)

VIRGINIA
Blue Ridge Poison Center
University of Virginia Hospital
Charlottesville, VA 22908
(800) 552-3723; (800) 222-5927 (TDD VA
only); (804) 924-5543

Central Virginia Poison Center
Medical College of Virginia

Richmond, VA 23298
(804) 786-9123 (24-hour emergency number)

WASHINGTON
Seattle Poison Center*
Children's Hospital and Medical Center
4800 Sand Point Way NE
PO Box C5371
Seattle, WA 98105
(206) 526-2121

WASHINGTON, DC
National Capital Poison Center*
Georgetown University Hospital
3800 Reservoir Rd. NW
Washington, DC 20007
(202) 625-3333

WEST VIRGINIA
West Virginia Poison Center
West Virginia University School of
  Pharmacy
3110 McCorckle Ave. SE
Charleston, WV 25304
(304) 348-4211;
(800) 642-3625 (West Virginia only)

WISCONSIN
Green Bay Poison Control Center
St. Vincent Hospital
PO Box 13508
Green Bay, WI 54307
(414) 433-8100

WYOMING
Wyoming Poison Center
Hathaway Bldg., Rm. 527
Cheyenne, WY 82001
(800) 442-2702

APPENDIX H
TOXICITY RATINGS OF
POISONS

To allow a quick estimate of the chance for recovery of poisoning victims, scientists have designed systems of toxicity based on six commonly used measures (such as a taste, a mouthful, etc.) and on the assumption that the victim is a 150- pound man. Substances so poisonous that a taste (less than seven drops) can kill a man are rated class "6" (or "supertoxic"); substance ratings range to class 1 ("practically nontoxic").

A few household products such as some insecticides and caustic cleaners carry a rating from 5 to 6; about 70 percent of consumer products are rated 3 or below, however. Most cosmetics are class 2 ("slightly toxic") while those with high concentrations of alcohol are rated class 3 (Moderately toxic).

It should be noted that the toxicity rating reflects an estimate of the probable lethal dose, not the minimal lethal dose. Because of idiosyncrasy or hypersensitivity among poisoning victims, minimal lethal doses recorded in the literature are usually considerably lower than those implied by the ratings.

For most corrosive agents (such as mineral acids, alkalies, bleaches, etc.) no toxicity rating is suggested. In these cases, death is usually the result of severe local tissue injury (with secondary complications). The intensity of the tissue damage is determined by the concentration of the corrosive substance; the dose is a secondary consideration. Therefore, for these corrosive compounds, no toxicity rating is appropriate to determine lethality.

Toxicity Rating	Probable Lethal Dose for a 150-Pound Man
6 Supertoxic	A taste (less than 7 drops)
5 Extremely toxic	Between 7 drops and 1 tsp.
4 Very toxic	Between 1 tsp. and 1 oz.
3 Moderately toxic	Between 1 oz. and 1 pt.
2 Slightly toxic	Between 1 pt. and 1 qt.
1 Practically nontoxic	More than 1 qt. (2.2 lb.)

TOXICITY 1
marijuana
MSG
pyrethrum
vitamin C
vitamin E

TOXICITY 2
ethyl alcohol
LSD
reglan
riboflavin (B2)
sea anemones
Tylenol
vitamin B1 (thiamine)

TOXICITY 3
Aldomet
ammonia
black widow spider
borax
caffeine
calcium
chloramine-T
chloroform
cimetidine
cinchophen
cortinarius mushrooms
diazepam
disulfiram
DDT
ethyl alcohol
ethylene glycol
fly agaric
formaldehyde
gasoline
Haldol
holly
isopropanol
isopropyl alcohol
jimsonweed
kerosene
lithium
methylene chloride
naloxone
niacin
nightshade, deadly
nutmeg
panther mushroom
phosphate esters
procaine
sodium bicarbonate

sodium chloride (table salt)
1,1,1-trichloroethane
turpentine
vitamin B3
vitamin B6
white snakeroot

TOXICITY 4
acetaminophen
acid
acrylamide
aniline
aspirin
benzene
benzene hexachloride
bloodroot
boric acid
bromates
bronchial tube relaxers
brown recluse spider
bryony
cadmium
caffeine
camphor
carbaryl
carbon tetrachloride
cationic detergents
chloral hydrate
chlorate salts
chlordane
cinchona bark
corn cockle
DDT
death camas
depakene
derris
digitalis
Dilantin
elderberry
fluoride
fool's parsley
grounsel
larkspur
Lasix
laudanum
lead
levallorphan
lidocaine
lindane
lomotil
malathion
mandrake
mescaline

methaldehyde
Mirex
monoamine oxidase inhibitors
naphthalene
nitroglycerin
nux-vomica
oxalates
pennyroyal oil
Persantine
petroleum distillates
peyote
phenobarbital
phenytoin
pokeweed
potassium
Psilocybe mexicana
pyrethrin
pyrethrum
quaalude
quinidine
quinine
rattlesnake
rhubarb
Rotenone
salicylates
sodium
spindle tree
squill
stibine
theophylline
Thyrolar
TNT
toads, *Bufo* species
tobacco
toluene
warfarin
wintergreen, oil of

TOXICITY 5
aconite
acrylamide
akee
aldrin
Amanita mushroom
amphetamines
amyl nitrite
aniline
apomorphine
arsenic
atropine
baneberry
barbiturates
beaked sea snake

betel nut seed
black hellebore
black locust
boric acid
botulin
bromates
cadmium
camphor
carbon monoxide
cassava
celendine
chloral hydrate
cinchophen
cocaine
colcocynth
cottonmouth
croton oil
Dalmane
daphne
dieldrin
digitoxin
dog mercury
Elavil
endrin
epinephrine
ergot
ether
ethylene chlorohydrin
false hellebore
fer-de-lance
formaldehyde
foxglove
gelsemium
geography cone
Gyromitra mushroom
Haldol
horse chesnut
hydrangea
Inderal
Indian tobacco
Inocybe mushroom
insulin
iodine
ipecac
jequirity bean
lead
lithium
meadow saffron
minipress
moonseed
mountain laurel
muscarine

muscimol
narcissus
nitrite
nitrous oxide
opium
paraquat
Percodan
phenol
phenylpropanolamine
physostigmine
potassium permanganate
potato
Preludin
privet
Procainamide
quaalude
scorpionfish
silver nitrate
Stelazine
speed
Tagamet
tansy
Thorazine
toxaphene
trichloroethane
Vacor
Valium
yellow jessamine
yohimbine

TOXICITY 6

adder
alder
alkalies
amatoxin
anectine
antimony
atophan
atropine
Barbados nut
belladonna
blue-ringed octopus
botulin antitoxin
cantharidin
carbon tetrachloride
castor bean
Catapres
chloramine-T
chlordane
cobra
codeine

coniine
croton oil
curare
cyanide
dieldrin
digitoxin
Digoxin
dimethyl sulfate
ethylene chlorohydrin
fluoroacetate
Gila monster
hemlock
heroin
hydrocyanic acid
hydrogen sulfide
jellyfish
jimsonweed
lily of the valley
LSD
monkshood
morphine
nicotine
nitroglycerin(e)
oleander
oxymorphone
paraquat
parathion
paternoster pea
Pavulon
PCP
phosgene
phosphine
phosphorus
physostigmine
pilocarpine
Procaine
pufferfish
quinidine
rhododendron
rhubarb
Ricin
savin
stonefish
strychnine
Tanghin
TEPP
tetrachlorethane
TNT
water hemlock
yew

---

* Gosselin, R. E., et al, *Clinical Toxicology of Commercial Products* (Baltimore: Williams & Wilkins, 1984).

REFERENCES

Aaron, James E.; Bridges, A. Frank; and Ritzel, Dale O. *First Aid and Emergency Care*. New York: Macmillan, 1972.

Albner, John I., and Albner, Delores M. *Baby-Safe Houseplants and Cut Flowers*. Highland, Ill.: Genus Books, 1991.

Allison, Malorye. "Not Just for Kids." *Harvard Health Letter* 17 (May 1992): 6–8.

American Academy of Pediatrics. *Handbook of Common Poisonings in Children*. Elk Grove Village, Ill.: American Academy of Pediatrics, 1983.

Anderson, Kathryn D.; Rouse, Thomas M.; and Randolph, Judson, G. "A Controlled Trial of Corticosteroids in Children with Corrosive Injury of the Esophagus." *New England Journal of Medicine* 323 (September 6, 1990): 637–40.

Angle, C. R. "Is Ipecac Obsolete?" *Journal of Toxicology and Clinical Toxicology* 29, no. 4 (1991): 513–14.

Arbuckle, J. G., etal. *Environmental Law Handbook*. 11th ed. Rockville, Md.: Government Institutes, Inc., 1991.

Arena, J. M. "Plants That Poison." *Emergency Medicine* 21, 30–35.

———. *Poisoning: Toxicology, Symptoms, Treatment*. Springfield, Ill.: Charles C. Thomas, 1986.

Arnold, E. N., and Burton, J. A. *A Field Guide to the Reptiles and Amphibians of Europe*. London: Collins, 1978.

Aspherheim, M. K. *Pharmacologic Basis of Patient Care*. 5th ed. Philadelphia: W. B. Saunders, 1985.

Auerbach, Paul S. "Marine Envenomations." *New England Journal of Medicine* 325 (August 15, 1991): 486–94.

Balint, G. A., et al. "Ricin: The Toxic Protein of Castor Oil Seeds." *Toxicology* 2 (1974): 77–102.

Baroff, L. J., et al. "Relationship of Poison Control Contact and Injuries to Children." *Annals of Emergency Medicine* 21, no. 2 (February 1992): 153–57.

Barone, Michael. "Chances Are. *U.S. News and World Report*, July 1, 1991, 19.

Baskin, E. *The Poppy and Other Deadly Plants*. New York: Delacorte Press, 1967.

Bayer, Marc J.; Rumack, Barry H.; and Wanke, Lee A. *Toxicologic Emergencies*. Bowie, Md.: Robert J. Brady, 1984.

Beal, Clifford F. "Poison Bomb Alert: Chemical Weapons." *World Monitor: The Christian Science Monitor Monthly*, September 1990, 62–67.

"Before You Head for the Raw Bar." *Tufts University Diet and Nutrition Letter* 9 (November 1991): 1.

Behler, John L. *Simon and Schuster's Guide to Reptiles and Amphibians of the World*. New York: Simon & Schuster, 1989.

Behler, John L., and King, F. Wayne. *The Audubon Society Field Guide to North American Reptiles and Amphibians*. New York: Alfred A. Knopf, 1991.

Benevich, Teri. "New Sources Add to Lead Poisoning Concerns." *Journal of the American Medical Association* 263 (February 9, 1990): 790–91.

Berkow, Robert, and Fletcher, A. J., eds. *The Merck Manual of Diagnosis and Therapy*. 15th ed. Rahway, N.J.: Merck & Co., 1987.

Beyer, Lisa. "Coping with Chemicals." *Time*, February 25, 1991, 47–48.

Bittman, Mark. "How to Buy and Eat Fish." *New York Times' Good Health Magazine*, April 26, 1992, S18.

Block, Bradford J. *Signs and Symptoms of Chemical Exposure*. Springfield, Ill.: Charles C. Thomas, 1980.

Bonar, Ann. *The Macmillan Treasury of Herbs*. New York: Macmillan, 1985.

Bosveld, Jane. "Food Poisoning: The Culprit Could Be in Your Kitchen." *McCall's*, March 1992, 32.

Bremness, Lesley. *Herbs*. London: Dorling Kindersley Ltd., for Reader's Digest Association, Inc., 1990.

Brobeck, Stephen, and Averyt, Anne C. *The Product Safety Book: The Ultimate Consumer Guide to Product Hazards*. New York: E. P. Dutton, 1983.

Browder, Sue. "Are You Allergic to the Modern World?" *Woman's Day*, April 1, 1992, 56, 102.

Calabrese, Edward J., and Dorset, Michael W. *Healthy Living in an Unhealthy World*. New York: Simon & Schuster, 1984.

Carr, Donald E. *The Deadly Feast of Life*. Garden City, N.Y.: Doubleday, 1971.

Casarett, L. M., and Doull, J. *Toxicology*. 2d ed. New York: Macmillan, 1980.

Castleman, Michael. "Lead Again." *Sierra*, July–August 1992, 25–26.

Chestnut, V. K. *Thirty Poisonous Plants of North America*. Seattle: Shorey, 1976.

Chiusoli, A., and Boriani, M. L. *Simon and Schuster's Guide to House Plants*. New York: Simon & Schuster, 1986.

Chollar, Susan. "The Poison Eaters: Some Cultivated Bacteria Are Finally Getting Down to Business, Gobbling Up Hazardous Pollutants." *Discover*, April 1990, 76–79.

Chugh, S. N. "Incidence and Outcome of Aluminum Phosphide Poisoning in a Hospital Study." *Journal of the American Medical Association* 267 (February 5, 1992): 642.

Clayman, Charles B., M.D. *The American Medical Association Encyclopedia of Medicine.* New York: Random House, 1989.

Clayton, L. T., ed. *Taber's Cyclopedic Medical Dictionary.* 16th ed. Philadelphia: F. A. Davis, 1985.

Clifford, Nathan J., and Nies, Alan S. "Organophosphate Poisoning from Wearing a Laundered Uniform Previously Contaminated with parathion." *Journal of the American Medical Association,* 262 (December 1, 1989): 3035–36.

Cloudsley-Thompson, John L. *Spiders and Scorpions.* New York: McGraw-Hill, 1980.

Cobb, Nathaniel, and Etzel, Ruth A. "Unintentional Carbon Monoxide–Related Deaths in the United States, 1979 through 1988." *Journal of the American Medical Association* 266 (August 7, 1991): 659–63.

Cooper, Peter. *Poisoning by Drugs and Chemicals, Plants and Animals.* Chicago: Alchemist Publications, 1974.

Cousteau, Jacques. "Attack and Defense." In *Jacques Cousteau: The Ocean World,* 103–26. New York: Harry N. Abrams, 1985.

Dadd, Debra Lynn. *The Nontoxic Home.* Los Angeles: Tarcher Press, 1986.

Dalvi, R. R., and Borvic, W. C. "Toxicity of Solanine: An Overview." *Veterinary and Human Toxicology* 23 (1983): 13–15.

Delaney, Lisa. "Dictionary of Healing Techniques and Remedies" (part 31). *Prevention,* December 1991, 26–30.

Der Marderosian, A. H., and Roia, F. C. *Toxic Plants.* New York: Columbia University Press, 1979.

De Wolf, G. P. *1987 Taylor's Guide to Houseplants.* New York: Houghton Mifflin, 1987.

Dipalma, J. R. "Poisonous Plants." *American Family Physician* 29 (1984): 252–54.

Dozier, Thomas A. *Dangerous Sea Creatures.* New York: Time-Life Films, 1977.

Dreisbach, R. H. *Handbook of Poisoning.* 11th ed. Los Altos, Calif.: Lange Medical Publications, 1983.

Duffy, David Cameron. "Land of Milk and Poison: A Mysterious Death Overtook Many of America's Pioneers." *Natural History,* July 1990, 4–7.

Duke, James A. *CRC Handbook of Medicinal Herbs.* Boca Raton, Fla.: CRC Press, 1985.

Dukes, M. N. G., ed. *Meyler's Side Effects of Drugs: An Encyclopaedia of Adverse Reactions and Interactions.* 9th ed. Amsterdam: Excerpta Medica, 1980.

Editors. *Handbook of Common Poisonings in Children.* Evanston, Ill.: American Academy of Pediatrics, 1983.

Edlow, Jonathan. "Gut Reactions: Preventing Food Poisoning." *American Health,* June 1992, 66–70.

Ellenhorn, Matthew J., and Barceloux, Donald G. *Medical Toxicology*. New York: Elsevier, 1988.

Ellis, M. D. *Dangerous Plants, Snakes, Arthropods and Marine Life*. Hamilton, Ill.: Drug Intelligence Publications, 1978.

Environmental Protection Agency. *Carcinogenic Assessment of Aldrin and Dieldrin*. Washington, D.C.: EPA, 1987.

Erickson, Deborah. "Demonic Toxin Found in Shellfish," *Scientific American*, May 1992, 129–30.

Everett, Thomas H. *The New York Botanical Garden Illustrated Encyclopedia of Horticulture*. New York: Garland, 1981.

Fackelmann, Kathy A. "Device Sounds Out Salmonella-Infected Eggs." *Science News*, March 7, 1992, 150.

———. "Painting a Perilous Picture of Mercury." *Science News*, October 20, 1990, 244.

Fatovich, D. M. "Aconite: A Lethal Chinese Herb." *Annals of Emergency Medicine* 21, no. 3 (March 1992): 309–11.

FDA. "Succimer (DMSA) Approved for Severe Lead Poisoning." *Journal of The American Medical Association* 265 (April 10, 1991): 1802.

Fischer, Arlene. "Would Your Kitchen Pass a Health Inspection?" *Family Circle*, August 11, 1992, 144–48.

Fleisher, G. R. "Gastric Decontamination in the Poisoned Patient." *Pediatric Emergency Care* 7, no. 6 (December 1991): 378–81.

Fogden, Michael. "A Tiff over Turf (Strawberry Poison Dart Frogs)." *Natural History*, June 1991, 76–77.

Foley, Denise. "Case of the 'Anemic' Diagnosis." *Prevention*, September 1991, 106–12.

Frame, P. *In Quick Reference to Clinical Toxicology*. Philadelphia: J. B. Lippincott, 1980.

Franklin, Deborah. "The Case of the Paralyzed Travelers." *In Health*, December–January 1992, 28–30.

———. "Lead: Still Poison After All These Years." *In Health*, September–October 1991, 38–50.

Freethy, Ron. *From Agar to Zenry: A Book of Plant Uses, Names and Folklore*. Dover, N.H.: Tanager Books, 1985.

Friberg, L.; Nordberg, G. F.; and Vouk, V. B., eds. *Handbook on the Toxicology of Metals*. New York: Elsevier, 1986.

Fritsch, Albert J., ed. *The Household Pollutants Guide*. Garden City, N.Y.: Anchor Press/Doubleday, 1978.

Fritz, Cheryl. "Household Hazards: Protecting Your Pets from Poisons." *Better Homes and Gardens*, August 1992, 116.

Gadd, L. *Deadly Beautiful: The World's Most Poisonous Animals and Plants*. New York: Macmillan, 1980.

Garrettson, L. K. "Ipecac Home Use." *Journal of Toxicology and Clinical Toxicology* 29, no. 4 (1991): 515–19.

Giannini, A. James; Slaby, Andrew E.; and Giannini, Matthew C. *Handbook of Overdose and Detoxification Emergencies.* New Hyde Park, N.Y.: New York Medical Examination Publishing Co., 1982.

Gibson, Janice T. "Beware of Poisonous Plants." *Parents,* October 1991, 160.

Gill, Paul. "Fatal Fumes: Preventing Carbon Monoxide Poisoning." *Outdoor Life,* June 1992, 94–96.

Goldfrank, L. R. *Toxicologic Emergencies.* New York: Appleton-Century-Crofts, 1982.

Goodman, A. G.; Gilman, L. S.; and Gilman, A. *The Pharmacological Basis of Therapeutics.* New York: Macmillan, 1980.

Gosselin, R. E.; Hodge, Harold; Smith, Roger P.; and Gleason, Marion N. *Clinical Toxicology of Commercial Products.* 5th ed. Baltimore: Williams & Wilkins, 1984.

Graf, A. B. *Tropica: A Color Encyclopedia of Exotic Plants.* East Rutherford, N.J.: Roehrs, 1985.

Greenberg, R. S., and Osterhout, S. K. "Diurnal Trends in Reported Poisonings." *Journal of Toxicology and Clinical Toxicology* 19 (1982): 167–72.

Griffith, H. Winter. *Complete Guide to Prescription and Non-Prescription Drugs.* New York: Putnam, 1992.

Griggs, Barbara. *Green Pharmacy: A History of Herbal Medicine.* New York: Viking Press, 1981.

Gutman, W. E. "A Poison in Every Cauldron: Chemical and Biological Weapons." *Omni,* February 1991, 42–51.

Guyton, Arthur C. *Textbook of Medical Physiology.* Philadelphia: W. B. Saunders, 1981.

Haddad, L. M., and Winchester, J. F., eds. *Clinical Management of Poisoning and Drug Overdose.* Philadelphia: W. B. Saunders, 1983.

Hardin, J., and Arena, J. M. *Human Poisoning from Native and Cultivated Plants.* Durham: Duke University Press, 1974.

Harris, Ben Charles. *The Compleat Herbal.* Barre, Mass.: Barre Publishers, 1972.

Harte, John, et al. *Toxics A to Z.* Berkeley and Los Angeles: University of California Press, 1991.

Hayes, W. J., Jr. *Pesticide Studies in Man.* Baltimore: Williams & Wilkins, 1982.

HealthFacts editors. "Susceptibility to Food Poisoning: Certain Foods, Certain People." *HealthFacts,* May 1992, 4.

Heiser, Charles B., Jr. *Nightshades.* San Francisco: W. H. Freeman and Co., 1969.

Hevesi, Dennis. "After New Testing, Parents Worry About Levels of Lead at School." *New York Times,* June 18, 1992, 83(L).

"Hidden Danger in the Home." *USA Today,* February 1991, 12.

Hoffman, R. S., et al. "Association Between Life-Threatening Cocaine Toxicity and Plasma Cholinesterase." *Annals of Emergency Medicine*, 21, no. 3 (March 1992): 247–53.

Hoffman, Robert S., and Barsan, William G. "Emergency Treatment of Acute Drug Ingestions." *Journal of the American Medical Association* 266 (November 27, 1991): 2831–32.

Holloway, Marguerite. "A Great Poison: Dioxin Helps Elucidate the Function of Genes." *Scientific American*, November 1990, 16–17.

Hoppu, Kalle; Tikanoja, Tero; Tapanainen, Paivi; Remes, Mikko; Saarenpaa-Heikkila, Outi; and Kouvalainen, Kauko. "Accidental Astemizole Overdose in Young Children." *Lancet* 338 (August 31, 1991): 538–40.

Horowitz, Janice; Lafferty, Elaine; and Thompson, Dick. "The New Scoop on Vitamins." *Time*, April 6, 1992, 59.

Huebner, Albert L. "Get the Lead Out." *American Baby*, August 1992, 32–37.

Hunter, Beatrice Trum. "Dietary Lead: Problems and Solutions." *Consumers' Research Magazine*, May 1992, 18–22.

————. "Paralytic Shellfish Poisoning: A Growing Problem." *Consumers' Research Magazine*, February 1992, 8–9.

————. "Short-Term Illness, Long-Term Health Disorders." *Consumers' Research Magazine*, September 1990, 8–9.

Hunter, Linda Mason. *The Healthy Home: An Attic-to-Basement Guide to Toxin-Free Living*. New York: Pocket Books, 1990.

Hutchens, Alma. *Indian Herbalogy of North America*. Boston and London: Shambhala, 1991.

Hyams, Jay. *Poisons*. Springhouse, Pa.: Springhouse Corporation, 1986.

"Iron Pills Lead the List in Killing of the Young." *New York Times*, June 9, 1992, 88(N).

"Japan's Fugu Is a Delicacy: But Is It Poisson or Poison?" *People*, January 22, 1990, 95.

Jaroff, Leon. "Is Your Fish Really Foul?" *Time*, June 29, 1992, 70–71.

Johnson, Howard M.; Russell, Jeffrey K.; and Pontzer, Carol H. "Superantigens in Human Disease." *Scientific American*, April 1992, 92–99.

Kaplan, Eugene. *A Field Guide to Coral Reefs*. Boston: Houghton Mifflin, 1982.

Kaye, Sidney. *Handbook of Emergency Toxicology*. Springfield, Ill.: Charles C. Thomas, 1988.

Keegan, H., and MacFarlane, L., eds., *Venomous and Poisonous Animals and Noxious Plants of the Pacific Region*. Oxford: Pergamon Press, 1963.

Kerstitch, Alex. "Primates of the Sea." *Discover*, February 1992, 34–37.

Kerstitch, Alex, and Kluger, Jeffrey. "Pretty Poison: Dart Poison Frog." *Discover*, July 1991, 68–71.

Khare, M., et al. "Poisoning in Children," *Journal of Postgraduate Medicine*, 36, no. 4 (October 1990): 203–6.

Kinghorn, A. D., ed. *Toxic Plants*. New York: Columbia University Press, 1979.

Kingsbury, J. M. *Deadly Harvest: A Guide to Common Poisonous Plants*. New York: Holt, Rinehart, 1965.

———. *Poisonous Plants of the United States and Canada*. Englewood Cliffs, N.J.: Prentice-Hall, 1964.

Klassen, C. D.; Amdur, M. O.; and Doull, J., eds. *Casarett and Doull's Toxicology: The Basic Science of Poisons*. 3d ed. New York: Macmillan, 1986.

Klein-Schwartz, W., et al. "Effect of Milk on Ipecac-induced Emesis." *Journal of Toxicology, Clinical Toxicology* 29, no. 4 (1991): 505–11.

———. "Poisoning in the Elderly." *Drugs and Aging* 1 (January 1991): 67–89.

Kohn, Howard. "Dial P-O-I-S-O-N-S." *Readers' Digest*, March 1992, 119.

———. "The Poison People." *In Health*, November 1991, 66–80.

Kopferschmidt, J., et al. "Acute Voluntary Intoxication by Ricin." *Human Toxicology* 2 (1983): 239–42.

Korn, Peter. "The Persisting Poison: Agent Orange in Vietnam." *Nation*, April 8, 1991, 440–45.

Kowalchik, Claire, and Hylton, William H., eds. *Rodale's Illustrated Encyclopedia of Herbs*. Emmaus, Pa.: Rodale Press, 1987.

Kozma, J. J. *Killer Plants: A Poisonous Plant Guide*. Jacksonville, Ill.: Milestone, 1969.

Lampe, K. F., and McCann, M. C. *AMA Handbook of Poisonous and Injurious Plants*. Chicago: American Medical Association, 1985.

"Lead Poisoning." *USA Weekend*, January 3, 1992, 8.

Lefferts, Lisa Y., and Schmidt, Stephen. "Molds: The Fungus Among Us." *Nutrition Action Healthletter*, November 1991, 1–3.

———. "Name Your (Food) Poison." *Nutrition Action Healthletter*, July/August 1991, 1–4.

Levy, C. K., and Primack, R. B. *A Field Guide to Poisonous Plants and Mushrooms of North America*. Brattleboro, Vt.: Stephen Greene Press, 1984.

Lewis, W. H., and Elvin-Lewis, M. *Medical Botany: Plants Affecting Man's Health*. New York: John Wiley and Sons, 1977.

Lichtenstein, Grace. "They're Poisoning Our Children." *Woman's Day*, November 27, 1990, 56–58.

Litovitz, T. L., et al. "1988 Annual Report of the American Association of Poison Control Centers National Data Collection System." *American Journal of Emergency Medicine* 7 (1988): 495–544.

Lovejoy, Frederick H., Jr. "Corrosive Injury of the Esophagus in Children:

Failure of Corticosteroid Treatment Re-emphasizes Prevention." *New England Journal of Medicine*, 323 (September 6, 1990): 668–70.

Lund, Barbara M. "Foodborne Disease due to Bacillus and Clostridium Species." *Lancet* 336 (October 20, 1990): 982–86.

McElvaine, M. D.; Harder, E. M; Johnson, L.; Baer, R. D.; and Satzger, R. D. "Lead Poisoning from the Use of Indian Folk Medicines." *Journal of the American Medical Association* 264 (November 7, 1990): 2212–13.

McKnight, Kent, and McKnight, Vera. *Peterson Field Guides to Mushrooms*. Boston: Houghton Mifflin, 1987.

McLeod, Michael. "Death on the Doorstep." *Reader's Digest*, August 1991, 135–40.

Malloy, Julia. "Straight Answers About Produce and Pesticides." *Better Homes and Gardens*, August 1992, 37–38.

Mayo Clinic. "Seafood Safety: Fish Is Low in Fat, but What About Pollutants?" *Mayo Clinic Health Letter* 9 (November 1991): 6–7.

Michaels, Evelyne. "Holiday Food Safety." *Chatelaine*, December 1991, 34.

Mills, Simon. *The Dictionary of Modern Herbalism: A Comprehensive Guide to Practical Herbal Therapy*. New York: Thorsons Publishers, 1985.

Minton, Sherman A., Jr. *Venomous Reptiles*. New York: Scribner's, 1980.

Mitchell, J., and Rook, A. *Botanical Dermatology: Plants and Plant Products Injurious to the Skin*. Vancouver: Greengrass, 1979.

Moll, Lucy. "Getting the Lead out of Dinner." *Vegetarian Times*, March 1992, 30.

Morrow, Jason D., and Jackson, L. "Was the Tuna a Red Herring? Scombroid Fish Poisoning Caused by Improper Storage." *Patient Care 26* May 15, 1992: 245–47.

Morrow, Jason D.; Margolies, Gary R.; Rowland, Jerry; and Roberts, L. Jackson. "Evidence that Histamine is the Causative Toxin of Scombroid-Fish Poisoning." *New England Journal of Medicine*, 324 (March 14, 1991): 716–20.

Mott, L., and Snyder, K. *Pesticide Alert*. San Francisco: Sierra Club Books, 1987.

Murray Mary. "Are You Serving Poison?" *Readers' Digest*, December 1990, 129–33.

New, Amy Hoffman. "Home (Sniff!) Home: Household Allergies Are Nothing to Sneeze At." *Better Homes and Gardens*, April 1992, 446.

"New Drug to Treat Lead Poisoning." *FDA Consumer*, June 1991, 2.

Olson, Kent R., et al. *Poisoning and Drug Overdose*. Norwalk, Conn.: Appleton & Lange, 1990.

Pantridge, Margaret. "Fish." *Boston Magazine*, April 1992, 62–69.

Pappas, Nancy. "Controlling Poison Ivy." *Country Journal* 17, July/August 1990, 15–16.

"Parasitic Strategy for Poison Control: How Plasmodium Falciparum Protects Itself from Toxins." *Science News*, February 9, 1991, 92.

Parker, H. W., and Grandison, A. G. C. Snakes—*A Natural History*. Ithaca, N.Y.: Cornell University Press, 1977.

Pennisi, Elizabeth. "Pharming Frogs: Chemist Finds Precious Alkaloids in Poisonous Amphibians." *Science News*, July 18, 1992, 40–42.

Perl, Trish M.; Bedard, Lucie; Kosatsky, Tom; Hockin, James C.; Todd, Ewen C. D.; and Remims, Robert S. "An Outbreak of Toxic Encephalopathy Caused by Eating Mussels Contaminated with Domoic Acid," *New England Journal of Medicine* 322 (June 21, 1990): 1775–80.

"Pesticide May Cause Allergy." *Science News*, February 15, 1992, 141.

Phelps, Tony. *Poisonous Snakes*. Poole, Dorset, England: Blandford Press, 1981.

"Poison Ivy Protection? (A Question of Health)." *Consumer Reports*, June 1991, 424.

Potterton, David, ed. *Culpeper's Color Herbal*. New York: Sterling, 1983.

Proctor, Nick H., and Hughes, James P. *Chemical Hazards of the Workplace*. Philadelphia: J. B. Lippincott, 1978.

Purdy, Candy. "Houseplants: What You Don't Know Can Hurt You." *Current Health*, December 1992, 24–25.

Rategan, Cathy. "Make Your Home Poison Proof." *Consumers' Research*, October 1990, 32–34.

Reitbrock, N., and Woodcock, B. G. "Two Hundred Years of Foxglove Therapy: *Digitalis purpurea*." *Trends of Pharmacology Science* 6 (1985): 277–84.

"Request for Assistance in Preventing Lead Poisoning in Construction Workers." *Journal of the American Medical Assocation* 267 (April 15, 1992): 2012.

Ricciuti, E. R. *The Devil's Garden: Fact and Folklore of Poisonous Plants*. New York: Walker, 1978.

Robinson, Arnold G. "Painful Mistakes: An Emergency-Room Doctor Tells How to Avoid the Common Blunders That Keep Him So Busy." *Men's Health*, April 1991, 32–33.

Rosenberg, Stephen N., M.D. *The Johnson & Johnson First Aid Book*. New York: Warner Books, 1985.

Rosenthal, Elizabeth. "Poison Berries." *Discover*, February 1990, 80–83.

Rowse, Arthur, ed. *Help: The Indispensable Almanac of Consumer Information 1980*. Washington, D.C.: Consumer News, 1979.

Rumack, B. H.; Sullivan, J. B.; and Peterson, R. G. *Management of Acute Poisoning and Overdose*. Denver: Rocky Mountain Poison Center, 1981.

Russell, F. E. *Snake Venom Poisoning*. Philadelphia: J. B. Lippincott, 1980.

Sacks, Jeffrey J. "Points of Potential IQ Lost from Lead." *Journal of the American Medical Association* 264 November 7, 1990: 1044–46.

Satchell, Michael. "A Vicious Circle of Poison: New Questions About American Exports of Powerful Pesticides." *U.S. News and World Report*, June 10, 1991, 31–32.

Schmidt, Karen F. "Puzzling over a Poison: On Closer Inspection, the Ubiquitous Pollutant Dioxin Appears More Dangerous Than Ever." *U.S. News and World Report*, April 6, 1992, 60–61.

"Scrambled: After 2,000 Food-Poisoning Cases, Fear of Salmonella Is No Yolk," *Time*, May 13, 1991, 50.

Segal, Marian. "Botulism in the Entire United States." *FDA Consumer*, January–February 1992, 27.

Sewell, B., and Whyatt, R. *Intolerable Risk: Pesticides in Our Children's Food*. New York: Natural Resources Defense Council, 1989.

Shannon, Michael, and Graef, John. "Hazard of Lead in Infant Formula." *New England Journal of Medicine*, 326 (January 9, 1992): 137.

"Should You Drink from Crystal?" *University of California, Berkeley Wellness Letter* 7 June 1991, 7.

Sittig, Marshall. *Handbook of Toxic and Hazardous Chemicals*. Park Ridge, N.J.: Noyes Publications, 1981.

Smith, Bradley, and Stevens, Gus. *The Emergency Book: You Can Save a Life*. New York: Simon & Schuster, 1978.

Snyder, Solomon. *Inhalants: The Toxic Fumes*. New York: Chelsea House, 1986.

———. *Prescription Narcotics, the Addictive Painkillers*. New York: Chelsea House, 1986.

Snyder, Solomon H., and Bredt, David S. "Biological Roles of Nitric Oxide." *Scientific American*, May 1992, 68–77.

Spencer, Peter L. "Poison Oak, Ivy." *Consumers' Research Magazine*, March 1990, 2.

Spongberg, Stephen A. "Deck the Halls: Poisonous Plants." *Harvard Health Letter* 17 (December 1991): 4.

Stephens, H. A. *Poisonous Plants of the Central United States*. Lawrence: University of Kansas, 1980.

Stevens, S. D., and Klarner, A. *Deadly Doses*. Cincinnati: Writer's Digest Books, 1990.

Stone, R. "Name Your Poison: Toxicologists Meet." *Science*, March 13, 1992, 1356–57.

Stoner, J. G., and Rasmussen, J. E. "Plant Dermatitis." *American Academy of Dermatology* 9 (1983): 1–14.

Street, Robin. "Safety First for Summertime Foods." *Better Homes and Gardens*, August 1991, 40–41.

Sunshine, I. *Methodology for Analytical Toxicology*. Boca Raton, Fla.: CRC Press, 1975.

Swain, T., ed. *Plants in Development of Modern Medicine*. Cambridge: Harvard University Press, 1972.

Swann, Lauren. "When Food Bites Back: Sage Advice on How to Savor Food Safely." *Weight Watchers Magazine*, July 1991, 16–17.

Telzak, Edward E.; Budnick, Lawrence D.; Zweig Greenberg, Michele S.;

Blum, Steve; Shayegani, Mehdi; Benson, Charles E.; and Schultz, Stephen. "A Nosocomial Outbreak of *Salmonella Enteritidis* Infection due to the Consumption of Raw Eggs." *New England Journal of Medicine* 323 (August 9, 1990): 394–97.

Tenenbein, Milton; Kowalski, Stephen; Sienko, Anna; Bowden, Drummon H.; and Adamson, Ian. "Pulmonary Toxic Effects of Continuous Desferrioxamine Administration in Acute Iron Poisoning." *Lancet* 339 (March 21, 1992): 699–71.

"Therapeutic Poison: Botulinum Toxin Used to Treat Blepharospasm and Strabismus." *Harvard Health Letter,* February 1991, 7–8.

Thygerson, Alton L. *The First Aid Book.* 2d ed. Englewood Cliffs, N.J.: Prentice-Hall, 1986.

Tranter, Howard S. "Foodborne Staphylococcal Illness." *Lancet* 336 (October 27, 1990): 1044–46.

Trestrail, J. H. *Mushrooms and Mushroom Poisoning.* Grand Rapids, Mich.: Blodgett Regional Poison Center, 1989.

"Two Agencies Look at Lead in Wine." *FDA, Consumer,* November 1991, 2–3.

Van Etten, C. *Toxic Constituents of Plant Foodstuffs.* New York: Academic Press, 1969.

Vickery, Donald M., M.D., and Fries, James F., M.D. *Take Care of Yourself: A Consumer's Guide to Medical Care.* Reading, Mass.: Addison-Wesley, 1976

Waldman, Steven. "Lead and Your Kids." *Newsweek,* July 15, 1991, 42–48.

Warrick, Sheridan. "The Milk Cow, the Rat Poison and the President: How Dicumerol and Warfarin Were Developed as an Anticoagulant." *In Health,* July–August 1990, 14.

Wasco, James. "Was It Something You Ate?" *Woman's Day,* July 21, 1992, 10.

Waters, Tom. "The Fine Art of Making Poison." *Discover,* August 1992, 29–32.

Wexler, Philip. *Information Resources in Toxicology.* New York: Elsevier, North Holland, 1982.

Williams, W. K. *A Handbook for Physicians and Mushroom Hunters.* New York: Van Nostrand Reinhold, 1977.

"Wine: Getting the Lead Out." *Science News,* September 21, 1991, 189.

Woodward, L. *Poisonous Plants: A Color Field Guide.* New York: Hippocrene Books, 1985.

Zamula, Evelyn. "Contact Dermatitis: Solutions to Rash Mysteries." *FDA Consumer,* May 1990, 28–32.

Zyla, Gail. "Vitamin Vigilance: Preventing Vitamin Poisoning." *Reader's Digest* (Canada), April 1992, 115–16.

INDEX

Boldface numbers
indicate main headings

AAPC National Data Collection 1
abortifacient 41, 50, 62, 79, 106, 134, 167, 211, 233, 241, 256-7, 283, 305, 311
Abrus prevatorius 176, **252**
absinthe 305
Acanthophis antarcticus **4**
Acanthophis pyrrhus **4**
acetaldehyde 83
acetaminophen **1**, 32, 78, 96, 214, 228, 254
acetazolamide 103
acetic acid (vinegar) **2**
acetone 272
acetylcholinesterase 249
acetylcysteine
  as antidote 172
acetylene workers 219
acetylsalicylic acid See *aspirin*
acids **2**, 9, 64, 134, 227
ack-ack 135
ackee 7
Acokanthera oblongifolia **311**
aconite 176; see also *monkshood*
aconitine **2**, 177
Aconitum 176
  A. columbianum **176**
  A. lutescens **176**
  A. uncinatum 176
Aconitus 176
acrylamide **2-3**
acrylamide monomer 2-3
acrylic amide 2-3
Actaea 34
  A. alba 34
  A. pachypoda 34
  A. rubra 34
  A. spicata 34
Actifed See *decongestants*
Actinia equinia 15
Actinodendron plumosum 15
adder **3**
adder, common **3-4**
adder, death **3-4**, 75
adder, desert death 4
adder, European 301; see also *adder, common*
adder, night 3, **4**
adder, puff 3, **5**, 297, 301
adhesives 123
adrenaline 21
adrenocortical steroids 153
  as treatment for poisoning 49
Advil See *anti-inflammatory drugs*
Aenas 175
aerosol propellants See *chlorofluorocarbons*
aescin 50
Aesculapian snake 4
Aesculapius 4
Aesculus 50
aflatoxins **5-6**, 31
African coffee tree 61
African lilac tree 64
African milk plant **6**
African violet 200

Afrin **7**
Agent Orange 102
Ageratine altissima 309-10
Agkistrodon 131, 221
Agkistrodon bilineatus 56
  A. contortrix 82
  A. piscivorus 308
  A. rhodostoma **298-9**
Agrostemma githago 86
Agrotect 294
Aipysurus laevis 262
akee 7
Aketedron 13
aki 7
Alar **7-8**
Alaskan butter clam 257, 266
alcohol 9, 17, 19, 20, 39, 63, 83, 88, 91, 96, 106, 141, 143, 147, 161, 178, 181, 189, 198, 205, 232, 287
  as antidote 20, 150, 217, 259
alcoholism 77
aldicarb **8-9**, 57
Aldomet **9**, 21
aldrin 9, 67, 140, 281
alkalies 11, 64, 134, 227, 240
alkali grass 93
alkaline corrosives **9-11**, 26, 163
alkaloid **11**, 32, 53, 77, 78, 80, 81, 125, 126, 128, 132, 135, 136, 140, 151- 2, 165, 180, 181, 190, 192, 194, 196, 241, 273, 284, 289
alphanaphthylthiourea 244
alprazolam 18
aluminum plant 200
Amanitaceae family **11-12**, 186-7
Amanita mushrooms **11-12**, 87, 93, 115-6, 141, 184, 186-7 (charts)
  A. bisporigera 12, 95-96, 186
  A. cokeri 12, 186
  A. cothurnata 12, 186
  A. gemmata 12, 186
  A. muscaria 11, **115-6**, 183, 186
  A. ocreata 12, 95-96, 186-7
  A. pantherina 12, 115, 183, 186-7, **208**
  A. phalloides 11-12, 93, 115, 185, 186-7
  A. suballiacae 12, 186
  A. tenuifolia 12, 186
  A. verna 12, 95-96, 186-7
  A. virosa 12, 186-7
amanitin 12, 93, 96
amatoxins **12**, 93, 158, 184, 186
amebiasis **120**
amebic dysentery **120**
American Dental Association 114, 170
American elder 105
American nightshade See *nightshade, black*
amiloride 103
amino benzol See *aniline*
aminophylline 181
ammonia 10, **13**, 66, 68, 113, 228
  as antidote 16, 99, 150, 232
ammonium chloride
  as antidote 215-6
ammonium hydroxide **13**
amobarbital See *Amytal*
amphetamines **13-14**, 77-78, 94, 178, 191, 235
  treatment for 154, 174, 194, 217, 236
amygdalin 61, 64, 89, 128, 236
amyl nitrite **14**
  as treatment for poisoning 71, 106
Amytal 35
anabasine 289

analgesics 22, 54, 138, 181
Anaprox (naproxen) See *nonsteroidal anti-inflammatory drugs*
Androctonus asutralis 258
andromedotoxin 103, 250
anectine **14-15**
  as antidote 15
anemone 146
anemone, sea **15-16**, 149
anesthesia 15, 89, 90, 91, 107
anesthetics, gaseous/volatile (general) **16**, 71, 90, 107, 198, 202
anesthetics, local **16-17**, 55-56, 77-78, **158**, 224, 232, 235
angel dust 215
angiotensin-converting enzyme inhibitors 21
aniline **17**
animal dip 88
anisakiasis **121**, 280
Anisakis marina 280
Antabuse **17-18**, 141
antacid 22, 199, 201
anthracenones 51
anthraquinone glycosides 251
antianxiety drugs **18**
antiarrhythmic drugs 18, 158, 235, 240, 272
antibiotics 201, 275
  as treatment for poisoning 161, 222, 245, 256
antichlorine compounds 26
anticoagulants 9, **18-19**, 21, 22, 199, 254, 307
anticonvulsant 91, 95
  as treatment for poisoning 93, 216
antidepressants **19**, 91, 158, 181, 211, 220, 235, 268, 272
antiemetic 171
antifreeze **19-20**, 171, 214, 228
  antidote for 107
antihistamines **20-21**, 73, 91, 94, 96, 102-3, 212, 222, 268
  as antidote 38, 49, 84, 98, 111, 150, 224, 257, 293
antihypertensive drugs 9, **21**, 48, 62, 91, 106, 174
anti-inflammatory drugs **21-22**, 199
antimicrobials **26**
antimony **22-23**, 142
  antidote for 34, 99-100
antimony hydride See *stibine*
antiperspirant 172
antipsychotic/psychometric drugs **23**
antipyretic 31
antiseptics and disinfectants 2, **23-24**, 44, 88, 123, 138, 143, 147, 169, 189, 216, 233
antispasmodic 14, 196
antivenin **24-25**, 57, 75
antivenin, Australian black snake 42
antivenin, black widow spider 24, **25**, 43, 273
antivenin, eastern coral snake **25**, 85-86, 271
antivenin, rattlesnake **25**, 166, 222, 245-9, 268
antivenin, sea wasp 265
antivenin, snake 271
antivenin, stonefish 261, 278
ant paste 22
ants 11
anuncena de Mejico 195
aphrodisiac 43, 56, 77, 165
apormorphine

as antidote **25-26**
appetite suppressant 94, 234-5
apple 128
apple juice 7
apple of Peru 151
apple of Sodom **26**
apricot pits See *prunus*
aquarium products 9-10, **26**, 201
aquarium salts **26**
Araceae family 97
Arachnida 258
arbre 7
Areca catechu 40
arecain 41
Aristotle 41
arrow-poison frogs **26-27**, 153
arrow poison frogs, boulenger's 27
arrow poison frogs, gold 27
arrow poison frogs, three-striped 27
arrow poison frogs, two-toned 27
arrow poison frogs, yellow-spotted 27
arrow poisons 6, 61, 89, 126, 153
arsenic 22, **28-29**, 64, 244, 297
  antidote for 30, 34, 99-100, 103, 211
arsenic compounds 142
arsenic hydride 29
arsenic trihydride 28-29
arsenic trioxide 28-29
arsenous oxide 28-29
arsine 22
arsine gas 22, **29**
artane See *trihexyphenidyl*
artificial sweetener See *sweeteners, artificial*
asbestos **29-30**, 267
ascorbic acid 2, **30**
  as antidote 72
Asian food 179
asp 75
aspartame **30-31**, 280-1
aspartic cid 30-31
Aspergillus flavus 5-6, **31**
Aspidelaps lubricus 85
aspidistra 200
aspirin 21, 22, **31-32**, 53, 78, 189, 199,
  207, 212, 227, 254, 285
aster 200
Asthenosoma jimoni 263
asthma weed 140
Atelopus boulengeri 27
  A. planispina 27
  A. zeteki 27
Ativan (lorazepam) 18, 39
Atropa belladonna L. **195-7**
atropine 11, 21, **32-33**, 40, 134, 152,
  165, 194, 195-6, 292
  as antidote 9, 41, 57, 58, 62, 71-72,
  79, 93, 99, 115, 141-2, 149, 155,
  174, 206, 211, 219, 238, 239, 250,
  285, 311
Atropos 195
Aunt Shawnee 310
auto 123
autumn crocus 167
azalea See *rhododendron*
Aztecs 180

baby food 6
baby oil 201
baby powder 44
baby's tears 200
bacillary dysentery **117**
Bacillus cereus bacterium 117
bacillus thuringiensis (Bt) **34**, 45
bacterial gastroenteritis 25, 60, 110,
  115, 151, 276

bacterial toxins
  antidote for 30
baking soda
  as antidote 38, 150, 232
BAL **34**
Balder 175
ball nettle 60
ball nightshade 60
banded krait See *krait, banded*
baneberry **34-35**
baneberry, red 34
baneberry, white 34
banewort 195
barba amarillo 110
Barbados lily 195
Barbados nut **35**, 84
barbiturates **35-36**, 135, 268, 287
  as treatment for poison 70, 73, 133,
  140, 160, 201, 235, 289-90
barium **36**
barium carbonate 244
barium nitrate 111
barium salts 36
barium sulfate 36
barley 5-6
barracuda 72
bass 112
bassinet 51
bastard acacia 41
batrachotoxin 11
batteries 9-10, 22, 156, 169
batteries, auto 2
batteries, disk 10
batteries, dry cell 201
batteries, nickel-cadmium 53
Baudelaire, Charles 154
bead tree 64
bead vine 252
beans 13
bear's foot 176
beech 256
bee stings **36-38**
begonia 200
belladonna 152, 176, 194-6; see also
  nightshade, deadly
belladonna lily 195
bellflower 140
bellyache bush **38**, 84
Benadryl 150
bendroflumethiazide 103
bennies 13
Benzedrine 13
benzene **38-39**, 70, 88, 137, 142
  antidote for 30
benzene hexachloride **39**
benzocaine
  as treatment for poison 224
benzodiazepines 18, **39-40**, 97, 174, 268
  antidote for 114, 216
benzoic acid 205
benztropine **40**
Betadine 144
beta adrenergic blockers 18, 21, **40**, 48,
  94, 106, 287
  antidote for 147
betel nut seed **40-41**
BHC 39
bicarbonate
  as antidote 20
biotoxins 290
bird's nest fern 200
birth control, botanical 41
birth control pills **41**, 91, 191, 201
bismuth
  antidote for 99-100

bismuth subcarbonate
  as treatment for poisoning 62
Bitis 5
  B. gabonica
bitter almonds 89
bitter apple 79
bitter cassava 60
bitter cucumber 79
bittersweet, European (woody nightshade) 195
black acacia 41
black beauties 13
black-eyed Susan 252
black mollies 13
black snake, American 42
black snake, Australian **41-42**, 75
black snakeroot 93
black widow spider **42-43**, 55, 75, 273
  treatment for 97, 170
bladderpod 140
bleach 2, 10, 68, 228, 272; see also *alkaline corrosives*
Blighia sapida 7
blister beetle **43**, 56
blister flower 51
bloodroot **43**
blotter acid 162
blowfish See *pufferfish*
bluefish 112, 257
blue-green algae 129
blue krait See *krait, blue*
bois joli 91
Boletus calopus 186
  B. luridus 186
  B. pulcherrimus 186
  B. satanas 186
boneset 310
boomslang **44**
borax 142
boric acid **44**
Boston fern 200
botanic insecticides 34, **45**, 60, 192, 238,
  239, 252
Bothrops 110, 298
  B. alternatus 110, 311-2
  B. nummifera 110
botulin **45**
botulin antitoxin **45**
botulin toxins 45
botulinum bacterium 45
botulism **45-47**, 116, 121, 137
botulism, infant 45, 137
botulus 46
brain fungi 130
Brazil nuts 5-6
breadfruit vine 218
brewer's yeast
  as antidote 47
British mandrake See *mandrake, British*
bromates **47-48**
bromate salts 47
bromide **48**
bromoacetone 284
bromocriptine
  as antidote 23
bromomethylethylketone 284
Bromo-Seltzer 48
bronchial tube dilators See *bronchial tube
  relaxers*
bronchial tube relaxers **48**, 104
  as treatment for poison 70
Browning, Elizabeth Barrett 154
brown recluse spider **48-49**, 273
brown snake, Australian **49-50**, 75
brown spider See *brown recluse spider*

brown spiders, South American   49
brown widow spider   42
Bryonia alba   50
    B. cretica   50
    B. dioica   50
bryonidin   50
bryonin   50
bryony   **50**
bubble bath   201
buckeye   **50-51**
buckhorn   **51**
bufencarb   57
Bufo marinus   288
bufogin   288
bufonin   288
bufotalin   288
Bufo toxin   288
bull nettle   60
bumetanide   103
Bunguras coeruleus   **153**
    B. fasciatus   153
burning bush   273
bushmaster   **51**
Buspirone   178
Buthus occitanus   258
butter clam, Alaskan   257, 266
buttercress   51
buttercup   34, **51-52**, 71, 146, 176
butter daisy   51
butterflower   51
butterfly cod   160
butterfly fish   260
butterweed   243
button spider   42
butylene   137
butyl nitrites   14

cadmium   34, **53**, 99
caffeine   **53-55**, 77, 78, 94, 136, 161, 212, 214, 285
    as antidote   9, 99, 236
caffeinism   54
Caladium   181
calamine lotion
    as treatment for poison   150, 224-6, 232
calcium   21, **54**
    as treatment for poisoning   54
calcium arsenate   170
calcium channel blocking drugs   18, 21, 106
calcium chloride
    as treatment for poisoning   115
calcium EDTA   **55**, 204, 211
calcium gluconate
    as treatment for poisoning   115, 251
calcium hydroxide (slaked lime)   240
calcium hypochlorite   281
calcium oxalate raphides   97, 181-2, 207, 218, 234, 251, 273, 307
calcium oxide   240
calfkill   154
calico bush   154
California fern   132
California mussel   **55**
California poppy   200
calla lily   97
Calla palustris L.   307
Calotropis gigantea   126
    C. procera   126
camellia   200
Campho-Phenique   305
camphor   **55-56**, 205, 224, 305
camphorated oil   55, 305
Campylobacter jejujni bacterium   117

campylobacterosis   **117**
cancer jalap   229
candles   201
canning   46, 116
cantharidin   43, **56**
cantil snake   **56-57**
capacitors   231
cape belladonna   195
cap pistol caps   201
Captain Bligh   7
carbamate   8-9, **57**, 142
    antidote for   234
carbamazepine   269
carbamic acid   57
carbaryl   **57**, 142
carbofuran   57
carbohydrate andromedotoxin   155
carbolic acid   **2**; see also *phenol*
carbon dioxide gas   227
carbonless copy paper   230
carbon monoxide   **58-59**, 64, 172, 236, 267
    treatment for poisoning by   207
carbon tetrachloride   **59**, 67
    antidote for   **1**
carbutol   See *barbiturate*
carcinogens, human/animal (possible)
    aflatoxins   **5-6**
    Alar   7-8,
    aldrin   9, 67, 281
    ammonia   13,
    asbestos   29-30
    benzene   38-39
    carbon tetrachloride   67
    chlordane   67, 140, 142, 281
    chlorinated water   69
    chloroform   67, 70-71, 107
    comfrey   80
    creosote   88, 216
    cyclamates   280
    dieldrin   67, 98, 140, 281
    dimethyl sulfate   100
    dioxin   102
    ethylene chlorohydrin   107-8
    formaldehyde   123, 137, 171, 182, 267
    heptachlor   67, 140, 281
    hexavalent compounds   72
    kepone   174, 281
    lindane   67, 159, 281
    methyl bromide   171
    methyl chloride   172
    mirex   174
    PCBs   231
    radiation poisoning   242
    radon   242-3
    saccharin   254
    toxaphene   67, 289
    trichloroethane   290-1
    vinyl chloride   67, 68
cardiac glycosides   **59-60**, 98, 99, 125, 126, 128, 197, 204, 273, 275, 311
cardiotoxin   75, 164
car exhaust   58, 156, 197, 267
carisoprodol   268-9
carneum   60, 238, 239
carocaine   16
Carolina horse nettle   **60**
Carolina jessamine   151
carp   62
carpet   123, 182, 267
Carroll, Lewis   169
cascabel   See *rattlesnake, cascabel*
cashews   224
cassava   **60-61**, 121, 128

cassava flour   60
castor bean   **61-62**, 89, 176, 220
castor oil   35, 55, 61, 201
    as treatment for poisoning   217, 257, 305
castor oil plant   61
Catapres (clonidine)   21, **62**
caterpillars   9, 34
catfish   **62-63**
cathartic oils   129
Causus   4
CD-68   66
cedar   41
ceiling materials   29
Celotin   269
Centers for Disease Control, The   47, 156, 160
centipedes   **63**
Centrax (prazepam)   18, 39
Centruroides exilicauda   258, **260**
    C. gertschii   **258**
    C. vittatus   **258**
Cephaelis ipecacuanha   144
ceramics   13, 22, 28, 156, 169
Cerberus   176
cereus   **117**
Ceylon creeper, golden   234
chalk   227
chalk, blackboard   201
chalice vine   292
charcoal, activated   **63-64**
charcoal briquettes   **64**
charcoal grill   58, 64
cheese   19, 66, 160, 178, 274, 310
chelating agent   55, **64**, 95, 103, 158, 166, 204, 211, 242
chelation therapy   53, 72
chemical pneumonitis   53, 197
chemical weapon   See *poison gas*
cherries, wild and cultivated   **64**, 90, 128
cherry pie filling   7
cherry pit   90; see also *cherries, wild and cultivated; Prunus*
chicken   6; see also *poultry*
children and poisons   1
child-resistant caps   32
chinaberry   **64-65**
China tree   64
chincherinchee   275
chinchonism   64
Chinese food   179
Chinese restaurant syndrome   179
Chironex fleckeri   264
Chiropsalmus quadrigatus   264
chloral hydrate   **65-66**, 268
    antidote for   196
chloramine gas   **66**, 68
chloramine-T   **66**
chlorate poisoning   66
chlorazepate   See *Tranxene*
chlordane   **66-67**, 140, 142, 281
chlordecone   281
chlordiazepoxide   See *Librium*
chlorinated biphenyl   216
chlorinated camphene   281, 289
chlorinated hydrocarbons   9, 67, 70, 92, 142, 172, 174, 230, 285
chlorinated hydrocarbon pesticides   **67-68, 98**, 105
chlorine   66, **68-69**, 112, 172, 228, 281
chlorine gas   68, **69-70**
chloroacetophenone   284
chlorobenzine derivatives   70, 231, 281
chlorofluorocarbons   68
chloroform   16, 65, 67, **70-71**, 107

antidote for **1**
chlorophyll 234
chloroquine 241
chlorothion 281
chlorpromazine See *Thorazine*
as treatment for poisoning 216
chlorpropham 57
chlorprothixene 23
chlorthion See *organophosphate insecti-cides*
chocolate 53, 191, 214
choke cherry pit 89; see *Prunus*
cholera **117**
Cholo Indians 153
Christmas cactus 200
Christmas rose **71-72**
Christmas tree lights 172
chromate salts 72
chromic acid 72
chromic anhydride 72
chromic oxide 72
chromic sulfate 72
chromium
antidote for 55, 99-100
chromium trioxide 72
chrysanthemum 60, 238, 252
Cicuta bolanderi 132-3
C. bulbifera 132-3
C. californica 132-3
C. curtissii 132
C. douglasii 132-3
C. maculata 132-3
C. occidentalis 132-3
C. vagans 132-3
cicutoxin 133
cigarettes 192, 194
ciguatera 72, 101, 113, 129
ciguatoxin 72
cimetidine **73**
as treatment for poisoning 96, 257, 293
cinchona bark 241
cinchophen (cinchonan-9-ol and others) 21, 65, **73**
Circe 165
citanest 16
citrate 55; see also *anticoagulants*
Citrullus colocynthis 79
clams 113, 209, 265-6
Claudius 176
Claviceps purpurea **106**
clay, modelling 201
cleaning solutions 2, 13, 66
cleansers 66
clematis **73-74**
Cleopatra 75
climbing lily **74**
Clinoril (sulindac) 199-200
Clitocybe family 183
C. cerrusata 183
C. clavipes 183
C. dealbata 183
C. illudens 149, 183
C. riuulosa 183
clonidine 189; see also *Catapres*
Clostridium botulinum A,B,E 45-46, 136
Clostridium perfringens **117**
cloth 123-4
clove cigarettes See *phenol*
clove oil 216
coal tar 189
cobra 3, 4, 50, **74-75**, 82, 85, 86, 153, 260, 271, 282, 288, 299, 300, 301, 302
cobra, African 75
cobra, Asian 75

cobra, black necked 75; see also *cobra, spitting*
cobra, blue
cobra, Egyptian **75**
cobra, Indian **75**
cobra, king **76**, 262, 269
cobra, spitting **76-77**, 251
cobra, tree 75
cobra venom 46, 75
coca bush alkaloids 16, 77, 158
Coca-Cola 77
cocaine 16, **77-78**, 94, 125, 158, 161, 191, 235
treatment for 154, 194, 217, 236
Cocculus ferrandianus 180
cocoa 54
cocoa beans 53
codeine **78-79**, 96, 136, 190, 205, 207
cod liver oil 55
coelenterates 15, 149-50
coffee 53-54, 169, 190, 279
Cogentin 276; see also *benztropine*
cohosh 34
cohosh, red 34
cola babies 231
cola nut, African 77
colchicine 74, 112, 167
Colchicum autumnale 167
C. speciosum 167
C. vernum 167
cold medicines 96
Coleridge, Samuel Taylor 154, 198
coleus 200
coliform bacteria **79**
colocynth **79**
colocynthin 79
Colubridae 44
columbine 176
comfrey **79-80**
comfrey-pepsin tablets 80
compound 118 9
Compound 269 105
compound 1080 **80-81**
cone shell **81**
coniine **81-82**, 132
Conium maculatum 81, **132**
Conocybe cyanopus 131
C. smithii 131
conocybes 131
conquerors 50
Conus 81
C. geographus 81
C. striatus 81
C. tulipa 81
Convallaria majalis **159**
convallatoxin 275, 311
convalloside 275
Convolvulaceae family 180-1
cooking oil sprays 198
coon tail rattler See *rattlesnake, western diamondback*
copilots 13
copper 125
antidote for 34, 99-100, 211
copperhead, Australian **82**
copperhead, North American 82, 269-71, 308
copperhead snake 24, **82-83**, 221, 269-71, 308
copper sulfate 26
coprine **83**, 141, 186-7
Coprinus 141
C. atramentarius 83, **141**, 186
C. comatus **141**
coral 277

coral, fire 84
coral, hydroid 84
coral, stinging 84
coral bead plant 252
coral plant 35, **83-84**
coral poisoning **84**
coral reef 81
coral snake 24, **85**, 269-70
coral snake, African 75, 85
coral snake, Arizona 75, **85-86**
coral snake, black-banded 75, 85
coral snake, Brazilian giant 75, 85
coral snake, eastern 25, 75, 85, **86**, 271
coral snake, Sonoran 25, 85
coral snake, Texas 25
coral snake, western 271
corn 5-6
corn cockle **86-87**, 256
corn and wart removers
cort family **87**, 141
corticosteroids 21-22, **87**, 135
as antidote 10, 43, 69, 94, 111, 158, 197, 224, 226
Cortinarius gentilis 126
C. orellanus 126
C. speciosissimus 126
cortinarius mushrooms **87**, 141
cottonmouth 24, 56, 221, 270; see also *water moccasin*
cottonseed meal 5-6
cottonseed oil 6
cough medicines 78, 96, 143, 228
cough suppressant 78, 94, 96, 190
cough syrup 17
Coumadin 19
coumarin 307
antidote for 305
crab's eyes 252
crack cocaine 77-78
crank 13
creeping Charlie 200
creosote **87-88**, 216
cresols 87, 216
crocus See *meadow saffron*
crossroads 13
Crotalinae 301-2
Crotalus genus 221, 249, 271
C. adamanteus **245**
C. atrox **248**
C. basiliscus **246**
C. cerastes **267**
C. durissus **245**
C. horridus atricaudatus 244, 247
C. horridus horridus 247
C. ruber **246**
crotamine 245, 249
croton **88-89**
croton oil 88
Croton tiglium 88
crow berry 229
crowfoot 51
crystal 13, 156
Cuban lily 274
cube jellies See *jellyfish*
curare 15, **89**, 101, 132, 193, 209, 237, 267
antidote for 105
curcin 129
curcus bean 35
cuticle remover 9-10
Cyanea capillata **149**
cyanide 61, 66, 80, **89-90**, 137, 138, 142, 162, 198, 236
antidote for 14, 64
cyanide antidote kit 90, 236

cyanogenic glycosides 61, 64, 89, **90**, 105, 128, 162, 236
cyclamate (sodium or calcium) 280
cyclohexane hexachloride **159-60**, 281
cyclopropane 16, 89, **90**
cytotoxic saponins 50

2,4-D **294-5**
daboia See *viper, Russell's*
dahlia 200
dairy products 140
Dalmane (flurazepam) 18, 39, **91**
daminozide (Alar) **7-8**
dandelion 200
dantrolene
  as treatment for poisoning **91**, 107
daphne **91-92**
Daphne mezereum 91
  D. laureola 91
daphnetoxin 91
dart poison frogs See *arrow poison frogs*
Darvon 190
Dasyatis longus **276**
datura See *jimsonweed*
Datura stramonium **151**
Davy, Sir Humphry 198
DBH 39
DDT 9, 67, 70, **92-93**, 137, 142, 159, 206, 281, 289
deadly cort **126**; see also *galerina mushrooms*
deadly galerina **126**; see also *galerina mushrooms*
deadly lawn galerina 126; see also *galerina mushrooms*
dead man's fingers 307
dead man's thimbles 124
Dead Sea apple 25
death angel 95
death camas **93**
death cap/death cup 11-12, **93**
decongestants 7, 48, **94-95**, 96
DEET 143
deferoxamine **95**
dehumidifying packets 201
Demansia textilis 49-50
Demerol See *meperidine; narcotics*
Dendroaspis angusticeps 164
  D. polylepis 164
Dendrobates auratus 27
  D. flavopictus **27**
  D. trivittatus **27**
Dendrobatidae 26
Denisonia superba 82
denture adhesives 201
deodorant 66, 201
Depakene **95**
depilatories 36, 47
derrin See *rotenone*
derris **95**; see also *rotenone*
destroying angel 11-12, 93, **95-96**
detergents 13, 228
devil's apple 165
devil's claws 51
devil's eye 133
devil's ivy 234
devil's trumpet 151
devil's turnip 50
dexies 13
dextromethorphan **96-97**, 178
DFDT 70, 281
DFP 281
diacetylmorphine **135**
Diadema setosum 263
diaper rash ointment 201

diapers 17
diarrhea See *traveller's diarrhea*
diazepam 44, **97**
  as treatment of poisoning 54, 56, 97, 129, 132, 139, 174, 183, 193, 201, 207, 208, 216, 306
diazinon 67, 142, 206, 281
dichlorodiphenyl methyl carbinol 281
dichlorodiphenyltrichloroethane (DDT) **92-93**, 281
dichlorphenamide 103
dichromate salts 72
Dicodid 190
dicumarol 19
dieffenbachia **97-98**, 207
Dieffenbachia amoena 97
  D. bausei 97
  D. candida 97
  D. exotica 97
  D. maculata 97
  D. segume 97
dieldrin 67, **98**, 140 , 281
diet aid 140
diethyltoluamide See *DEET*
diet pills 13-14
diflunisal (Dolobid) 22, 199
difluorodiphenyltrichloroethane 281
digitalis 18, 59, 71, **98-99**, 124-5, 126, 134, 159, 175, 204, 257, 273, 288-9, 311
Digitalis purpurea 59, 98-99, 124-5
digitoxin 59, 98, **99**, 125
digoxin 98, **99**, 158, 235
digoxin specific antibodies 99
7-dihydroxypropyltheophylline 104
diisopropylfluorophosphate 281
diisopropylphosphate 190
dilan 70, 281
Dilantin See *phenytoin*
Dilaudid See *hydromorphone*
dimercaprol **99-100**; see also *BAL*
  as antidote 23, 29, 158, 169, 172, 211
2,3-dimercaptopropanol 103; see also *BAL*
dimethyl sulfate **100**
dimethyl sulfoxide (DMSO) **100**
dimite dichlorodiphenylethanol 281
dinitrophenol derivatives 134, 216
dinoflagellates 55, 72, **100-102**, 208, 257, 266, 280, 292
dioxins **102**
diphenhydramine
  as treatment for poisoning **102-103**
diphtheria 109
dipotassium 204
diquat 134, 209
dishwasher detergent 10; see also *alkaline corrosives*
disinfectants See *antiseptics and disinfectants*
disopyramide (Norpace) 18
Dispholidus typus 44
disulfiram 91, 141; see also *Antabuse*
diuretics 21, **103**, 169, 196
  as antidote 20
DMC 70, 281
DMSA **103**
DMSO See *dimethyl sulfoxide*
dogbane 60
dog button plant 201
dog fennel 310
dog hobble **103**
Dolantin 190
doll's eyes 34
Dolobid See *diflunisal*
dolphinfish 72

Doriden 269
dose-response curve
doublecross 13
Doubleday, Sir Henry 80
dove's dung 275
Dowklor 66
downers 35
doxapram
  as antidote 17
Doyle, Sir Arthur Conan 77
drain cleaners 9-10, 163, 228; see also *alkaline corrosives*
drinking water 66, 71, 79, 88, 114
Dr. Miles Nervine 48
druids 175
dry cleaned clothes 59, 183
Dubonnet 241
Dumas, Alexandre 154
dumbcane 97
dumb plant 97
duplicating fluid 171
duranest 16
Duranta repens 128
dust 47
dwarf bay 91
dwale **104**, 195
dye 17, 66, 100, 143, 169, 171, 216, 218
dye removers 9-10
dyphylline **104**
dysentery See *shigellosis; amebic dysentery; bacillary dysentery*

Easter lily 200
E. coli 79, 119
edetate calcium disodium 158
edrophonium chloride **105**
  as antidote 238
eggs 118, 255
Elapidae family 74, 85
Elastonon 13
elderberry, black and scarlet elders **105**
electroplating solution 90
elves 165
emetine 144, 278
enamels 22, 28
endosulfan 67
endotoxin 290
endrin **105-6**, 140, 281
Enhydrina schistosa 262
Entamoeba histolytica 120
enterotoxin 274-5, 290
Environmental Protection Agency 6, 8, 9, 88, 98, 102, 159, 205, 213, 231, 243
ephedrine 78, 94, 135, 178, 217
  as antidote 93, 103, **106**, 155, 236, 250
epidural block 16,
epinephrine 21, 48, 93, 94, 107, 313
  as treatment for poisoning 38, **106**, 144, 263, 273
Epipremnum aureum **234**
EPN 281
Equal See *aspartame*
ergot 41, **106**, 162
  antidote for 14, 194, 198
Eriobotrya japonica 161
erythematous shellfish poisoning **265**
erythromycin 91
Escherichia coli 79, 119
essential oils **305**
estrogen 41
ethacrynic acid 103
ethanol 83, 141, 189
  as treatment for poisoning **106**, 107, 171

ether 16, 77, **107**
ethinamate 269
ethopropazine See *Trilafon*
ethosuximide 269
Ethotoin 269
ethyl alcohol 147, 268
  as treatment for poisoning **107**
ethylan (perthane) 67
ethylbromoacetate 284
ethylchlorvynol 269
ethylene 16, 137
ethylene chlorohydrin **107**
ethylene dibromide **107**
ethylene glycol **19**, 147; see also *anti-freeze*
  antidote for 116, 272, 287, 303
eucalyptol 108
eucalyptus **108-9**, 305
Eucalyptus globulus Labill. 108-9
eucalyptus oil 108
eugenol 216
Euonymus atropurpureus 273
  E. europaeus 273
Eupatorium rugosum 309-10
Euphorbia 6
  E. candelabrum 6
  E. giomgiecpstata 6
  E. grantii 6
  E. neglecta 6
  E. pulcherrima **222**
  E. systyloides 6
  E. tirucalli 6
European baneberry 34
Euthymus pelamis 293
Eutonyl 178
evomonoside 273
evonine 274
exotoxin **109**, 290
explosives 13, 47, 66, 123, 169, 292
Exuviaella mariaelebouriae 101
eyebright 140
eye makeup 201

fabric cleaners 290
fabric sizing 123
fabric softener 183, 201
fairy bells 124
fairy cap 124
fairy finger 124
fairy glove 124
fairy thimbles 124
fall crocus 167
false acacia 41
false Jerusalem cherry **110**
false morel 11-12, 130, 293
false sycamore 64
February daphne 91
Feldene (piroxicam) 199-200
female water dragon 307
fenoprofen 199-200
fentanyl See *narcotics*
fer-de-lance 25, **110**, 131, 298, 301, 311
fertilizers 13, **111**, 120, 216, 219
fetterbush 103
fiddleback spider 48
fierce snake 282
figwort 51, 60, 124
filefish 72
fire ant **111**, 174
fire coral See *coral, fire*
fire extinguishers 59, 171
fire fighters 218, 219
firefish 160
fireworks 36, **111**, 169, 219
fish 179, 279

fish contamination **111-3**, 117, 120-21
fish poison (buckeye) 50, 72
fish poisoning 24
fish spoilage 113
flat-spined Atelopus **27**
flax 128
flax olive 91
flea killer 206, 214, 238, 252
fleas 39
flooring 123
floor polish and wax 2, 228; see also *petroleum distillates*
Florida diamondback 45-6
Flumazenil
  as antidote 40, **114**
fluoride 55, **114-5**, 142
fluoride toothpaste 114
fluoroacetate 80; see also *Compound 1080; sodium fluoroacetate*
fluoroacetic acid 80
Fluoxetine 178
flurazepam See *Dalmane*
fly agaric (yellow or red) 11-12, **115-6**, 183, 208
flying ointment 196
flying saucer 180
fly mushroom See *fly agaric*
fly poison 115
foil 22
folic acid **116**, 171
folk's gloves 124
food additives 30-31
Food and Drug Administration 6, 13, 30, 46, 55, 100, 112, 134, 140, 156, 170, 179, 213, 231, 254, 279, 303
food handling, proper **118**
food poisoning 59, 79, **116-123**, 185, 237
food preservative 44
food storage, safe **122**
fool's angel 95
formaldehyde **123-4**, 137, 171, 182, 267
formalin See *formaldehyde*
formic acid 116
foxes glofa 124
foxglove 59-60, 98, **124-5**, 134
Franklin, Benjamin 124
free base cocaine 77, 125
Freon 59, 70
Freud, Sigmund 77
friar's cap 176
fricasse 7
frogs, poisonous 11, 26, 285
frogs, tree 26
fruit salad plant 218
fuel oil 88
fugu 237
fumigants 90, 142, 169, 171-2
fungicide 112, **125**, 212
Fungicide and Rodenticide Act, U.S. 98
fungus fruit 184
furazolidone (Furoxone) 178
furniture 123
furniture polish 2, 228
furosemide 103
Furoxone 178

Galen 205
Galerina autumnalis 12, 126
  G. marginata 12
  G. venenata 126
galerina mushrooms **126**, 186-7
Gambierdiscus toxicus 72
gammahexane 39
Ganymede 282

gardenia 200
gas chambers 90
gasoline 38, 58, 107, 228; see also *petroleum distillates*
Gautier, Theophile 154
gelsamine 11, **126**, 151
gelsemicine 151
Gelsemium sempervirens **151**
Generally Recognized As Safe (GRAS) 134, 279
geography cone 81
giant milkweed **126**
Giardia lamblia protozoa 120, **127**
giardiasis 120, **127**
Gila monster **127-8**, 173
githagin 87
glass 22, 36
Gloriosa rothschildiana 74
  G. superba 74
glory lily 74
glucose
  as antidote 12, 94, 143, 158
glucose-6-phosphate dehydrogenase, deficiency of 189
glucosides See *glycoside*
glue See *solvent abuse*
glutamate 179
glutethimide 269
glycerin 201
glyceryl trinitrate **198**
glycoproteins 230
glycoside 50, 71, 87, 91, 125, **128**, 136, 165, 204, 274
gold
  antidote for 34, 99-100
goldballs 51
golden bough 175
golden dewdrop **128-9**
goldweed 51
Gonyaulax 209, 266
Gonyaulax acatenella 100
  G. breve 100
  G. catenella 100
  G. polyedra 100
  G. tamarensis 100
gourd 61
gout stalk **129**
grape juice 7
grapes, wild 180
graphite 157, 201
GRAS See *Generally Recognized As Safe*
grass snakes 50
grayanotoxin 103
Great Lakes 112
ground cherry **129**
groundsel 243
groundsel, common 244
grouper 72
grouper, spotted **129**
grouper, yellowfin See *grouper, spotted*
grubs 9
guanethidine 178
guitar varnish 35
gum plant 79
gum tree 108-9
gunpowder 111
Gymnothorax javanicus **180**
Gyromitra ambigua 186
  G. brunnea 186
  G. caroliniana 186
  G. esculenta 186, 293
  G. fastigiata 186
  G. helvella 187
  G. infula 186, 293
Gyromitra family **130**, 179, **186-7**, **293**

antidote for 303
gyromitrin 130, 179. 186

habu, Okinawa 110, **131**
hair bleach 13, 138, 169
hair dyes 13, 228
hair spray 172, 228
hair straighteners 13
Halcion 18, 39-40, 269; see also
   benzodiazepines; sleeping pills
Haldol 9, 23, 216; see also *antipsy-
   chotic/psychometric drugs*
   antidote for 292
hallucinogenic mushrooms **131-2**
hallucinogenic plants 180-1
haloperidol See *Haldol*
Haltrain See *ibuprofen*
hamadryad 76
hand creams and lotions 201
Hapalochlaena maculosa **203**
   H. lunulata 203
Hardwicke's sea snake 262-3
harlequin snake 86; see also *coral snake,
   eastern*
hatters 169
haze 162
HCCH 39
HCH 39
healing herb 79
hearts 13
heater fuel 170
heavenly blue 180
Hecate 196
Hedera 147
   H. helix 147
hederin 148
hellebore, black 71
helleborin 71
Helleborus niger 71
   H. orientalis 71
hell's fire sea anemone 15,
helmet flower 176
Heloderma horridum 173
   H. suspectum 127
Hemachatus hemachatus **251**
hemlock 305
hemlock, deadly See *hemlock, poison*
hemlock, ground See *yew*
hemlock, lesser See *hemlock, poison*
hemlock, poison 81, **132**
hemlock, spotted See *hemlock, poison*
hemlock, water **132-3**, 308
hemlock water dropwort 307
henbane **133-4**
henbell 133
hepatitis A 119, 266
heptachlor 67, 140, 281
herbal cigarettes 135
herbal tea 135
herb bonnett 132
herb-Christopher 34
herbicides 13, 102, 111, **134**, 212, 294
herbs 51, 79-80
Hercules 176
Hermes 3
heroin **135-6**, 190
herring 72
hexachlorobenzene 67, 125
1,2,3,4,5,6-hexachlorocyclohexane 39
hexachlorophene 216
hexavalent compounds 72
hexylresorcinol 24
highland moccasin 82
histamine 20, 293
histidine 293

hog apple 165
hog bush 64
hognose snake 3
hog's bean 133
hog's potato 93
holly **136**
Holmes, Sherlock 77
holothurin 262
Holothurioidea family 261
home permanents See *permanent wave
   lotions; permanent wave neutralizers*
honey 47, **136-7**, 151, 154
hook heller 154
hornets **36-38**
horse chestnut 50
horse gold 51
horse nettle See *California horse nettle*
horse protein 24
horseradish 146
horse serum allergy See *serum sickness*
hot water heaters 58
household cleaners 10, 66
hunger weed 51
hunter's robe, golden 234
hurricane plant 218
hyacinth **137**
hyacinth-of-Peru 274
Hyacinthus orientalis 137
Hycodan 190
hydrangea 128, **137**
Hydrangea macrophylla 137
hydrangin 137
hydrazine 303
hydrocarbon 38, 48, **137**
hydrochloric acid 2, 12, 48, 68, 73, **137-
   8**, 218
hydrochloride 125
hydrochlorothiazide 103
hydrocortisone 100, 144
hydrocyanic acid 61, 64, 89, 90, 128,
   142, 236
hydrofluoric skin burns 115
hydrogen bromate 48
hydrogen chloride **137**, 172
hydrogen cyanide 89
hydrogen peroxide 24, **138**
   as treatment for poisoning 84
hydrogen sulfide 80, **138**
hydroid 232
hydromorphone **138-9**, 190
Hydrophidae family 262
Hydrophis cyanocinctus 262
   H. spiralis 262
hydroquinone 216
hydroxocobalamin
   as antidote 198
hyoscine 152, 194, 196
hyoscyamine 134, 151, 165, 194, 196
Hyoscyamus niger 133
hypochlorite 66, 68; see also *alkaline corrosives*
hypnotic drugs 65

ibotenic acid 12, 115, 183, 186-7, 208
ibuprofen 5, 21-22, 199-200; see also
   nonsteroidal anti-inflammatory drugs
Ilex 136
   I. aquifolium 136
   I. opaca 136
impatiens 200
indane derivatives **140**, 281, 305
Inderal 40,
Indian apple 165
Indian licorice 252
Indian lilac 64

Indian polk 229
Indians, North American 180, 211, 283
Indian tobacco **140-1**
indole 186
indomethacin See *nonsteroidal anti-inflammatory drugs*
infant botulism See *botulism, infant*
ink 169, 229
inkberry 229
inky cap 83, **141**
Inocybe fastigiata 141, 186
   I. geophylla 186
   I. lilacina 186
   I. napipes 141
   I. patouillardii 186
   I. purica 186
   I. rimosus 186
Inocybe mushrooms **141-2**, 149, 183
inorganic chemical insecticides 45, **147**,
   170, 219
insane root 133
insect growth regulators 142
insecticides 9, 28, 45, 57, 59, 70, 79, 90,
   92, 95, 111, 121, 140, **142**, 164, 169,
   174, 182, 205, 210-12, 219, 238-9, 252,
   284, 289, 290
insect repellants **142-3**
insulation 29, 123
insulin **143**
Inversine See *mecamylamine*
iodine 63, **143-4**
   antidote for 191
iodochlorhydroxyquin 143
iodoform 143
ipecac syrup 63, **144-5**, 227
ipecacuanha **144**
iris 41
iron 63, 64, 95, 99, 145-6
   antidote for 191
iron supplements 34, **145-6**
irradiation (of food) 255-6
irritant oils **146**
isobutyl nitrites 14
isocarboxazid (Marplan) 178
isogermidine 93
isolan 57
isopropanol See *isopropyl alcohol*
isopropyl alcohol **147**
isoproterenol
   as antidote **147**
ivy **147-8**, 256
ivy arum 234
ivy bush 154

jack-in-the-pulpit 97
jack'o lantern fungus **149**
jade plant 200
Jamestown weed 151
Japanese bead tree 64
Japanese medlar 161
Japanese mercury poisoning 112
Japanese PCB poisoning 231
Japanese plum 161
jasmine 151
Jasminum 151
Jatropha curcas **35**
   J. gossypiifolia **38**
   J. multifida 83
   J. podagrica **129**
   J. stimulosus 274
jatrophin 35, 83, 129
jellyfish 24, **149-50**, 232, 264
jequirity bean 252
Jericho rose 203
Jerusalem cherry **150-1**, 195

jessamine, yellow 126, **151**
jimsonweed 32, 135, **151-2**
joe-pye weed 310
juca 60
jumping spider 273
Juniperus sabina 256-7
jupiter bean 133

kalanchoe 200
Kalmia augustifolia 154
  K. latifolia 154
  K. microphylla 154
kaolin 201
  as antidote 84
karakurt 42
Karwinskia humboldtiana 51
katipo 42
kepone 67, 140, 174, 281
kerosene 70, 142, 182, 228, 281; see also *petroleum distillate*
kerosene heaters 58, 182
kill cow 132
kingfish 64
knitbone 79
knockout drops 65
kokoi frog **153**
kola nuts 53
koli 61
krait, banded
krait, blue 75, **153**
krait, yellow-lipped sea 262
kufah 131
kukui haole 35

labetalol
  as treatment for poisoning **154**
laccine 230
Lachesis muta 51
lacquer 294
lacquer trees, Chinese/Japanese 224
Lactoria cornutus 292
ladybugs 11
lambkill 154
lanolin 201
Lanoxin See *digoxin*
lanthopine 181
Lapemis hardwickii 262
larkspur 176
Laticauda colubrina 262
  L. semifasciata 262
Latrodectus 273
laudanoisine See *morphine*
laudanum **154**, 181, 204-5
laughing gas See *nitrous oxide*
laundry starch 60
laurel 250
laurel, alpine 154; see also *laurel, mountain*
laurel, American
laurel, copse 91
laurel, dog 103
laurel, dwarf See *laurel, mountain*
laurel, lady 91
laurel, mountain **154-5**
laurel, narrow leafed See *laurel, mountain*
laurel, pale See *laurel, mountain*
laurel, poison See *laurel, mountain*
laurel, sheep See *laurel, mountain*
laurel, spurge 91
laurel, swamp See *laurel, mountain*
laurel, wood 91
lauric acid 201
Lawn-keep 294
laxatives **155**

l-dopa 178
lead 53, 64
lead crystal 156
lead foil 156
lead poisoning **155-8**
  antidote for 30, 34, 55, 99-100, 103, 211
lead removal 157
lead salts 135
lectin 41, 61, 84, 129, 175
Legionnaires' disease 267
lemon
  as antidote 16, 150
Lenten rose 71
Lepiota brunneoincarnata **158**
  L. helveola **158**
  L. josserandii **158**
  L. subincarnata **158**
Lepiota mushrooms 12, **158**
leptophos 281
lesser celandine 51
Leucothoe 103
levallorphan 190
Levo-Dromoran 190
levorphanol See *Levo-Dromoran*
Librium 18, 39; see also *benzodiazepines*
licorice vine 252
lidocaine 16, **158-9**
  as treatment for poison 241, 250
lighter fluid See *petroleum distillate*
ligustrin 235
Ligustrum vulgare **235**
lily family 59-60, 93, 167
lily-of-the-valley 60, **159**, 275
lima beans 128
lime, slaked 240
lime, unslaked 240
linamarin 61
Lincoln, Nancy Hanks 309
lindane 39, 67, 142, **159-60**, 281
liniments 55
lionfish **160**, 260
lion's mane jellyfish 149; see also *jellyfish*
lipstick 201
lipstick plant 200
Liquid Paper 290
Liquid Paper Thinner 290
lirio 195
Listeria monocytogenes bacterium 117, 160
listeriosis 117, **160-1**
lithium 9, 48, 63, **161**
liver cancer 6
lizards, poisonous 127
L'Obel, Matthais 140
lobelamine 140
lobelia 140
Lobelia Inflata 140
lobeline 140
lobster 209, 265
Locker Room 14
locust, black **41**, 220
locust, green 41
locust tree 41
Lopressor 40
loquat 161
lorazepam See *Ativan*
lorchel See *turbantop*
Lorfan See *levallorphan*
lotaustralin 61
love bean 252
loxapine 23
Loxosceles recluse **48-49**, 273
Lpomoea **180**
LSD **162**, 174, 178, 180, 215

lubricant 88, 229
lucky bean 252
Luminal See *phenobarbital*
lunchmeats 160
lycorine 190
lye **9-11**, 26, **163**
lysergic acid diethylamide See *LSD*
Lytta vesicatoria 43

Macbeth 177
mace 201
mackerel 121, 257, 293
mad apple 151
magnesium sulfate
  as antidote 41, 51, 241
magnesium trisilicate
  as treatment for poisoning 62
magnolia 200
mahi mahi 121, 257, 293
mainlining 135
malathion 67, 142, **164**, 206, 281
Malayan moccasin 299
malmignatte 42
mamba, black 75, 164
mamba, green 75, 164
mambas **164-5**
mandragorin 165
mandrake 135
mandrake, American **165-6**
mandrake, British 50
maneb 57
manganese **166**
  antidote for 55
mangos 224
Manihot esculenta 60
manioc/manioc tapioca 60
man's motherwort 61
marcaine 16
marigold 200
marijuana 215
Marplan 178
massasauga **166-7**, 249
Matamalu samasama 15-16
matches 22, 66, **167**, 219
Matulane 178
Maya 60
mayapple 88, 165
mayonnaise 118
meadow saffron **167**
meat 6, 117, 140, 179, 255
meat tenderizer
  as antidote 16, 38, 150, 232
mecamylamine 193, 194
meclofenamate See *nonsteroidal anti-inflammatory drugs; ibuprofen*
Meclomen See *nonsteroidal anti-inflammatory drugs; ibuprofen*
meconidine 181
Medea 176
medications as poisons 1, 103, 104, 143, **168**
de Medici, Catherine 289
medicinal soap 143
Medipren See *ibuprofen*
Meixner test 12
Melia azedarach 64
Mellaril 23
Meloidae 43
meningitis 117, 161
Menispermum canadense **180**
Mentha pulegium **211**
menthol 305
Mentholatum 305
meperidine **168-9**, 178
mephenytoin 269, 307

mercury 13, 63, 64, 112-113, 125, 142, **169**, 287
  antidote for 34, 99-100, 103, 191, 211
mercury chloride 169
mercury and dental fillings **169-70**
mercury salts 135
mercury vapor 169-70
mersalyl 103
Mesantoin 269
mescaline 215
metacide 281
metal cleaner 2, 90; see also *alkaline corrosives*
metaldehyde 142, **170**
metallic arsenic 28-29
metal salts 135
metaraminol 178
meth 13
methacholine 210
methanol **19**, 100, 123, 147, 171; see also *methyl alcohol*
  antidote for 116, 272
methaqualone See *quaalude*
methazolamide 103
methemoglobinemia 14, 30, 111, 294
methocarbamol **170**
methoxychlor 67, 281
methsuximide 269
methyclothiazide 103
methyl alcohol **171**
methyl bromide **171-2**
methyl chloroform See *trichloroethane*
methyldopa 178; see also *Aldomet*
methylene blue
  as antidote 14, 30
methylene chloride 137, **172-3**
methyl mercury 112; see also *fish contamination; mercury*
  antidote for 103
methyl mercury chloride 112
methylmorphine 78
methylphenidate 251
methyl phenol 87-88
4-methylpyrazole
  as antidote 171
methyl sulfate 100
methyprylon 269
metoclopramide **173**
Metopium toxiferum **229**
metronidazole
  as treatment for poisoning 127
Mexican beaded lizard 127, **173**
Mexican breadfruit 218
Mexican hallucinogenic mushroom **173-4**
Mexican moccasin 56; see also *cantil snake*
Mexico weed 61
mezerein 91
Mickey Finn 65, 88
microdots 162
Micruroides euryxanthus euryxanthus 25, 85
Micrurus fulvius 25, 85, 86
  M. frontalis 85
  M. fulvius tenere 25
  M. nigrocinctus 85
midazolam **174**; see also *Versed*
mienie-mienie Indian bean 252
migraine drugs 54
mildew removers 183
milk sickness 309
millipedes 11
Milontin 269

minibennies 13
Minipress (prazosin hydrochloride) 21, **174**
minnows 62
minoxidil 106
mirex 67, **174**
mistletoe **175**
mobile homes 123
Mogadon (nitrazepam) 268
mold 119
molindone 23
mollusks 55, 81, 101, 266
monkeyflower 124
monkshood 2, **176-8**
monoamine oxidase (MAO) inhibitors 9, 19, 91, 94, 96, 168, **178-9, 251**
  antidote 198
monocaine 16
monomethylhydrazine 130, **179**, 184, 186-7, 293
monosodium glutamate 31, **179**
Monstera deliciosa **218**
Montezuma's revenge See *traveller's diarrhea*
moon jellyfish 150
moonseed **180**
moray eel 72, **180**, 257
morning glory **180**
morphine 25, 78, 135-6, 168, **181**, 190, 205, 207, 212
  as treatment for poisoning 133, 144, 233, 259
mosquito repellant 61, 142, 164
mothballs 55, 142, 189, 208, 231; see also *camphor; naphthalene*
mother-in-law plant 97, **181-2**
motor oil 231
Motrin See *ibuprofen; nonsteroidal anti-inflammatory drugs*
Motrin IB See *ibuprofen; nonsteroidal anti-inflammatory drugs*
mountain ivy 154
mountain laurel See *laurel, mountain*
mouthwash 66, 138
MSG See *monosodium glutamate*
mugwort 41
mulga 42
multiple chemical sensitivity **182-3**
muscarine 115, 141-2, 149, **183**, 186-7, 211
  antidote for 196
muscimol 12, 115, **183**, 186-7, 208
muscle relaxants 39-40, 89, 91, 132,
  as treatment for poisoning 49, 170, 202, 232
mushroom identification 185
mushroom poisoning 83, 87, 94, 95-96, 115-6, 121, 126, 130, 141, 149, 158, 183, **184-7**, 208, 293-4
mushroom toxins 12, 87, 183, 186, **187-8**
muskie 112
muskrat weed 132
mussels 101, 113, 209, 265
mustard 146
mycetismus 187
mycotoxins 290
Myristica fragrans **201**
myrtle 108
Mysoline 269
myster grass 93
Mytilus californianus 55

nail polish 201, 228
nail polish remover 228

Naja haje 75
  N. hannah 76
  N. naja 75
  N. nigricollis 76
naked lady 167
naked lady lily 195
Nalfon (fenoprofen) See *nonsteroidal anti-inflammatory drugs; ibuprofen*
naloxone **189**, 205, 207
  as antidote 26, 79, 96-97, 136, 139, 181, 212
nap at noon 275
naphthalene 142, **189**, 208
Naprosyn (naproxen) See *nonsteroidal anti-inflammatory drugs*
naproxen See *nonsteroidal anti-inflammatory drugs*
narcissus **190**
Narcissus jonquilla 190
  N. pseudonarcissus 190
narcotics 77, 78, 91, 154, 181, 189, **190**, 196, 204, 212
narcotine 181, 205
Nardil 178
nasturtium 200
National Animal Poison Control Center 20, **190-1**, 214-5
National Organic Standards Board 213
Navane 23
Nazi experiments 97
Nebraska fern 132
necklaceweed 34
nematocyst 150
Nembutal 35; see also *parasympathomimetic drugs*
neogermidine 93
neostigmine 210
neotrane 70, 281
nerioside 204
Nerium oleander 59, **203**
Nero 176
nerve gas 196, 205, 210-11
nesacaine 16
neuroleptic malignant syndrome 23
neuromuscular blocking agents 14-15, **191**
neurotoxic shellfish poisoning 113, **265**
neurotoxin 3, 42, 65, 76, 81, 86, 164, 257, 258
neutralizers **191**
niacin **305**
nialamide (Niamid) 178
Niamid 178
nickel
  antidote for 34, 55, 99-100
Nicorette 192, **193**; see also *nicotine gum*
Nicot de Villemain, Jean 289
Nicotiana 288
  N. tabacum 289
nicotinamide 192, **297**
nicotine 11, 45, 63, 140-1, 142, **192-3**
  antidote for 30, 191, 233
nicotine gum 192, **193**
nicotine patch 192, **193**
nicotine polacrilex See *nicotine gum*
nifedipine 106, **194**
nightshade 32, 133, 150, 288
nightshade, bittersweet **194-5**
nightshade, black (American nightshade) 195
nightshade, Brazilian 276
nightshade, deadly 32, 104, 134, 194, **195-7**, 234
nightshade, English 195
nightshade, fetid 133

nightshade, sleeping 195
nightshade, stinking 133
nightshade, woody (European bitter-sweet) 195
nightshade, yellow 197
nipbone 79
nitrazepam 268
nitric acid 2
nitric oxide 197-8
nitrogen dioxide 197-8
nitrogen oxide 197-8
nitroglycerin 198
nitroprusside 198
  as treatment for poisoning 94, 198
nitrous oxide 16, 70, 107, 198-7
Noludar 269
nonsteroidal anti-inflammatory drugs (NSAIDs) 21-22, 199-200
nontoxic plants 200
nontoxic substances 201
norepinephrine 49, 53
Norfolk Island pine 200
Norpace 18
Norwalk virus 119
Notechis scutatus 288
novocaine 16
NSAIDs See nonsteroidal anti-inflamma-tory drugs
Numorphan See oxymorphone
nupercaine 16
Nuprin See ibuprofen
nutmeg 134, 201, 305
NutraSweet See aspartame
nux-vomica 201-2, 278
nuzhenids 235

Oak Ridge Radiation Emergency Assis-tance Center 242
Octa-Klor 66
octalene 9
octopus, Australian spotted 203
octopus, blue ringed 203
Octopus apollyon 203
Oenanthe crocata 307
oenanthotoxin 308
oil burners 58
oldendrin 204
oleander 60, 203-4
olive 41, 151
onion juice 41
Ophiophagus hannah 76
opiates/opiods 181
opium 78, 135, 154, 181, 190, 204-5
  antidote for 196
oracaine 16
oral contraceptives See birth control pills
Oregon State Hospital fluoride overdose 114
orellanin 87, 126
organic insecticides 45, 70, 142, 159-60, 174
organochlorine pesticides, synthetic 66
organophosphate insecticides 57, 142, 205-6
  antidote for 234
organophosphates 67
Ornithogalum thyrsoides 275, 311
  O. umbellatum 275
Orthedrine 13
orthochlorobenzylidene malononitril 284
Ortho-Klor 66
ouabain 311
oven cleaner See alkaline corrosive
ovotran 70, 281

oxalates 55, 206-7, 218
oxalate salts 207
oxalic acid 2, 206, 251
Oxalidaceae family 206
oxazepam See Serax
oxycodone 207, 212
oxycodone hydrochloride 207
oxycodone terrephthalate 207
oxygen 48, 59, 72, 166, 174, 207
oxymetazoline 7
oxymorphone 190, 207
oxyphenbutazone 199
Oxyuranus scutellatus 282
oyster poisoning 101, 209, 265-6

painkiller 73, 78, 100, 154, 158, 168, 181, 199, 212, 254
paint 17, 28, 156, 169, 216, 229
paintbrush 124
paint removers 17, 171, 172, 216, 228, 290; see also hydrocarbons
paint thinner 172, 182, 228, 294; see also petroleum distillate
palma Christi 61
pama 75, 153
Panadol 1
pancuronium 191
panther mushroom 11-12, 115, 208
papaverine 205
Papaver somniferum 204-5
Paracelsus 154
Parademansia microlepidotus 269, 282
paradichlorobenzene 189, 208
paradise tree 64
paralytic shellfish poisoning (PSP) 55, 101, 113, 208-9, 257, 265
para-oxon 281
paraquat 134, 209-10
parasympathomimetic drugs 210
parathion 58, 205, 210-11, 281
paregoric 190, 204-5
pargyline (Eutonyl) 178
Parnate 178
paternoster pea 252
pavulon See neuromuscular blocking agents
Paxina 186
PCB 113, 137; see also polychlorinated biphenyls
PCP See phencyclidine
peace plant 273
peach pit See Prunus
pea flower locust 41
peanut butter 7
peanuts 5-6, 121
pearly gates 180
peganone 269
Pelamis platurus 262
pen, marking 182
pencils 157, 201
penicillamine
  as antidote 29, 158, 211
penicillin
  as antidote 12, 94, 96, 158, 211
pennyroyal plant 41, 211, 305
pennyroyal oil 211, 305
pentachlorophenol 125, 216
pentazocine 190
pentobarbital 193; see also Nembutal
Pentothol 35
pepperbush 103
pepperomia 200
pep pills 13; see also amphetamines
peptide toxins 93
perch 112

Percodan 207, 212
perfume 100, 171, 216
permanent wave lotions 13,
permanent wave neutralizers 2, 47
Persian lilac 64
perthane See ethylan
pesticides 7, 8, 9-10, 13, 28, 34, 57, 68, 100, 107-8, 112, 183, 191, 212, 218, 238, 267, 286
  how to use (chart) 212
pethidine See Dolantin
petroleum based insecticides 214
petroleum distillates 64, 134, 214, 227
petroleum jelly 201
pets and poisoning 20, 214-5
petunia 200
phalloidin(e) 12, 93, 96
phallotoxins 12, 186
pheasant's eye 60
phenacemide 269
phenacetin 53, 212
Phenamine 13
phencyclidine (PCP) 78, 173, 191, 215-6
  as treatment for 194
Phenedrine 13,
phenelzine (Nardil) 178
phenindione 19
phenmetrazine hydrochloride See Pre-ludin
phenobarbital 35, 44, 181, 216
  as treatment for poisoning 55, 70, 140, 160, 174, 216, 272
phenol 2, 87, 216-7, 224
phenothiazine 287
  as treatment for poisoning 132, 216
phenothiazine-type antihistamines 21,
phenprocoumon 19,
phensuximide 269
phentolamine
  as treatment for poisoning 49, 94, 217, 251
Phenurone See sleeping pills
phenylalanine 30,
phenylbutazone 135, 199-200
phenylephrine 94, 178
phenylketonuria (PKU) 31,
phenylpropanolomine 78, 94, 178; see also decongestants
  antidote for 194, 217
phenytoin 181, 212, 217, 311
  as treatment for poisoning 241, 250
Phidippus 273
philodendron 97, 207, 217-8
philodendron, cut leaf See philodendron, split leaf
philodendron, split leaf 218
philodendron, variegated 234
pH indicators 26
Phoradendron rubrum 175
  P. serotinum 175
  P. tomentosum 175
phoratoxins 175
phosgene 172, 218
phosphate 55,
phosphate detergent 287
phosphate esters 219, 281
phosphide 220
phosphine 219
phosphoric acid 2, 164
phosphorus 142, 219-20, 244
phosphorus oxide 164
phossy jaw 220
photo film 143
Phyllobates 26

P. bicolor 27
P. horribilius 27
Physalia palagica **232-3**
Physalis 129
physic nut 35
physostigmine 115, 134, 152, 183, 195, 196, 208, 210, **220**, 292
physostigmine salicylate
   as antidote 19
Phytolacca americana **229-30**
phytonadione See *vitamin K₁*
phytotoxins 41, **220**, 290
pickerel 112
pie plant 250
Pierce, Anna 310
pigeon berry 128, 229
pike 112
pilewort 51
pilocarpine 183; see also *parasympatho-mimetic drugs*
   as treatment for poisoning 195, 196, 210
pirimicarb 57
piroxicam (Feldene) 199-200
pistachios 5-6, 224
pit viper See *viper, pit*
Placidyl 269
plant growth regulator 8
plastics 53, 68, 69
Plotosus lineatus 62
plum cherry pit See *Prunus*
plywood 123
pocan bush 229
podophylloresin 165
Podophyllum pelatum 165
Poe, Edgar Allan 154
poinsettia 6, 191, 200, **222**
poison gas 29, 68, 196, 205, 218, 219
poison hemlock See *hemlock, poison*
poisoning **226-8**
poisoning, how to prevent (chart) **228**
poison ivy **222-5**, 296
poison oak 223-4, **225-6, 296**
poison parsley 132
poison root 132
poison sego 93
poison sumac 223-4, **226, 296**
poison tobacco 133
poisonwood **229**
pokeberry 229
pokeweed **229-30**, 256
polyacrylamide 2
polychlorinated biphenyls (PCB) **230-2**
polythiazide 103
pompano 72
poppers 14
popping, skin 135
poppy plant 78, 135, 181, 204
porcupine fish 237, 285
portland cement 240
Portuguese man-of-war 149, **232-3**
post locust 41
potassium 161
potassium bromate 47-48
potassium chlorate 167
potassium chloride
   as antidote 36, 125
potassium cyanate 134
potassium cyanide 89
potassium hydroxide 9-10; see also *alka-line corrosives*
potassium iodide 143
potassium permanganate **233**
   as antidote 11, 191
potassium sulfite 292

potassium thiocyanate 233
potato 121, 133, 151, **234**
potato famines, Irish 80
pothos 97, **234**
pothos, golden See *pothos*
potosan 281
pottery 53,
poultry 117, 140, 179, 255
povidone 144
pralidoxime
   as antidote 72, 129, 206, **234**
prayer bean 252
prayer plant 200
prazepam See *Centrax*
prazosin hydrochloride See *Minipress*
precatory bean 252
prednisone
   as antidote 10
Preludin **234-5**
preservatives 2
pride of India 64
primary air quality standards
primidone 269
printing 17
privet **235**
procainamide 18, 21, 107
procaine 16, **236-7**
procarbazine (Matulane) 178
prochlorperazine 23
progesterone 41
promethazine 23
Pronestyl 18
propane **236**
propanolol
   as treatment for poisoning 106, **236**, 287
propenamide 2
propoxur 57, 142
propoxyphene See *Darvon*
propylene 137
proteolytic enzymes 97
protoanemonin 51, 71, 74
protopine 181
protoveratridine 93
protozoa **120**
Prunus 89, **236**
Prussian blue
   as treatment for poison 286
prussic acid See *hydrogen cyanide; hydrocyanic acid*
Pseudeschis australis 42
   P. guttatus 42
   P. porphyriacus 41-42
pseudoephedrine 94
psilocin 131, 173, 186
Psilocybe baeocystis 131, 186
   P. caerulescens 131, 186
   P. cubensis 131, 186
   P. cyanescens 131, 186
   P. fimentaria 186
   P. Mexicana 131, **173**, 186
   P. pelluculosa 186
   P. semilanceata 186
   P. silvatica 186
psilocybin 131, 173, 186-7, 215
Pterosis **160**
ptomaine poisoning **236-7**
pufferfish 113, 121, 153, **237**, 285
purgative 79
purge nut 35
purple haze 162
purple passion 200
putty 201
pygmy rattlesnake 166, 249
pyrethrin 45, 142, **238-9**

pyrethroid 142
pyrethrum 45, 60, 238, **239**, 252
pyridostigmine 238
pyridoxine (vitamin B₆); see also *vitamins*
   as antidote 130, 179, 294, **303**
pyrrolizidine alkaloid 80, 244

quaalude **240**
quicklime 228, **240**
quinacrine
   as treatment for poisoning 127
quinethazone 103
quinidine 18, 21, **240-1**, 295
quinine 63, 65, **241**
   antidote for 191. 233

rabbits 196
raccoon berry 165
Radianthus paumotensis 15-16
radiation poisoning **242**
radioisotopes, heavy
   antidote for 55
radish 146
radon **242-3**
ragweed 239
ragwort **243-4**
ram's claws 51
Ranunculus 51
rape 305
rat poison 28, 36, 47, 80, 90, 105, 192, 214, 220, 228, **244**, 249, 278, 285, 297, 307
rattlesnake, Brazilian 249
rattlesnake, canebrake **244-5, 249, 270**
rattlesnake, cascabel 25, **245**, 249
rattlesnake, eastern diamondback 25, **245-6**, 249, 270
rattlesnake, Florida diamondback See *rattlesnake, eastern diamondback*
rattlesnake, horned See *sidewinder*
rattlesnake, Mexican west coast **246**, 249
rattlesnake, Mojave 249, 270
rattlesnake, Pacific 249
rattlesnake, pygmy 166
rattlesnake, red diamondback **246-7**
rattlesnake, South American See *rattle-snake, cascabel*
rattlesnake, timber **247-8**, 249, 270
rattlesnake, tropical See *rattlesnake, cascabel*
rattlesnake venom 45
rattlesnake, western diamondback 25, 247, 249, 270
rattlesnakes 24, 166, 221, 244-5, **248-9**, 269-71
Recommended Daily Allowance 303
red bean vine 252
red ink plant 229
red pepper 134
reds 35
Red Sea 266
red snapper 72, 120
red squill 244, **249-50**
red tide 100, 113, 209, 266, 280
red weed 229
refrigerants 13
regional block 16
reserpine 178
resins **250**
Restoril 269
restricted pesticides
Reyes syndrome 6, 32
Rheum rhabarbarum **250**
Rhodactis howesii 15-16

rhododendron 154-5, **250**
rhubarb **250-1**
rice 5-6
ricin 61
Ricinus communis 61, 176
Rider 294
ringhals 75, **251**
Ritalin **251**
roach poison 44, 114, 228, 286
robin 41
Robinia pseudoacacia 41
rocket fuel 130, 179, 303
rockfish 260-1
rock perch 160
Roget, Peter 198
Romeo and Juliet 176, 196
roofing 29
Rosaceae 128
rosary bean 252
rosary pea 176, 220, **252**
rose dust 228
roses 13, 200
roseum 238, 239, **252**
rosy anemone 15
rotenone 45, 95, **252-3**
rubbing alcohol 147, 228; see also *isopro-pyl alcohol*
rue 41, 305
Rufen See *ibuprofen*
rust remover See *alkaline corrosive*
rye grain 106

sabadilla 45
saccharin **254**, 280
Sagarita elegans 15
salicylate acid 31-32
salicylates 65, 73, 135, **254-5**
antidote for 272, 305
salmon 112
Salmonella 117, **255**
  S. aertrycke 255
  S. choleraesius 255
  S. cubana 255
  S. enteritidis 255
salmonellosis 117, 121, **255-56**
salt water (as antidote) 227, 232, 296
Sambucus canadensis 105
  S. mexicana 105
  S. pubens 105
sandbriar 60
sand corn 93
Sanguinaria canadensis 43
sanguinarine 43,
saponin 50, 71, 87, 125, 128, 129, 136, 147, 230, **256**
sarsaparilla, Texas
sarsaparilla, yellow
saurine 257, 293
savin **256-7**, 305
Saxidomus giganteus 257
saxitoxin 102, 209, **257**, 266
Schedule II drug 79, 207
Scilla 274
scoke 229
Scolopendra gigas 63
scombroid poisoning 113, **257**, 293
scopolamine 134, 194, 196
Scorpaenidae family 260, 277
scorpion 24, **258-9**
scorpion, brown 258, **259**
scorpion, common striped 258, **259-60**
scorpion, sculpturatus 258, **260**
scorpionfish 160 **260-1**, 277
Scrophulariaceae 124
sea cucumber **261-2**

sea krait, yellow-lipped 262
sea onion 274
sea snake **262-3**
sea snake, beaked 262
sea snake, Hardwicke's 262-3
sea snake, olive brown 262
sea snake, pelagic 262-3
sea snake, yellow 262-3
sea squab 237
sea urchin **263-4**
sea wasp **264-5**
seaweed 179
secobarbital See *Seconal; barbiturates*
secoiridoid glucosides 235
Seconal 35; see also *barbiturates*
sedative 20, 48, 65, 91, 154, 181, 196, 212
selenium 34, 99, 142, **265**
Seminole bead 252
Senecio 243
  S. longilobus 243
  S. vulgaris 244
sensitive plant 200
sensory reversal 72
Serax (oxazepam) 18, 39
Sernyl 215
Serranidae 129
serum sickness 24, 103
Sevin 57
sex hormones
  as treatment for poisoning 94, 158
shaggy cap 141
shaggy mane 141
shaving cream 201
shaving lotion 147
shellac 171
shellfish 279
shellfish poisoning 55, 72, 101, 117, 119, 209, **265-7**
Shigella bacterium 117
shigellosis **117**
shingle plant 218
shingles 29,
shoe polish 17, 228
sick building syndrome **267**
sidewinder 249, **267-8**
siding 29
Siluriformes 62
silver 13
  antidote for 34
silver chain 41
silver nitrate **268**
silver polish 90
Simpson, Dr. James 70
Sistrurus catenatus 166
Sistrurus genus 221
sitfast 51
skin creams 13
skyflower 128
slaked lime 240
slaves, punishment for 97
sleeping pills 65, 91, 181, 212, 240, **268-9**
slippery root 79
Slo-Phyllin 286
slug bait 170; see also *metaldehyde*
smooth-scaled snake **269**, 282
snakeberry 34,
snake charmers 75
snakes, poisonous 49, 50, 51, 56-57, 74, 75, 76, 82, 110, 131, 153, 164-5, 166, 244-9, 267-8, **269-272**, 282, 288, 297-302, 308
  treatment for snakebite **271-2**
  precautions **271-2**

snake weed 132
snapdragon 124
snuff 289
soap 201, 227
soap plant 93
Socrates 82, 132
sodium arsenite 134
sodium bicarbonate 48, 181, 191, 202, 227, 241, 255, **272**
sodium borate 142
sodium carbonate 10
sodium chlorate 134
sodium cyanide 89
sodium fluoride 114
sodium fluoroacetate 80, 244; see also *compound 1080*
sodium formaldehyde sulfoxylate 191
sodium hydroxide 9-11, 26, **163**
sodium hypochlorite **272**; see also *alka-line corrosives*
sodium iodide 143
sodium nitrate 66, 198
sodium nitrite 9
sodium phosphate 10
sodium *p*-toluenesulfochloramine 66
sodium salicylate 31
sodium sulfate
  as treatment for poisoning 163, 214
sodium thiocyanate 21 **233**
sodium thiosulfate 26, 66
  as antidote 48, 61, 64, 144, 162, 198, 236
Solanaceae family 133, 195
Solandra 292
solanine glycoalkaloid 25, 60, 110, 129, 151, 195, 234, 276
solanine poisoning 60, 129, 151, 195,
Solanum carolinense 60
  S. pseudocapsicum 110, **150**
  S. sodomeum 26
Solanum family 60
Solanum seaforthianum **276**
soldier's cap 176
Solenopsis 111
Solomon Island ivy 234
solvent 38-39, 59, 70, 100, 147, 171, 172, 181, 218, 285, 290-1, 294
solvent abuse **272-3**
Soma 115, 268
Sonoran coral snake See *coral snake, Sonoran*
sorrel 134
Southey, Robert 198
soybeans 5-6, 179
Spanish fly 43, 56
sparklers, gold 111
sparklers, green 111
spathiphyllum **273**
spearwort 51
speed 13-14
speedball 77
speedwell 124
spider plant 200
spiders, poisonous 24, **273**
spinal block 16
spindle tree **273-4**
spironolactone 103
spoonwood 154
spotted black snake 42
spotted parsley 132
spurge family 60, 61
spurge nettle **274**
spurge olive 91
squaw weed 243
squill 274

squirrel food 93
stain removers 13
stamp pads 17
St. Anthony's fire 106
St. Anthony's turnip 51
staph infection 118
staphylococcal poisoning 237
staphylococcus aureus **117**
staphylococcus enterotoxin **274-5**
star hyacinth 274
star of Bethlehem **275**
star-potato vine **276**
starve-acre 51
stearic acid 201
Stelazine 23, **276**
steroid, topical 224
stibine (antimony hydride) **22-23**
stimulants, over-the-counter 54
stinging coral See *coral, stinging*
stingray **276-7**
stinking willie 243
stinkweed 151
stonefish 260, **277-8**
stoves 29, 58
Streunex See *benzene hexachloride*
striated cone 81
stropharias 131
strychnine 63, 75, 151, 191, 201, 233, 244, **278**
    antidote for 15, 97, 191
Strychnos 89, **278**
    S. nux-vomica 201
    S. toxifera 89
Sublimaze (fentanyl) See *narcotics*
sucaryl 280
succinylcholine 191, 220, 278; see also *anectine; neuromuscular blocking agents*
sugar
    as antidote 16, 150
sugar beets 179
sulfide ores 53
sulfites 30, **278-9**
sulfuric acid 2, 100
sulfuric acid dimethyl ester 100
sulindac See *Clinoril*
summer snowflake 275
sun fish 285
superantigens **279-80**
Super D Weedone 294
surgeonfish 72, **280**
sushi 121, 179, **280**
Swedish ivy 200
sweet bells 103
sweet elder 105
sweeteners, artificial 254, **280-1**
Sweet-N-Low See *saccharin*
sweet potato plant 60
swimming pool disinfectants 68, **281**
Swiss cheese plant 218
switch ivy 103
swordfish 112, 257, 293
Symphytum officinale 79
Synanceja horrida 277
Syndenham, Thomas 205
synthetic organic insecticides **281**, 289
synthetic pesticides 57
syringin 235
systox 281

table salt (sodium chloride) 68
    as poison treatment 48
Tagamet **73**; see also *cimetidine*
taipan 75, 269, **282**
talcum powder 44
tallow 201

Talwin 190
tanacetin 283
Tanacetum vulgare **282-3**
tansy **282-3**, 305
tansy ragwort 243
tapioca 60
tarantellas 283
tarantula 258, 273, **283**
taro vine 234
taxine 11, **284**
Taxus 284
    T. baccata 313
    T. brevifolia 313
    T. canadensis 313
    T. cuspidata 313
TDE 70, 281
tea leaves 53
    as treatment for poisoning 99, 169, 190
tear gas **284**
teething gels 32
teething rings 201
Tegretol 269
temazepam 269
Tempra 1
Tenormin 40
TEPP 206, 281, **284-5**
teratogen **285**
terbutaline 94
terpenoids 136
tetanus 15, 109, 128, 222, 245, 277
tetrachlorodiphenylethane 281
tetrachloroethane **285**
tetraethyl pyrophosphate See *TEPP*
tetrahydrocannabinol See *THC*
tetramethylthiuram disulfide 125
tetranortriterpene 65
Tetraodontidae family 237
tetrodotoxin 113, 237, **285**
Texas sarsaparilla 180
Texas umbrella tree 64
textiles 22, 36, 72, 216
thallium 47, 142, 244, **285**
thallium sulfate 244
THC 215
thebaine 205
Theobid 286
theobromine 136, 215
Theo-Dur 286
Theophrastus 204
theophylline 158, **286-7**
    antidote for 235, 236
thermometers 169, **287**
Thevetia peruviana **204**
thiamine (Vitamin B₁) **287**, 305
thief ant 111
thioctic acid
    as antidote 12, 94, 158
thiocyanate 198
thiopental See *Pentothal*
thioridazine See *Mellaril*
thio-TEPP 281
thiothixene See *Navane*
thiram 57
Thorazine 23, **287-8**, 292
thornapple 135, 151
threadleaf groundsel 243
thrombolytics See *anticoagulants*
thrusters 13
thujone 283
thyme 41
tick killer 206, 214, 238
ticks 39
tic polonga See *viper, Russell's*
tiger lily 200

tiger snake 75, **288**
Tityus bahiensis 258
    T. serulatus 258
TNT See *trinitrotoluene*
toad, marine 288
toads 11
toads, Bufo 288
toadstool 11, 187
tobacco 192, 267, **288-9**
toilet cleaners 10, 189, 208, 228; see also *alkaline corrosives*
tolbutamide 9
Tolectin (tolmetin) 199-200
tolmetin (Tolectin) 199-200
toluene 38, 137, 272, 287
tommygoff 110, **298**
tonic water 241
tooth fillings 169
toothpaste 254
toothpaste, fluoride 114
toxalbumins 41, 61, 84, 129, 175, 220; see also *phytotoxins*
toxaphene 67, 281, **289-90**
Toxichlor 66
Toxicodendron diversilobum **225-6**
    T. radicans **222-5**
    T. vernix[L]Kuntzel(=Rhus vernix L) 226
toxin **290**
toxoid **290**
Toxpneustes elegans 263
Trachinus 309
    T. araneus 309
    T. draco 309
tranquilizers 91, 181, 212; see also *anti-anxiety drugs*
transformers 231
Tranxene (chlorazepate) 18, 39
tranylcypromine (Parnate) 178
traveler's diarrhea **119**
trazodone 178
tread softly 60
treesail 41
Trendar See *ibuprofen*
triamterene 103
triazolam 269
trichlormethane 70
trichlormethiazide 103
trichloroethane **290-1**
trichloroethylene 290, 291
tricyclic antidepressants 9, **19**
trifluoperazine See *Stelazine*
trifluralin 134
triggerfish 72
trihexyphenidyl **292**
Trilafon 23
Trimeresurus 110
    T. flavoviridis 110, **131**
    T. okinavesis 131
    T. Wagleri 110, **301**
trimethobenzamide 23
trinitrotoluene (TNT) **292**
trisodium phosphate 157, 255-6
trivalent chromium compounds 72
truck drivers 13
trumpet plant **292**
trunkfish **292-3**
tryptophan 178
tubocurarine 89
tuftroot 97
tulip cone 81
tuna 112-113, 121, 257, **293**
tungsten
    antidote for 99-100
tung tree 256

turbantop **293-4**
turkeyfish 160
turpentine 214, 281, 294
turtles 255
Tylenol 1, 254; see also *acetaminophen*
typewriter correction fluid 182, 290-1

umbrella leaf 165
umbrella tree 200
unacaine 16
universal antidote **296**
unslaked lime 240
uppers 13
Urechites lutea 197
urechitoxin 197
urine 309
Urobatis halleri **276**
urushiol 223-6, **296**

Vacor 192, 244, **297**
Valium 18, 39, 91; see also *diazepam*
  as treatment for poisoning 14, 141,
    162, 278
Valmid 269
valproic acid See *Depakene*
varnish 294
vecuronium 191
vegetal 7
Velsicol 1068 66
venin de crapaud **297**
Venus 124
verapamil 106
  as treatment for sting 150, 233
veratrine 93
Versed (midazolam) 39-40
vetch seed 128
Vibrio cholera bacterium 117
Vicks Vaporub 305
Victoria, Queen 70
vinegar 2, 137
  as antidote 150, 227
vine-maple 180
vinyl chloride 67
vinyl floor tile 29
violet wandering jew 200
violin spider 48
viper, desert 269
viper, European 3
viper, gaboon **297-8**
viper, jumping 110, **298**
viper, Malayan pit **298-9**
viper, pit 24, 51, 56-57, 82, 110, 131,
  221-2, 245, 249, 301, 308, 311
viper, Palestine **299**
viper, Russell's **299-300**, 302
viper, sawscaled **300-1**
viper, South American pit 51
viper, Wagler's pit 110, **301**
Vipera berus 3-4
  V. palestinae 299
  V. russelli 299-300
Viperidae family 82, 110, 166, 249, 267,
  300, 301-2
Viperinae 301-2
vipers 3, 4, 5, 110, 248, 271, 300, **301-2**
viral types of food poisoning 119-20
viscotoxins 175
Viscum album **175**
viscumin 175

Visken 40
vitamin A **303-4**
vitamin B_1 (thiamine) 305
vitamin B_6 **305**
vitamin C 2, **30**, 254, 289, 305
vitamin D **304**
vitamin E **304-5**
vitamin-fluoride tablets 114
vitamin K 19, 254
  as antidote **305**, 307
vitamin K_1
  as antidote 244
vitamin-and-mineral supplements with
  iron 146
vitamins 26, **302-3**
  as treatment for poison 94, 158
vitamins, multiple without iron 201
vitamins, water soluble **305**
volatile oils **305-6**

wakeups 13
wallpaper 28
warfarin 19, 22, 199, 244, **307**
warfarin sodium 19
wart remover 43, 56
waspfish 260
wasps **36-38**
water arum **307**
watercolor paint 201
water crowfoot 51
water disinfectant 66, 143
water dragon 307
water dropwort **307-8**
water lily 93; see also *death camas*
watermelons 8-9
water moccasin 56, 269, 271, **308-9**
water pipes 53, 155
waterproofing material 88
wax plant 200
weather plant 252
Weed-B-Gone 294
weedkiller 28, 66, 228
Weedol 209
Weedone 294
weever fish **309**
welding 53, 72, 166, 197, 218
well water 48
werewolves 177
western baneberry 34
western monkshood 176
West Indian lilac 65
wheat 5-6
white cedar 65
white clover 128
white honey flower 41
white locust 41
white osier 103
whites 13
white snakeroot **309-310**
wild calla 307
wild jalap 165
wild lemon 165
wild licorice 252
wild monkshood 176
wild onion 93
wild pepper 91
wild strawberry 200
willow bark 31
Wills, Horace 70

window cleaner 147
windowleaf 218
window panes 162
window plant 218
windshield washing liquid 171
wine 178, 279
wine bottles, lead foil around 156-7
wine plant 250
winter daphne 91
wintergreen, oil of 254
winter rose 71
wintersweet **311**
witch (associated with poison) 165, 176-
  7, 195-6, 282
wode whistle 132
wolfsbane 176
wolf spider 283
wood alcohol 171; see also *methyl alcohol*
wood preservative 87, 169; see also *petroleum distillates*
wood sorrel 206
wonder flower 275, **311**
wonder flower, African 275
worms, hook 6
worms, round 8
worms, wire 9
wormwood 283
wrasses 72
wutu 110, **311-2**

Xanax (alprazolam) 18, 39-40
xanthine 136
Xenophon 154, 250
xylene 137, 287
xylocaine 16

yellow jackets **36-38**, 174
yellow locust 41
yellow monkshood 176
yellow sarsaparilla 180
Yersinia enterocolitica 116
yew 284, **313**
yew, American 313
yew, English 41, 313
yew, ground 313
yew, Japanese 313
yew, Pacific 313
yew, western 313
yuca 60

Zarotin 269
zebrafish 260-1
zebra plant 200
Zectran 57
zetek's frog **27**
Zeus 282
Zigadenus venenosus 93
zinc 53
  antidote for 55, 99-100
zinc oxide 167
zinc phosphide 244
zineb 57
ziram 57
zombie 237
zootoxins 290
zygacine 93
zygadenine 93